H·C·P·C·S

Health Care Procedure Coding System

National Level II Medicare Codes

Color Coded

2024

PMIC
CODING & COMPLIANCE

ISBN 978-1-57066-742-8 (Perfect Bound)
ISBN 978-1-57066-741-1 (Spiral Bound)
ISBN 978-1-57066-435-9 (Digital Book)

Practice Management Information Corporation (PMIC)
4727 Wilshire Boulevard
Los Angeles, California 90010
1-800-633-7467
http://pmiconline.com

Additional copies of this book may be purchased from any medical book store, from PMIC by mail to the above address, by visiting our web site at http://pmiconline.com or by calling 1-800-633-7467.

FOREWORD

The Health Care Procedure Coding System (HCPCS), National Level II, is a listing of codes and descriptive terminology used for reporting the provision of supplies, materials, injections and certain services and procedures to Medicare. HCPCS 2022 is the most recent revision of the HCPCS National Level II codes. The changes that appear in this revision have been prepared by our editorial staff using the HCPCS revisions released by the Center for Medicare and Medicaid Services (CMS), which is overseen by the Department of Health and Human Services (DHHS).

HCPCS 2024 codes must be used to report supplies, materials, injections and some quality measures on your Medicare claims for items and services provided from January 1, 2024 through December 31, 2024.
The proper selection and reporting of HCPCS codes can improve your reimbursement and reduce your audit liability.

James B. Davis, President

DISCLAIMER

This publication is designed to offer basic information regarding coding and billing of medical services, supplies and procedures using the HCPCS coding system. The information presented is based upon material obtained from the Center for Medicare and Medicaid Services (CMS), and the experience and interpretations of the editors and publisher. Though all of the information has been carefully researched and checked for accuracy and completeness, the publisher accepts no responsibility or liability with regard to errors, omissions, misuse or misinterpretation.

CONTENTS

INTRODUCTION

HCPCS is an acronym for Health Care Procedure Coding System. This coding system was developed in 1983 by the Health Care Financing Administration (HCFA) for the purpose of standardizing the coding systems used to process Medicare claims. In 2001, HCFA changed its name to the Center for Medicare and Medicaid Services (CMS) to reflect its increased emphasis on improving Medicare and Medicaid beneficiary services and information.

The HCPCS coding system is primarily used to bill Medicare for supplies, materials and injections. It is also used to bill for certain services and procedures which are not defined in CPT. HCPCS codes must be used when billing Medicare carriers, and in some states, Medicaid carriers. Some private insurance carriers also allow or mandate the use of HCPCS codes, mostly those that are processing Medicare claims.

STRUCTURE OF HCPCS

HCPCS is a systematic method for coding supplies, materials, injections and services performed by health care professionals. Each supply, material, injection or service is identified with a five digit alphanumeric code. With the HCPCS coding system, the supplies, materials and injections can be accurately identified and properly reimbursed. There are three levels of codes within the HCPCS coding system.

LEVEL I CPT CODES

The major portion of the HCPCS coding system, referred to as Level I, is CPT. Most of the procedures and services you perform, even for Medicare patients, are billed using CPT codes. However, one of the major deficiencies of CPT is that it has limited code selections to describe supplies, materials and injections.

LEVEL II NATIONAL CODES

HCPCS National Level II codes are alphanumeric codes which start with a letter followed by four numbers. The range of HCPCS National Level II codes is from A0000 through V0000. There are also HCPCS National Level II modifiers. HCPCS National Level II codes are uniform in description throughout the United States. However, due to what is known as "carrier discretion" the processing and reimbursement of HCPCS National Level II codes is not necessarily uniform.

There are over 7,700 HCPCS National Level II codes covering supplies, materials, injections and services. A fundamental understanding of when and how to use HCPCS National Level II or Local Level III codes can have a significant impact on your Medicare reimbursement. The majority of health care professionals use codes from the Medical and Surgical Supplies section and Drugs Administered by Other Than Oral Method, commonly referred to as "A" codes and "J" codes.

HCPCS CODE OVERLAP

As may be expected, there is some overlap among the HCPCS code levels. On occasion you may have a coding situation where a specific code exists at all three levels for the same service or material. When faced with this situation, the general rule is that Local Level II codes have the highest priority, followed by CPT codes. You should consult your local Medicare carrier if you have any questions regarding HCPCS code overlap.

SECTIONS

The main body of HCPCS National Level II codes is divided into sections. The supplies, materials, injections and services are presented in alphanumeric order within each section. The sections of HCPCS National Level II are:

SECTION	CODE SERIES
Transportation Services	A0000–A0999
Medical And Surgical Supplies	A4000–A8999
Miscellaneous And Experimental	A9000–A9999

SECTION	CODE SERIES
Enteral And Parenteral Therapy	B0000–B9999
Temporary Hospital Outpatient PPS	C0000–C9999
Durable Medical Equipment (DME)	E0000–E9999
Temporary Procedures & Professional Services	G0000–G9999
Rehabilitative Services	H0000–H9999
Drugs Administered Other Than Oral Method	J0000–J8999
Chemotherapy Drugs	J9000–J9999
Temporary Codes For DMERCS	K0000–K9999
Orthotic Procedures	L0000–L4999
Prosthetic Procedures	L5000–L9999
Medical Services	M0000–M9999
Pathology and Laboratory	P0000–P9999
Temporary Codes	Q0000–Q9999
Diagnostic Radiology Services	R0000–R9999
Private Payer Codes	S0000–S9999
State Medicaid Agency Codes	T0000–T9999
Corona Virus Diagnostic Panel	U0001–U0005
Vision Services	V0000–V2999
Hearing Services	V5000–V5999

INSTRUCTIONS FOR USE OF HCPCS NATIONAL LEVEL II CODES

A health care professional using the HCPCS National Level II codes selects the name of the material, supply, injection, service or procedure that most accurately identifies the service performed or supply delivered. Most often, HCPCS National Level II codes will be used instead of, or in addition to, CPT codes for visits, evaluation and management services, or other procedures performed at the same time or during the same visit. All services, procedures, supplies, materials and injections should be properly documented in the medical record.

The listing of a supply, material, injection or service and its code number in a specific section of HCPCS does not usually restrict its use to a specific profession or specialty group. However, there are some HCPCS National Level II codes that are by definition, profession or specialty specific.

GUIDELINES

Specific GUIDELINES are presented at the beginning of most of the sections. These GUIDELINES define items that are necessary to appropriately interpret and report the supplies, materials, injections, services and procedures listed in that section.

HCPCS MODIFIERS

A modifier provides the means by which the health care professional can indicate that a service or procedure that has been performed has been altered by some specific circumstance but not changed in its definition or code. HCPCS modifiers may be used to indicate the following:

- A service was supervised by an anesthesiologist

- A service was performed by a specific health care professional, for example, a clinical psychologist, clinical social worker, nurse practitioner, or physician assistant.

- A service was provided as part of a specific government program
- A service was provided to a specific side of the body
- Equipment was purchased or rented
- Single or multiple patients were seen during nursing home visits

It is important to note that HCPCS National Level II modifiers can be combined with CPT codes when reporting services to Medicare.

An example of the use of HCPCS National Level II modifiers is:

E1280-NR Heavy duty wheelchair; detachable arms (desk or full length) elevating leg rests - new when rented

A listing of modifiers pertinent to each section of HCPCS National Level II are located in the GUIDELINES of each section. A complete listing of HCPCS National Level II modifiers is found in APPENDIX A.

UNLISTED PROCEDURE OR SERVICE

A service or procedure may be provided that is not listed in this edition of HCPCS National Level II. When reporting such a service, the appropriate "unlisted procedure" code may be used to indicate the service, identifying it by "special report" as defined below. HCPCS National Level II terminology is inconsistent in defining unlisted procedures. The procedure definition may include the term(s) "unlisted," "not otherwise classified," "unspecified," "unclassified," "other" and "miscellaneous." Prior to using these codes, try to determine if a Local Level III or CPT code is available. When an unlisted procedure code is used, the supply, material, injection, service or procedure must be described. Each of these unlisted procedure codes relates to a specific section of HCPCS National Level II and is presented in the GUIDELINES of that section.

SPECIAL REPORT

A supply, material, injection, service or procedure that is rarely provided, unusual, variable or new may require a special report for reimbursement purposes. Pertinent information should include an adequate definition or description of the nature, extent, and need for the supply, material, injection, service or procedure.

HCPCS CODE CHANGES

Each year numerous codes are added, changed or deleted. A summary of revisions to HCPCS 2024 is found in APPENDIX B. The following symbols, identical to those used in CPT, are used to indicate additions, changes and deletions in HCPCS National Level II.

CODES ADDED TO HCPCS

New HCPCS National Level II codes are identified with a small black circle placed to the left of the code number. An example of a new code in HCPCS 2024 is:

● **C7540** Removal of permanent pacemaker pulse generator with replacement of pacemaker pulse generator, dual lead system, with insertion of pacing electrode, cardiac venous system, for left ventricular pacing, at time of insertion of implantable defibrillator or pacemaker pulse generator (e.g., for upgrade to dual chamber system)

DESCRIPTIONS REVISED IN HCPCS

Changes in HCPCS National Level II code definitions are identified with a small black triangle placed to the left of the code number. An example of a changed code in HCPCS 2024 is:

▲ **T1026** Intensive, extended multidisciplinary services provided in a clinic setting to children with complex medical, physical, mental and psychosocial impairments, per hour

CODES DELETED FROM HCPCS

Deleted HCPCS National Level II codes are enclosed within parentheses, along with an italicized reference to replacement codes when available. An example of a deleted code in HCPCS 2024 is:

(**C9788** Opto-acoustic imaging, breast (including axilla when performed), unilateral, with image documentation, analysis and report, obtained with ultrasound examination
Code deleted effective 12/31/2023, no HCPCS/CPT cross-reference provided.)

SPECIAL COVERAGE SYMBOLS

NOT PAYABLE BY MEDICARE

There are codes listed in HCPCS which are not payable by Medicare. These codes are identified by a red bar over the HCPCS code. These codes should not be used to report services to Medicare

NON-COVERED BY MEDICARE

There are numerous supplies, materials, injections, services and procedures which are not covered by Medicare, either by program definition or by legislative statute. Examples of non-covered services include routine services and appliances, foot care and supportive devices for feet, custodial care, personal comfort items, and cosmetic surgery. These codes are identified by an orange bar over the HCPCS code. These codes should not be used to report services to Medicare; however, in most cases, you may bill the patient directly for non-covered services.

SPECIAL COVERAGE INSTRUCTIONS

Your local Medicare carrier has specific coverage instructions for processing certain HCPCS codes. These codes are identified by a yellow bar over the HCPCS code. While these codes are covered by the Medicare program, the use of these codes does not guarantee payment. If you have a question about a specific code in this category, review your Medicare provider manual or consult with your local Medicare carrier.

CARRIER JUDGMENT

Processing and payment for these codes is done at the discretion of each insurance carrier. These codes are identified by a blue bar over the HCPCS code. For codes in this category, you should check with your Medicare carrier for proper billing instructions prior to filing an insurance claim.

DURABLE MEDICAL EQUIPMENT MEDICARE ADMINISTRATIVE CONTRACTORS (DME-MACs)

All Medicare claims for durable medical equipment (DME), prosthetics, orthotics and supplies go to one of four durable medical equipment Medicare administrative contractors, or DME-MACs (formerly known as DMERCs).

MEDICARE SUPPLIER NUMBER

Before submitting claims to DME-MACs, you must apply for a supplier number. You must use this number when submitting claims to all four carriers. To find out more information, go to the Medicare website at http://www.cms.gov.

REGIONALIZATION OF CLAIM PROCESSING

Listed below are the contracted carriers and the states that they serve. The residence of the beneficiary is what determines which regional carrier processes the claim.

REGION A: STATES	REGION A: CONTRACTOR
Connecticut, Delaware, District of Columbia, Maine, Maryland, Massachusetts, New Hampshire, New Jersey, New York - Entire State, Pennsylvania, Rhode Island, Vermont	**Noridian Healthcare Solutions, LLC** PO Box 6727 900 42nd Street South Fargo, ND 58108-6727 https://med.noridianMedicare.com/web/jddme

REGION B: STATES	REGION B: CONTRACTOR
Illinois, Indiana, Kentucky, Michigan, Minnesota, Ohio, Wisconsin	**CGS Administrators, LLC** 2 Vantage Way - Metro Center Nashville, TN 37228- www.cgsMedicare.com/jb

REGION C: STATES	REGION C: CONTRACTOR
Alabama, Arkansas, Colorado, Florida, Georgia, Louisiana, Mississippi, New Mexico, North Carolina, Oklahoma, Puerto Rico, South Carolina, Tennessee, Texas, Virgin Islands, Virginia, West Virginia	**CGS Administrators, LLC** 2 Vantage Way - Metro Center Nashville, TN 37228- www.cgsMedicare.com/jc

REGION D: STATES	REGION D: CONTRACTOR
Alaska, American Samoa, Arizona, California - Entire State, Guam, Hawaii, Idaho, Iowa, Kansas, Missouri - Entire State, Montana, Nebraska, Nevada, North Dakota, Northern Mariana Islands, Oregon, South Dakota, Utah, Washington, Wyoming	**Noridian Healthcare Solutions, LLC** PO Box 6727 900 42nd Street South Fargo, ND 58108-6727 https://med.noridianMedicare.com/web/jddme

CHANGE OF CLAIM JURISDICTION

Prior to October 1, 1993, Medicare carriers processed durable medical equipment (DME), prosthetics, and orthotics claims based on where the transaction for the sale or rental took place. This is called the point of sale. Beginning October 1, 1993 and according to the state by state transfer schedule, regional processing of supplier claims began using beneficiary residence to determine which regional carrier had claim jurisdiction.

ELECTRONIC CLAIM FILING

The Center for Medicare and Medicaid Services is strongly encouraging electronic claims submission to DME-MACs. Suppliers submitting claims electronic must use the designated National Standard Format which meets all Medicare billing requirements and is accepted by other third-party insurance carriers. The regional carriers will assist you in converting to electronic claims submission. You can contact the Electronic Media Coordinator (EMC) at the DME-MACs listed above.

APPENDICES

APPENDIX A: **MODIFIERS:** Lists all National Level II modifiers, ambulance service, and PET scan modifiers.

APPENDIX B: **SUMMARY OF CHANGES**: Includes a summary of official additions, changes, and deletions to the current edition of HCPCS.

APPENDIX C: **TABLE OF DRUGS**: Includes drug names, cross references along with selected dosage, administration route, and HCPCS codes from the official HCPCS Table of Drugs.

HCPCS 2024 DATA CONTENT FILES

HCPCS data content is available via file transfer or CD-ROM. The HCPCS data file includes all official HCPCS codes with short, medium and full descriptions. The data file can be uploaded to your PC for inclusion in billing programs. For more information regarding the HCPCS data content call PMIC at 1-800-633-7467 or visit http://pmiconline.com.

TRANSPORTATION SERVICES

Guidelines

In addition to the information presented in the INTRODUCTION, several other items unique to this section are defined or identified here:

1. **VEHICLE AND CREW REQUIREMENTS:** The ambulance must be designed and equipped for transporting the sick or injured and include patient care equipment, such as a stretcher, clean linens, first aid supplies, oxygen equipment and other safety and lifesaving equipment required by state or local authorities. The ambulance crew must have two members, one of which has medical training equivalent to the standard and advanced Red Cross training. The vehicle and personnel supplier must provide a statement that describes the first-aid, safety and other patient-care items in the vehicle, the extent of first-aid training of the personnel and the supplier's agreement to notify Medicare of any changes that could affect coverage.

2. **AIR AMBULANCE SERVICE:** Air ambulance services are covered when the point of pick-up is inaccessible by land vehicle; distances or other obstacles are involved in getting the patient to the nearest hospital with appropriate facilities; and all other conditions of coverage are met.

3. **AMBULANCE SERVICE CLAIMS:** Reimbursement may be made for expenses incurred for ambulance services when specific conditions have been met and the appropriate medical documentation is provided.

4. **MATERIALS SUPPLIED BY AMBULANCE SERVICE:** Reusable devices, such as back boards, neck boards and inflatable leg and arm splints, are considered part of general ambulance services and included in the charge for the trip. A separate reasonable charge may be recognized for non-reusable items and disposable supplies, such as oxygen, gauze and dressings, which are required for patient care during the trip.

5. **UNLISTED SERVICE OR PROCEDURE:** A service or procedure may be provided that is not listed in this edition of HCPCS. When reporting such a service, the appropriate "unlisted procedure" code may be used to indicate the service, identifying it by "special report" as defined below. HCPCS terminology is inconsistent in defining unlisted procedures. The procedure definition may include the term(s) "unlisted", "not otherwise classified", "unspecified", "unclassified", "other" and "miscellaneous". Prior to using these codes, try to determine if a Local Level III code or CPT code is available. The "unlisted procedures" and accompanying codes for TRANSPORTATION SERVICES are as follows:

   A0999 Unlisted ambulance service

6. **SPECIAL REPORT:** A service, material or supply that is rarely provided, unusual, variable or new may require a special report in determining medical appropriateness for reimbursement purposes. Pertinent information should include an adequate definition or description of the nature, extent, and need for the service, material or supply.

7. **MODIFIERS:** Listed services may be modified under certain circumstances. When appropriate, the modifying circumstance is identified by adding a modifier to the basic procedure code. CPT and HCPCS National Level II modifiers may be used with CPT and HCPCS National Level II procedure codes. One digit codes are to be used in combination. The first digit should indicate the origin; the second digit should indicate the destination.

   The Level II modifiers commonly used with TRANSPORTATION codes are as follows:

   -GM Multiple patients on one ambulance trip

   -QM Ambulance service provided under arrangement by a provider of services

-QN Ambulance services furnished directly by a provider of services

AMBULANCE SERVICE MODIFIERS

For ambulance service, one-digit modifiers are combined to form a two-digit modifier that identifies the ambulance's place of origin with the first digit, and ambulance's destination with the second digit. They are used in items 12 and 13 on the CMS Form 1491.

One digit ambulance modifiers:

-D Diagnostic or therapeutic site other than -P or -H when these are used as origin codes

-E Residential, domiciliary, custodial facility (other than an 1819 facility)

-G Hospital-based dialysis facility (hospital or hospital related)

-H Hospital

-I Site of transfer (for example, airport or helicopter pad) between types of ambulance

-J Non-hospital-based dialysis facility

-N Skilled nursing facility (SNF) (1819 facility)

-P Physician's office (includes HMO non-hospital facility, clinic, etc.)

-R Residence

-S Scene of accident or acute event

-X (Destination code only) Intermediate stop at physician's office on the way to the hospital (includes HMO non-hospital facility, clinic, etc.)

8. **CPT CODE CROSS-REFERENCE:** Unless specified otherwise, there is no equivalent CPT code for listings in this section.

Transportation Services Including Ambulance

A0021 Ambulance service, outside state per mile, transport (Medicaid only)

Ambulance Waiting Time Table			
Units	**Time (Hrs)**	**Units**	**Time (Hrs)**
1	1/2 to 1	6	3 to 3 ½
2	1 to 1 ½	7	3 ½ to 4
3	1 ½ to 2	8	4 to 4 ½
4	2 to 2 ½	9	4 ½ to 5
5	2 to 3	10	5 to 5 ½

A0080 Non-emergency transportation, per mile - vehicle provided by volunteer (individual or organization), with no vested interest

A0090 Non-emergency transportation, per mile - vehicle provided by individual (family member, self, neighbor) with vested interest

A0100 Non-emergency transportation; taxi

A0110	Non-emergency transportation and bus, intra or inter state carrier
A0120	Non-emergency transportation: mini-bus, mountain area transports, or other transportation systems
A0130	Non-emergency transportation: wheelchair van
A0140	Non-emergency transportation and air travel (private or commercial) intra or inter state
A0160	Non-emergency transportation: per mile - case worker or social worker
A0170	Transportation ancillary: parking fees, tolls, other
A0180	Non-emergency transportation: ancillary: lodging-recipient
A0190	Non-emergency transportation: ancillary: meals-recipient
A0200	Non-emergency transportation: ancillary: lodging escort
A0210	Non-emergency transportation: ancillary: meals-escort
A0225	Ambulance service, neonatal transport, base rate, emergency transport, one way
A0380	BLS mileage (per mile)
A0382	BLS routine disposable supplies
A0384	BLS specialized service disposable supplies; defibrillation (used by ALS ambulances and BLS ambulances in jurisdictions where defibrillation is permitted in BLS ambulances)
A0390	ALS mileage (per mile)
A0392	ALS specialized service disposable supplies; defibrillation (to be used only in jurisdictions where defibrillation cannot be performed in BLS ambulances)
A0394	ALS specialized service disposable supplies; iv drug therapy
A0396	ALS specialized service disposable supplies; esophageal intubation
A0398	ALS routine disposable supplies
A0420	Ambulance waiting time (ALS or BLS), one half (1/2) hour increments
A0422	Ambulance (ALS or BLS) oxygen and oxygen supplies, life sustaining situation
A0424	Extra ambulance attendant, ground (ALS or BLS) or air (fixed or rotary winged); (requires medical review)
A0425	Ground mileage, per statute mile
A0426	Ambulance service, advanced life support, non-emergency transport, level 1 (ALS 1)
A0427	Ambulance service, advanced life support, emergency transport, level 1 (ALS 1 - emergency)
A0428	Ambulance service, basic life support, non-emergency transport, (BLS)
A0429	Ambulance service, basic life support, emergency transport (BLS-emergency)
A0430	Ambulance service, conventional air services, transport, one way (fixed wing)
A0431	Ambulance service, conventional air services, transport, one way (rotary wing)
A0432	Paramedic intercept (pi), rural area, transport furnished by a volunteer ambulance company which is prohibited by state law from billing third party payers
A0433	Advanced life support, level 2 (ALS 2)
A0434	Specialty care transport (SCT)
A0435	Fixed wing air mileage, per statute mile
A0436	Rotary wing air mileage, per statute mile

A0888 Noncovered ambulance mileage, per mile (e.g., for miles traveled beyond closest appropriate facility)

A0998 Ambulance response and treatment, no transport

A0999 Unlisted ambulance service

MEDICAL AND SURGICAL SUPPLIES

Guidelines

In addition to the information presented in the INTRODUCTION, several other items unique to this section are defined or identified here:

1. **SUBSECTION INFORMATION:** Some of the listed subheadings or subsections have special needs or instructions unique to that section. Where these are indicated, special "notes" will be presented preceding or following the listings. Those subsections within the MEDICAL AND SURGICAL SUPPLIES section that have "notes" are as follows:

Subsection	Code Numbers
External urinary supplies	A4356–A4358
Tracheostomy supplies	A4622–A4626
Supplies for ESRD	A4650–A4927

2. **UNLISTED SERVICE OR PROCEDURE:** A service or procedure may be provided that is not listed in this edition of HCPCS. When reporting such a service, the appropriate "unlisted procedure" code may be used to indicate the service, identifying it by "special report" as defined below. HCPCS terminology is inconsistent in defining unlisted procedures. The procedure definition may include the term(s) "unlisted", "not otherwise classified", "unspecified", "unclassified", "other" and "miscellaneous". Prior to using these codes, try to determine if a Local Level III code or CPT code is available. The "unlisted procedures" and accompanying codes for MEDICAL AND SURGICAL SUPPLIES are as follows:

HCPCS	HCPCS Description
A4335	Incontinence supply; miscellaneous
A4421	Ostomy supply; miscellaneous
A4649	Surgical supply; miscellaneous
A4913	Miscellaneous dialysis supplies, not otherwise specified
A5507	For diabetics only, not otherwise specified modification (including fitting) of off-the-shelf depth-inlay shoe or custom-molded shoe, per shoe
A6261	Wound filler, gel/paste, per fluid ounce, not otherwise specified
A6262	Wound filler, dry form, per gram, not otherwise specified
A9579	Injection gadolinium-based magnetic resonance contrast agent, not otherwise specified (nos), per ml
A9900	Miscellaneous DME supply, accessory, and/or service component of another HCPCS code
A9999	Miscellaneous DME supply or accessory, not otherwise specified
E1399	Durable medical equipment, miscellaneous
G9012	Other specified case management service not elsewhere classified
G9055	Oncology; primary focus of visit; other, unspecified service not otherwise listed (for use in a Medicare-approved demonstration project)
G9055	Oncology; primary focus of visit; other, unspecified service not otherwise listed (for use in a Medicare-approved demonstration project)
L8499	Unlisted procedure for miscellaneous prosthetic services
L8608	Miscellaneous external component, supply or accessory for use with the argus ii retinal prosthesis system
L8698	Miscellaneous component, supply or accessory for use with total artificial heart system
Q0181	Unspecified oral dosage form, FDA approved prescription anti-emetic, for use as a complete therapeutic substitute for a iv anti-emetic at the time of chemotherapy treatment, not to exceed a 48 hour dosage regimen
Q0507	Miscellaneous supply or accessory for use with an external ventricular assist device

HCPCS	HCPCS Description
Q0508	Miscellaneous supply or accessory for use with an implanted ventricular assist device
Q0509	Miscellaneous supply or accessory for use with any implanted ventricular assist device for which payment was not made under Medicare part a
Q4051	Splint supplies, miscellaneous (includes thermoplastics, strapping, fasteners, padding and other supplies)
Q5009	Hospice or home health care provided in place not otherwise specified (nos)
S0590	Integral lens service, miscellaneous services reported separately
T2025	Waiver services; not otherwise specified (nos)
T2032	Residential care, not otherwise specified (nos), waiver; per month
T2033	Residential care, not otherwise specified (nos), waiver; per diem
V2799	Vision item or service, miscellaneous
V5090	Dispensing fee, unspecified hearing aid
V5299	Hearing service, miscellaneous

3. **SPECIAL REPORT:** A service, material or supply that is rarely provided, unusual, variable or new may require a special report in determining medical appropriateness for reimbursement purposes. Pertinent information should include an adequate definition or description of the nature, extent, and need for the service, material or supply.

4. **MODIFIERS:** Listed services may be modified under certain circumstances. When appropriate, the modifying circumstance is identified by adding a modifier to the basic procedure code. CPT and HCPCS National Level II modifiers may be used with CPT and HCPCS National Level II procedure codes. Modifiers commonly used with MEDICAL AND SURGICAL SUPPLIES are as follows:

   -CC Procedure code change (use "CC" when the procedure code submitted was changed either for administrative reasons or because an incorrect code was filed)

   -LT Left side (used to identify procedures performed on the left side of the body)

   -RT Right side (used to identify procedures performed on the right side of the body)

5. **CPT CODE CROSS-REFERENCE:** Unless specified otherwise, the equivalent CPT code for all listings in this section is 99070.

6. **DURABLE MEDICAL EQUIPMENT REGIONAL CARRIERS (DMERCS):** Effective October 1, 1993 claims for supplies must be billed to one of four regional carriers depending upon the residence of the beneficiary. The transition dates for DMERC claims is from November 1, 1993 to March 1, 1994, also depending upon the state you practice in. See the Introduction for a complete discussion of DMERCs.

MEDICAL AND SURGICAL SUPPLIES

A2001 Innovamatrix ac, per square centimeter

A2002 Mirragen advanced wound matrix, per square centimeter

A2004 Xcellistem, 1 mg

A2005 Microlyte matrix, per square centimeter

A2006 Novosorb synpath dermal matrix, per square centimeter

A2007 Restrata, per square centimeter

A2008 Theragenesis, per square centimeter

A2009 Symphony, per square centimeter

A2010	Apis, per square centimeter
A2011	Supra sdrm, per square centimeter
A2012	Suprathel, per square centimeter
A2013	Innovamatrix fs, per square centimeter
A2014	Omeza collagen matrix, per 100 mg
A2015	Phoenix wound matrix, per square centimeter
A2016	Permeaderm b, per square centimeter
A2017	Permeaderm glove, each
A2018	Permeaderm c, per square centimeter
A4100	Skin substitute, FDA cleared as a device, not otherwise specified
A4206	Syringe with needle, sterile, 1 cc or less, each
A4207	Syringe with needle, sterile 2 cc, each
A4208	Syringe with needle, sterile 3 cc, each
A4209	Syringe with needle, sterile 5 cc or greater, each
A4210	Needle-free injection device, each
A4211	Supplies for self-administered injections
A4212	Non-coring needle or stylet with or without catheter
A4213	Syringe, sterile, 20 cc or greater, each
A4215	Needle, sterile, any size, each
A4216	Sterile water, saline and/or dextrose, diluent/flush, 10 ml
A4217	Sterile water/saline, 500 ml
A4218	Sterile saline or water, metered dose dispenser, 10 ml
A4220	Refill kit for implantable infusion pump
A4221	Supplies for maintenance of non-insulin drug infusion catheter, per week (list drugs separately)
A4222	Infusion supplies for external drug infusion pump, per cassette or bag (list drugs separately)
A4223	Infusion supplies not used with external infusion pump, per cassette or bag (list drugs separately)
A4224	Supplies for maintenance of insulin infusion catheter, per week
A4225	Supplies for external insulin infusion pump, syringe type cartridge, sterile, each
A4226	Supplies for maintenance of insulin infusion pump with dosage rate adjustment using therapeutic continuous glucose sensing, per week
A4230	Infusion set for external insulin pump, non needle cannula type
A4231	Infusion set for external insulin pump, needle type
A4232	Syringe with needle for external insulin pump, sterile, 3 cc
A4233	Replacement battery, alkaline (other than j cell), for use with medically necessary home blood glucose monitor owned by patient, each
A4234	Replacement battery, alkaline, j cell, for use with medically necessary home blood glucose monitor owned by patient, each

	A4235	Replacement battery, lithium, for use with medically necessary home blood glucose monitor owned by patient, each
	A4236	Replacement battery, silver oxide, for use with medically necessary home blood glucose monitor owned by patient, each
	A4238	Supply allowance for adjunctive, non-implanted continuous glucose monitor (cgm), includes all supplies and accessories, 1 month supply = 1 unit of service
•	A4239	Supply allowance for non-adjunctive, non-implanted continuous glucose monitor (cgm), includes all supplies and accessories, 1 month supply = 1 unit of service
	A4244	Alcohol or peroxide, per pint
	A4245	Alcohol wipes, per box
	A4246	Betadine or phisohex solution, per pint
	A4247	Betadine or iodine swabs/wipes, per box
	A4248	Chlorhexidine containing antiseptic, 1 ml
	A4250	Urine test or reagent strips or tablets (100 tablets or strips)
	A4252	Blood ketone test or reagent strip, each
	A4253	Blood glucose test or reagent strips for home blood glucose monitor, per 50 strips
	A4255	Platforms for home blood glucose monitor, 50 per box
	A4256	Normal, low and high calibrator solution / chips
	A4257	Replacement lens shield cartridge for use with laser skin piercing device, each
	A4258	Spring-powered device for lancet, each
	A4259	Lancets, per box of 100
	A4261	Cervical cap for contraceptive use
	A4262	Temporary, absorbable lacrimal duct implant, each
	A4263	Permanent, long term, non-dissolvable lacrimal duct implant, each
	A4264	Permanent implantable contraceptive intratubal occlusion device(s) and delivery system
	A4265	Paraffin, per pound
	A4266	Diaphragm for contraceptive use
	A4267	Contraceptive supply, condom, male, each
	A4268	Contraceptive supply, condom, female, each
	A4269	Contraceptive supply, spermicide (e.g., foam, gel), each
	A4270	Disposable endoscope sheath, each
	A4280	Adhesive skin support attachment for use with external breast prosthesis, each
	A4281	Tubing for breast pump, replacement
	A4282	Adapter for breast pump, replacement
	A4283	Cap for breast pump bottle, replacement
	A4284	Breast shield and splash protector for use with breast pump, replacement
	A4285	Polycarbonate bottle for use with breast pump, replacement
	A4286	Locking ring for breast pump, replacement

- • **A4287** Disposable collection and storage bag for breast milk, any size, any type, each
- **A4290** Sacral nerve stimulation test lead, each

Vascular Catheters

- **A4300** Implantable access catheter, (e.g., venous, arterial, epidural subarachnoid, or peritoneal, etc.) external access
- **A4301** Implantable access total catheter, port/reservoir (e.g., venous, arterial, epidural, subarachnoid, peritoneal, etc.)
- **A4305** Disposable drug delivery system, flow rate of 50 ml or greater per hour
- **A4306** Disposable drug delivery system, flow rate of less than 50 ml per hour

Incontinence Appliances and Care Supplies

- **A4310** Insertion tray without drainage bag and without catheter (accessories only)
- **A4311** Insertion tray without drainage bag with indwelling catheter, foley type, two-way latex with coating (Teflon, silicone, silicone elastomer or hydrophilic, etc.)
- **A4312** Insertion tray without drainage bag with indwelling catheter, foley type, two-way, all silicone
- **A4313** Insertion tray without drainage bag with indwelling catheter, foley type, three-way, for continuous irrigation
- **A4314** Insertion tray with drainage bag with indwelling catheter, foley type, two-way latex with coating (Teflon, silicone, silicone elastomer or hydrophilic, etc.)
- **A4315** Insertion tray with drainage bag with indwelling catheter, foley type, two-way, all silicone
- **A4316** Insertion tray with drainage bag with indwelling catheter, foley type, three-way, for continuous irrigation
- **A4320** Irrigation tray with bulb or piston syringe, any purpose
- **A4321** Therapeutic agent for urinary catheter irrigation
- **A4322** Irrigation syringe, bulb or piston, each
- **A4326** Male external catheter with integral collection chamber, any type, each
- **A4327** Female external urinary collection device; meatal cup, each
- **A4328** Female external urinary collection device; pouch, each
- **A4330** Perianal fecal collection pouch with adhesive, each
- **A4331** Extension drainage tubing, any type, any length, with connector/adaptor, for use with urinary leg bag or urostomy pouch, each
- **A4332** Lubricant, individual sterile packet, each
- **A4333** Urinary catheter anchoring device, adhesive skin attachment, each
- **A4334** Urinary catheter anchoring device, leg strap, each
- **A4335** Incontinence supply; miscellaneous
- **A4336** Incontinence supply, urethral insert, any type, each
- **A4337** Incontinence supply, rectal insert, any type, each
- **A4338** Indwelling catheter; foley type, two-way latex with coating (Teflon, silicone, silicone elastomer, or hydrophilic, etc.), each
- **A4340** Indwelling catheter; specialty type, (e.g., coudé, mushroom, wing, etc.), each

A4344 Indwelling catheter, foley type, two-way, all silicone, each

A4346 Indwelling catheter; foley type, three way for continuous irrigation, each

A4349 Male external catheter, with or without adhesive, disposable, each

A4351 Intermittent urinary catheter; straight tip, with or without coating (Teflon, silicone, silicone elastomer, or hydrophilic, etc.), each

A4352 Intermittent urinary catheter; coudé (curved) tip, with or without coating (Teflon, silicone, silicone elastomeric, or hydrophilic, etc.), each

A4353 Intermittent urinary catheter, with insertion supplies

A4354 Insertion tray with drainage bag but without catheter

A4355 Irrigation tubing set for continuous bladder irrigation through a three-way indwelling foley catheter, each

External Urinary Supplies

A4356 External urethral clamp or compression device (not to be used for catheter clamp), each

A4357 Bedside drainage bag, day or night, with or without anti-reflux device, with or without tube, each

A4358 Urinary drainage bag, leg or abdomen, vinyl, with or without tube, with straps, each

Ostomy Supplies

A4360 Disposable external urethral clamp or compression device, with pad and/or pouch, each

A4361 Ostomy faceplate, each

A4362 Skin barrier; solid, 4 x 4 or equivalent; each

A4363 Ostomy clamp, any type, replacement only, each

A4364 Adhesive, liquid or equal, any type, per oz

A4366 Ostomy vent, any type, each

A4367 Ostomy belt, each

A4368 Ostomy filter, any type, each

A4369 Ostomy skin barrier, liquid (spray, brush, etc.), per oz

A4371 Ostomy skin barrier, powder, per oz

A4372 Ostomy skin barrier, solid 4 x 4 or equivalent, standard wear, with built-in convexity, each

A4373 Ostomy skin barrier, with flange (solid, flexible or accordion), with built-in convexity, any size, each

A4375 Ostomy pouch, drainable, with faceplate attached, plastic, each

A4376 Ostomy pouch, drainable, with faceplate attached, rubber, each

A4377 Ostomy pouch, drainable, for use on faceplate, plastic, each

A4378 Ostomy pouch, drainable, for use on faceplate, rubber, each

A4379 Ostomy pouch, urinary, with faceplate attached, plastic, each

A4380 Ostomy pouch, urinary, with faceplate attached, rubber, each

A4381 Ostomy pouch, urinary, for use on faceplate, plastic, each

A4382 Ostomy pouch, urinary, for use on faceplate, heavy plastic, each

A4383 Ostomy pouch, urinary, for use on faceplate, rubber, each

A4384 Ostomy faceplate equivalent, silicone ring, each

A4385 Ostomy skin barrier, solid 4 x 4 or equivalent, extended wear, without built-in convexity, each

A4387 Ostomy pouch, closed, with barrier attached, with built-in convexity (1 piece), each

A4388 Ostomy pouch, drainable, with extended wear barrier attached, (1 piece), each

A4389 Ostomy pouch, drainable, with barrier attached, with built-in convexity (1 piece), each

A4390 Ostomy pouch, drainable, with extended wear barrier attached, with built-in convexity (1 piece), each

A4391 Ostomy pouch, urinary, with extended wear barrier attached (1 piece), each

A4392 Ostomy pouch, urinary, with standard wear barrier attached, with built-in convexity (1 piece), each

A4393 Ostomy pouch, urinary, with extended wear barrier attached, with built-in convexity (1 piece), each

A4394 Ostomy deodorant, with or without lubricant, for use in ostomy pouch, per fluid ounce

A4395 Ostomy deodorant for use in ostomy pouch, solid, per tablet

A4396 Ostomy belt with peristomal hernia support

A4397 Irrigation supply; sleeve, each

A4398 Ostomy irrigation supply; bag, each

A4399 Ostomy irrigation supply; cone/catheter, with or without brush

A4400 Ostomy irrigation set

A4402 Lubricant, per ounce

A4404 Ostomy ring, each

A4405 Ostomy skin barrier, non-pectin based, paste, per ounce

A4406 Ostomy skin barrier, pectin-based, paste, per ounce

A4407 Ostomy skin barrier, with flange (solid, flexible, or accordion), extended wear, with built-in convexity, 4 x 4 inches or smaller, each

A4408 Ostomy skin barrier, with flange (solid, flexible or accordion), extended wear, with built-in convexity, larger than 4 x 4 inches, each

A4409 Ostomy skin barrier, with flange (solid, flexible or accordion), extended wear, without built-in convexity, 4 x 4 inches or smaller, each

A4410 Ostomy skin barrier, with flange (solid, flexible or accordion), extended wear, without built-in convexity, larger than 4 x 4 inches, each

A4411 Ostomy skin barrier, solid 4 x 4 or equivalent, extended wear, with built-in convexity, each

A4412 Ostomy pouch, drainable, high output, for use on a barrier with flange (2 piece system), without filter, each

A4413 Ostomy pouch, drainable, high output, for use on a barrier with flange (2 piece system), with filter, each

A4414 Ostomy skin barrier, with flange (solid, flexible or accordion), without built-in convexity, 4 x 4 inches or smaller, each

A4415 Ostomy skin barrier, with flange (solid, flexible or accordion), without built-in convexity, larger than 4 x 4 inches, each

A4416 Ostomy pouch, closed, with barrier attached, with filter (1 piece), each

A4417	Ostomy pouch, closed, with barrier attached, with built-in convexity, with filter (1 piece), each
A4418	Ostomy pouch, closed; without barrier attached, with filter (1 piece), each
A4419	Ostomy pouch, closed; for use on barrier with non-locking flange, with filter (2 piece), each
A4420	Ostomy pouch, closed; for use on barrier with locking flange (2 piece), each
A4421	Ostomy supply; miscellaneous
A4422	Ostomy absorbent material (sheet/pad/crystal packet) for use in ostomy pouch to thicken liquid stomal output, each
A4423	Ostomy pouch, closed; for use on barrier with locking flange, with filter (2 piece), each
A4424	Ostomy pouch, drainable, with barrier attached, with filter (1 piece), each
A4425	Ostomy pouch, drainable; for use on barrier with non-locking flange, with filter (2 piece system), each
A4426	Ostomy pouch, drainable; for use on barrier with locking flange (2 piece system), each
A4427	Ostomy pouch, drainable; for use on barrier with locking flange, with filter (2 piece system), each
A4428	Ostomy pouch, urinary, with extended wear barrier attached, with faucet-type tap with valve (1 piece), each
A4429	Ostomy pouch, urinary, with barrier attached, with built-in convexity, with faucet-type tap with valve (1 piece), each
A4430	Ostomy pouch, urinary, with extended wear barrier attached, with built-in convexity, with faucet-type tap with valve (1 piece), each
A4431	Ostomy pouch, urinary; with barrier attached, with faucet-type tap with valve (1 piece), each
A4432	Ostomy pouch, urinary; for use on barrier with non-locking flange, with faucet-type tap with valve (2 piece), each
A4433	Ostomy pouch, urinary; for use on barrier with locking flange (2 piece), each
A4434	Ostomy pouch, urinary; for use on barrier with locking flange, with faucet-type tap with valve (2 piece), each
A4435	Ostomy pouch, drainable, high output, with extended wear barrier (one-piece system), with or without filter, each
A4436	Irrigation supply; sleeve, reusable, per month
A4437	Irrigation supply; sleeve, disposable, per month

Supplies

A4450	Tape, non-waterproof, per 18 square inches
A4452	Tape, waterproof, per 18 square inches
A4453	Rectal catheter for use with the manual pump-operated enema system, replacement only
A4455	Adhesive remover or solvent (for tape, cement or other adhesive), per ounce
A4456	Adhesive remover, wipes, any type, each
• A4457	Enema tube, with or without adapter, any type, replacement only, each
A4458	Enema bag with tubing, reusable
A4459	Manual pump-operated enema system, includes balloon, catheter and all accessories, reusable, any type
A4461	Surgical dressing holder, non-reusable, each
A4463	Surgical dressing holder, reusable, each

	A4465	Non-elastic binder for extremity
	A4466	Garment, belt, sleeve or other covering, elastic or similar stretchable material, any type, each
	A4467	Belt, strap, sleeve, garment, or covering, any type
•	A4468	Exsufflation belt, includes all supplies and accessories
	A4470	Gravlee jet washer
	A4480	Vabra aspirator
	A4481	Tracheostoma filter, any type, any size, each
	A4483	Moisture exchanger, disposable, for use with invasive mechanical ventilation
	A4490	Surgical stockings above knee length, each
	A4495	Surgical stockings thigh length, each
	A4500	Surgical stockings below knee length, each
	A4510	Surgical stockings full length, each
	A4520	Incontinence garment, any type, (e.g., brief, diaper), each
•	A4540	Distal transcutaneous electrical nerve stimulator, stimulates peripheral nerves of the upper arm
•	A4541	Monthly supplies for use of device coded at E0733
•	A4542	Supplies and accessories for external upper limb tremor stimulator of the peripheral nerves of the wrist
	A4550	Surgical trays
	A4553	Non-disposable under pads, all sizes
	A4554	Disposable underpass, all sizes
	A4555	Electrode/transducer for use with electrical stimulation device used for cancer treatment, replacement only
	A4556	Electrodes, (e.g., apnea monitor), per pair
	A4557	Lead wires, (e.g., apnea monitor), per pair
	A4558	Conductive gel or paste, for use with electrical device (e.g., tens, NMES), per oz
	A4559	Coupling gel or paste, for use with ultrasound device, per oz
	A4561	Pessary, rubber, any type
	A4562	Pessary, non rubber, any type
	A4563	Rectal control system for vaginal insertion, for long term use, includes pump and all supplies and accessories, any type each
	A4565	Slings
	A4566	Shoulder sling or vest design, abduction restrainer, with or without swathe control, prefabricated, includes fitting and adjustment
	A4570	Splint
	A4575	Topical hyperbaric oxygen chamber, disposable
	A4580	Cast supplies (e.g., plaster)
	A4590	Special casting material (e.g., fiberglass)
	A4595	Electrical stimulator supplies, 2 lead, per month, (e.g., tens, NMES)
	A4596	Cranial electrotherapy stimulation (CES) system supplies and accessories, per month

Supplies for Oxygen and Related Respiratory Equipment

A4600 Sleeve for intermittent limb compression device, replacement only, each

Supplies for Other Durable Medical Equipment

A4600 Sleeve for intermittent limb compression device, replacement only, each
A4601 Lithium ion battery, rechargeable, for non-prosthetic use, replacement
A4602 Replacement battery for external infusion pump owned by patient, lithium, 1.5 volt, each
A4604 Tubing with integrated heating element for use with positive airway pressure device
A4605 Tracheal suction catheter, closed system, each
A4606 Oxygen probe for use with oximeter device, replacement
A4608 Transtracheal oxygen catheter, each
A4611 Battery, heavy duty; replacement for patient owned ventilator
A4612 Battery cables; replacement for patient-owned ventilator
A4613 Battery charger; replacement for patient-owned ventilator
A4614 Peak expiratory flow rate meter, hand held
A4615 Cannula, nasal
A4616 Tubing (oxygen), per foot
A4617 Mouth piece
A4618 Breathing circuits
A4619 Face tent
A4620 Variable concentration mask
A4623 Tracheostomy, inner cannula
A4624 Tracheal suction catheter, any type other than closed system, each
A4625 Tracheostomy care kit for new tracheostomy
A4626 Tracheostomy cleaning brush, each
A4627 Spacer, bag or reservoir, with or without mask, for use with metered dose inhaler
A4628 Oropharyngeal suction catheter, each
A4629 Tracheostomy care kit for established tracheostomy
A4630 Replacement batteries, medically necessary, transcutaneous electrical stimulator, owned by patient
A4633 Replacement bulb/lamp for ultraviolet light therapy system, each
A4634 Replacement bulb for therapeutic light box, tabletop model
A4635 Underarm pad, crutch, replacement, each
A4636 Replacement, handgrip, cane, crutch, or walker, each
A4637 Replacement, tip, cane, crutch, walker, each.
A4638 Replacement battery for patient-owned ear pulse generator, each
A4639 Replacement pad for infrared heating pad system, each
A4640 Replacement pad for use with medically necessary alternating pressure pad owned by patient

Supplies for Radiological Procedures

A4641 Radiopharmaceutical, diagnostic, not otherwise classified

A4642 Indium in-111 Satumomab pendetide, diagnostic, per study dose, up to 6 millicuries

A4648 Tissue marker, implantable, any type, each

A4649 Surgical supply; miscellaneous

Supplies for ESRD

A4650 Implantable radiation dosimeter, each

A4651 Calibrated microcapillary tube, each

A4652 Microcapillary tube sealant

A4653 Peritoneal dialysis catheter anchoring device, belt, each

A4657 Syringe, with or without needle, each

A4660 Sphygmomanometer/blood pressure apparatus with cuff and stethoscope

A4663 Blood pressure cuff only

A4670 Automatic blood pressure monitor

A4671 Disposable cycler set used with cycler dialysis machine, each

A4672 Drainage extension line, sterile, for dialysis, each

A4673 Extension line with easy lock connectors, used with dialysis

A4674 Chemicals/antiseptics solution used to clean/sterilize dialysis equipment, per 8 oz

A4680 Activated carbon filter for hemodialysis, each

A4690 Dialyzer (artificial kidneys), all types, all sizes, for hemodialysis, each

A4706 Bicarbonate concentrate, solution, for hemodialysis, per gallon

A4707 Bicarbonate concentrate, powder, for hemodialysis, per packet

A4708 Acetate concentrate solution, for hemodialysis, per gallon

A4709 Acid concentrate, solution, for hemodialysis, per gallon

A4714 Treated water (deionized, distilled, or reverse osmosis) for peritoneal dialysis, per gallon

A4719 "y set" tubing for peritoneal dialysis

A4720 Dialysate solution, any concentration of dextrose, fluid volume greater than 249 cc, but less than or equal to 999 cc, for peritoneal dialysis

A4721 Dialysate solution, any concentration of dextrose, fluid volume greater than 999 cc but less than or equal to 1999 cc, for peritoneal dialysis

A4722 Dialysate solution, any concentration of dextrose, fluid volume greater than 1999 cc but less than or equal to 2999 cc, for peritoneal dialysis

A4723 Dialysate solution, any concentration of dextrose, fluid volume greater than 2999 cc but less than or equal to 3999 cc, for peritoneal dialysis

A4724 Dialysate solution, any concentration of dextrose, fluid volume greater than 3999 cc but less than or equal to 4999 cc, for peritoneal dialysis

A4725 Dialysate solution, any concentration of dextrose, fluid volume greater than 4999 cc but less than or equal to 5999 cc, for peritoneal dialysis

A4726 Dialysate solution, any concentration of dextrose, fluid volume greater than 5999 cc, for peritoneal dialysis

A4728 Dialysate solution, non-dextrose containing, 500 ml

A4730 Fistula cannulation set for hemodialysis, each

A4736 Topical anesthetic, for dialysis, per gram

A4737 Injectable anesthetic, for dialysis, per 10 ml

A4740 Shunt accessory, for hemodialysis, any type, each

A4750 Blood tubing, arterial or venous, for hemodialysis, each

A4755 Blood tubing, arterial and venous combined, for hemodialysis, each

A4760 Dialysate solution test kit, for peritoneal dialysis, any type, each

A4765 Dialysate concentrate, powder, additive for peritoneal dialysis, per packet

A4766 Dialysate concentrate, solution, additive for peritoneal dialysis, per 10 ml

A4770 Blood collection tube, vacuum, for dialysis, per 50

A4771 Serum clotting time tube, for dialysis, per 50

A4772 Blood glucose test strips, for dialysis, per 50

A4773 Occult blood test strips, for dialysis, per 50

A4774 Ammonia test strips, for dialysis, per 50

A4802 Protamine sulfate, for hemodialysis, per 50 mg

A4860 Disposable catheter tips for peritoneal dialysis, per 10

A4870 Plumbing and/or electrical work for home hemodialysis equipment

A4890 Contracts, repair and maintenance, for hemodialysis equipment

A4911 Drain bag/bottle, for dialysis, each

A4913 Miscellaneous dialysis supplies, not otherwise specified

A4918 Venous pressure clamp, for hemodialysis, each

A4927 Gloves, non-sterile, per 100

A4928 Surgical mask, per 20

A4929 Tourniquet for dialysis, each

A4930 Gloves, sterile, per pair

A4931 Oral thermometer, reusable, any type, each

A4932 Rectal thermometer, reusable, any type, each

Additional Ostomy Supplies

A5051 Ostomy pouch, closed; with barrier attached (1 piece), each

A5052 Ostomy pouch, closed; without barrier attached (1 piece), each

A5053 Ostomy pouch, closed; for use on faceplate, each

A5054 Ostomy pouch, closed; for use on barrier with flange (2 piece), each

A5055 Stoma cap

A5056 Ostomy pouch, drainable, with extended wear barrier attached, with filter, (1 piece), each

A5057 Ostomy pouch, drainable, with extended wear barrier attached, with built in convexity, with filter, (1 piece), each

A5061 Ostomy pouch, drainable; with barrier attached, (1 piece), each

A5062 Ostomy pouch, drainable; without barrier attached (1 piece), each

A5063 Ostomy pouch, drainable; for use on barrier with flange (2 piece system), each

A5071 Ostomy pouch, urinary; with barrier attached (1 piece), each

A5072 Ostomy pouch, urinary; without barrier attached (1 piece), each

A5073 Ostomy pouch, urinary; for use on barrier with flange (2 piece), each

A5081 Stoma plug or seal, any type

A5082 Continent device; catheter for continent stoma

A5083 Continent device, stoma absorptive cover for continent stoma

A5093 Ostomy accessory; convex insert

Additional Incontinence Appliances/Supplies

A5102 Bedside drainage bottle with or without tubing, rigid or expandable, each

A5105 Urinary suspensory with leg bag, with or without tube, each

A5112 Urinary drainage bag, leg or abdomen, latex, with or without tube, with straps, each

A5113 Leg strap; latex, replacement only, per set

A5114 Leg strap; foam or fabric, replacement only, per set

Supplies for Either Incontinence or Ostomy Appliances

A5120 Skin barrier, wipes or swabs, each

A5121 Skin barrier; solid, 6 x 6 or equivalent, each

A5122 Skin barrier; solid, 8 x 8 or equivalent, each

A5126 Adhesive or non-adhesive; disk or foam pad

A5131 Appliance cleaner, incontinence and ostomy appliances, per 16 oz.

A5200 Percutaneous catheter/tube anchoring device, adhesive skin attachment

Shoe Supplies for Diabetics

A5500 For diabetics only, fitting (including follow-up), custom preparation and supply of off-the-shelf depth-inlay shoe manufactured to accommodate multi-density insert(s), per shoe

A5501 For diabetics only, fitting (including follow-up), custom preparation and supply of shoe molded from cast(s) of patient's foot (custom molded shoe), per shoe

A5503 For diabetics only, modification (including fitting) of off-the-shelf depth-inlay shoe or custom-molded shoe with roller or rigid rocker bottom, per shoe

A5504 For diabetics only, modification (including fitting) of off-the-shelf depth-inlay shoe or custom-molded shoe with wedge(s), per shoe

A5505 For diabetics only, modification (including fitting) of off-the-shelf depth-inlay shoe or custom-molded shoe with metatarsal bar, per shoe

A5506 For diabetics only, modification (including fitting) of off-the-shelf depth-inlay shoe or custom-molded shoe with off-set heel(s), per shoe

A5507 For diabetics only, not otherwise specified modification (including fitting) of off-the-shelf depth-inlay shoe or custom-molded shoe, per shoe

A5508 For diabetics only, deluxe feature of off-the-shelf depth-inlay shoe or custom-molded shoe, per shoe

A5510 For diabetics only, direct formed, compression molded to patient's foot without external heat source, multiple-density insert(s) prefabricated, per shoe

A5512 For diabetics only, multiple density insert, direct formed, molded to foot after external heat source of 230 degrees Fahrenheit or higher, total contact with patient's foot, including arch, base layer minimum of 1/4 inch material of shore a 35 durometer or 3/16 inch material of shore a 40 durometer (or higher), prefabricated, each

A5513 For diabetics only, multiple density insert, custom molded from model of patient's foot, total contact with patient's foot, including arch, base layer minimum of 3/16 inch material of shore a 35 durometer (or higher), includes arch filler and other shaping material, custom fabricated, each

A5514 For diabetics only, multiple density insert, made by direct carving with cam technology from a rectified cad model created from a digitized scan of the patient, total contact with patient's foot, including arch, base layer minimum of 3/16 inch material of shore a 35 durometer (or higher), includes arch filler and other shaping material, custom fabricated, each

Wound Dressings

A6000 Non-contact wound warming wound cover for use with the non-contact wound warming device and warming card

A6010 Collagen based wound filler, dry form, sterile, per gram of collagen

A6011 Collagen based wound filler, gel/paste, per gram of collagen

A6021 Collagen dressing, sterile, size 16 sq. in. or less, each

A6022 Collagen dressing, sterile, size more than 16 sq. in. but less than or equal to 48 sq. in., each

A6023 Collagen dressing, sterile, size more than 48 sq. in., each

A6024 Collagen dressing wound filler, sterile, per 6 inches

A6025 Gel sheet for dermal or epidermal application, (e.g., silicone, hydrogel, other), each

A6154 Wound pouch, each

A6196 Alginate or other fiber gelling dressing, wound cover, sterile, pad size 16 sq. in. or less, each dressing

A6197 Alginate or other fiber gelling dressing, wound cover, sterile, pad size more than 16 sq. in. but less than or equal to 48 sq. in., each dressing

A6198 Alginate or other fiber gelling dressing, wound cover, sterile, pad size more than 48 sq. in., each dressing

A6199 Alginate or other fiber gelling dressing, wound filler, sterile, per 6 inches

A6203 Composite dressing, sterile, pad size 16 sq. in. or less, with any size adhesive border, each dressing

A6204 Composite dressing, sterile, pad size more than 16 sq. in. but less than or equal to 48 sq. in., with any size adhesive border, each dressing

A6205 Composite dressing, sterile, pad size more than 48 sq. in., with any size adhesive border, each dressing

A6206 Contact layer, sterile, 16 sq. in. or less, each dressing

A6207 Contact layer, sterile, more than 16 sq. in. but less than or equal to 48 sq. in., each dressing

A6208 Contact layer, sterile, more than 48 sq. in., each dressing

A6209 Foam dressing, wound cover, sterile, pad size 16 sq. in. or less, without adhesive border, each dressing

A6210 Foam dressing, wound cover, sterile, pad size more than 16 sq. in. but less than or equal to 48 sq. in., without adhesive border, each dressing

A6211 Foam dressing, wound cover, sterile, pad size more than 48 sq. in., without adhesive border, each dressing

A6212 Foam dressing, wound cover, sterile, pad size 16 sq. in. or less, with any size adhesive border, each dressing

A6213 Foam dressing, wound cover, sterile, pad size more than 16 sq. in. but less than or equal to 48 sq. in., with any size adhesive border, each dressing

A6214 Foam dressing, wound cover, sterile, pad size more than 48 sq. in., with any size adhesive border, each dressing

A6215 Foam dressing, wound filler, sterile, per gram

A6216 Gauze, non-impregnated, non-sterile, pad size 16 sq. in. or less, without adhesive border, each dressing

A6217 Gauze, non-impregnated, non-sterile, pad size more than 16 sq. in. but less than or equal to 48 sq. in., without adhesive border, each dressing

A6218 Gauze, non-impregnated, non-sterile, pad size more than 48 sq. in., without adhesive border, each dressing

A6219 Gauze, non-impregnated, sterile, pad size 16 sq. in. or less, with any size adhesive border, each dressing

A6220 Gauze, non-impregnated, sterile, pad size more than 16 sq. in. but less than or equal to 48 sq. in., with any size adhesive border, each dressing

A6221 Gauze, non-impregnated, sterile, pad size more than 48 sq. in., with any size adhesive border, each dressing

A6222 Gauze, impregnated with other than water, normal saline, or hydrogel, sterile, pad size 16 sq. in. or less, without adhesive border, each dressing

A6223 Gauze, impregnated with other than water, normal saline, or hydrogel, sterile, pad size more than 16 sq. in., but less than or equal to 48 sq. in., without adhesive border, each dressing

A6224 Gauze, impregnated with other than water, normal saline, or hydrogel, sterile, pad size more than 48 sq. in., without adhesive border, each dressing

A6228 Gauze, impregnated, water or normal saline, sterile, pad size 16 sq. in. or less, without adhesive border, each dressing

A6229 Gauze, impregnated, water or normal saline, sterile, pad size more than 16 sq. in. but less than or equal to 48 sq. in., without adhesive border, each dressing

A6230 Gauze, impregnated, water or normal saline, sterile, pad size more than 48 sq. in., without adhesive border, each dressing

A6231 Gauze, impregnated, hydrogel, for direct wound contact, sterile, pad size 16 sq. in. or less, each dressing

A6232 Gauze, impregnated, hydrogel, for direct wound contact, sterile, pad size greater than 16 sq. in., but less than or equal to 48 sq. in., each dressing

A6233 Gauze, impregnated, hydrogel, for direct wound contact, sterile, pad size more than 48 sq. in., each dressing

A6234 Hydrocolloid dressing, wound cover, sterile, pad size 16 sq. in. or less, without adhesive border, each dressing

A6235 Hydrocolloid dressing, wound cover, sterile, pad size more than 16 sq. in. but less than or equal to 48 sq. in., without adhesive border, each dressing

A6236 Hydrocolloid dressing, wound cover, sterile, pad size more than 48 sq. in., without adhesive border, each dressing

A6237 Hydrocolloid dressing, wound cover, sterile, pad size 16 sq. in. or less, with any size adhesive border, each dressing

A6238 Hydrocolloid dressing, wound cover, sterile, pad size more than 16 sq. in. but less than or equal to 48 sq. in., with any size adhesive border, each dressing

A6239	Hydrocolloid dressing, wound cover, sterile, pad size more than 48 sq. in., with any size adhesive border, each dressing
A6240	Hydrocolloid dressing, wound filler, paste, sterile, per ounce
A6241	Hydrocolloid dressing, wound filler, dry form, sterile, per gram
A6242	Hydrogel dressing, wound cover, sterile, pad size 16 sq. in. or less, without adhesive border, each dressing
A6243	Hydrogel dressing, wound cover, sterile, pad size more than 16 sq. in. but less than or equal to 48 sq. in., without adhesive border, each dressing
A6244	Hydrogel dressing, wound cover, sterile, pad size more than 48 sq. in., without adhesive border, each dressing
A6245	Hydrogel dressing, wound cover, sterile, pad size 16 sq. in. or less, with any size adhesive border, each dressing
A6246	Hydrogel dressing, wound cover, sterile, pad size more than 16 sq. in. but less than or equal to 48 sq. in., with any size adhesive border, each dressing
A6247	Hydrogel dressing, wound cover, sterile, pad size more than 48 sq. in., with any size adhesive border, each dressing
A6248	Hydrogel dressing, wound filler, gel, per fluid ounce
A6250	Skin sealants, protectants, moisturizers, ointments, any type, any size
A6251	Specialty absorptive dressing, wound cover, sterile, pad size 16 sq. in. or less, without adhesive border, each dressing
A6252	Specialty absorptive dressing, wound cover, sterile, pad size more than 16 sq. in. but less than or equal to 48 sq. in., without adhesive border, each dressing
A6253	Specialty absorptive dressing, wound cover, sterile, pad size more than 48 sq. in., without adhesive border, each dressing
A6254	Specialty absorptive dressing, wound cover, sterile, pad size 16 sq. in. or less, with any size adhesive border, each dressing
A6255	Specialty absorptive dressing, wound cover, sterile, pad size more than 16 sq. in. but less than or equal to 48 sq. in., with any size adhesive border, each dressing
A6256	Specialty absorptive dressing, wound cover, sterile, pad size more than 48 sq. in., with any size adhesive border, each dressing
A6257	Transparent film, sterile, 16 sq. in. or less, each dressing
A6258	Transparent film, sterile, more than 16 sq. in. but less than or equal to 48 sq. in., each dressing
A6259	Transparent film, sterile, more than 48 sq. in., each dressing
A6260	Wound cleansers, any type, any size
A6261	Wound filler, gel/paste, per fluid ounce, not otherwise specified
A6262	Wound filler, dry form, per gram, not otherwise specified
A6266	Gauze, impregnated, other than water, normal saline, or zinc paste, sterile, any width, per linear yard
A6402	Gauze, non-impregnated, sterile, pad size 16 sq. in. or less, without adhesive border, each dressing
A6403	Gauze, non-impregnated, sterile, pad size more than 16 sq. in. less than or equal to 48 sq. in., without adhesive border, each dressing
A6404	Gauze, non-impregnated, sterile, pad size more than 48 sq. in., without adhesive border, each dressing
A6407	Packing strips, non-impregnated, sterile, up to 2 inches in width, per linear yard

A6410	Eye pad, sterile, each
A6411	Eye pad, non-sterile, each
A6412	Eye patch, occlusive, each
A6413	Adhesive bandage, first-aid type, any size, each
A6441	Padding bandage, non-elastic, non-woven/non-knitted, width greater than or equal to three inches and less than five inches, per yard
A6442	Conforming bandage, non-elastic, knitted/woven, non-sterile, width less than three inches, per yard
A6443	Conforming bandage, non-elastic, knitted/woven, non-sterile, width greater than or equal to three inches and less than five inches, per yard
A6444	Conforming bandage, non-elastic, knitted/woven, non-sterile, width greater than or equal to 5 inches, per yard
A6445	Conforming bandage, non-elastic, knitted/woven, sterile, width less than three inches, per yard
A6446	Conforming bandage, non-elastic, knitted/woven, sterile, width greater than or equal to three inches and less than five inches, per yard
A6447	Conforming bandage, non-elastic, knitted/woven, sterile, width greater than or equal to five inches, per yard
A6448	Light compression bandage, elastic, knitted/woven, width less than three inches, per yard
A6449	Light compression bandage, elastic, knitted/woven, width greater than or equal to three inches and less than five inches, per yard
A6450	Light compression bandage, elastic, knitted/woven, width greater than or equal to five inches, per yard
A6451	Moderate compression bandage, elastic, knitted/woven, load resistance of 1.25 to 1.34 foot pounds at 50% maximum stretch, width greater than or equal to three inches and less than five inches, per yard
A6452	High compression bandage, elastic, knitted/woven, load resistance greater than or equal to 1.35 foot pounds at 50% maximum stretch, width greater than or equal to three inches and less than five inches, per yard
A6453	Self-adherent bandage, elastic, non-knitted/non-woven, width less than three inches, per yard
A6454	Self-adherent bandage, elastic, non-knitted/non-woven, width greater than or equal to three inches and less than five inches, per yard
A6455	Self-adherent bandage, elastic, non-knitted/non-woven, width greater than or equal to five inches, per yard
A6456	Zinc paste impregnated bandage, non-elastic, knitted/woven, width greater than or equal to three inches and less than five inches, per yard
A6457	Tubular dressing with or without elastic, any width, per linear yard
A6460	Synthetic resorbable wound dressing, sterile, pad size 16 sq. in. or less, without adhesive border, each dressing
A6461	Synthetic resorbable wound dressing, sterile, pad size more than 16 sq. in. but less than or equal to 48 sq. in., without adhesive border, each dressing
A6501	Compression burn garment, bodysuit (head to foot), custom fabricated
A6502	Compression burn garment, chin strap, custom fabricated
A6503	Compression burn garment, facial hood, custom fabricated
A6504	Compression burn garment, glove to wrist, custom fabricated
A6505	Compression burn garment, glove to elbow, custom fabricated

A6506 Compression burn garment, glove to axilla, custom fabricated

A6507 Compression burn garment, foot to knee length, custom fabricated

A6508 Compression burn garment, foot to thigh length, custom fabricated

A6509 Compression burn garment, upper trunk to waist including arm openings (vest), custom fabricated

A6510 Compression burn garment, trunk, including arms down to leg openings (leotard), custom fabricated

A6511 Compression burn garment, lower trunk including leg openings (panty), custom fabricated

A6512 Compression burn garment, not otherwise classified

A6513 Compression burn mask, face and/or neck, plastic or equal, custom fabricated

Gradient Compression Supplies

- ● A6520 Gradient compression garment, glove, padded, for nighttime use, each
- ● A6521 Gradient compression garment, glove, padded, for nighttime use, custom, each
- ● A6522 Gradient compression garment, arm, padded, for nighttime use, each
- ● A6523 Gradient compression garment, arm, padded, for nighttime use, custom, each
- ● A6524 Gradient compression garment, lower leg and foot, padded, for nighttime use, each
- ● A6525 Gradient compression garment, lower leg and foot, padded, for nighttime use, custom, each
- ● A6526 Gradient compression garment, full leg and foot, padded, for nighttime use, each
- ● A6527 Gradient compression garment, full leg and foot, padded, for nighttime use, custom, each
- ● A6528 Gradient compression garment, bra, for nighttime use, each
- ● A6529 Gradient compression garment, bra, for nighttime use, custom, each

- ● A6520 Gradient compression garment, glove, padded, for nighttime use, each
- ● A6521 Gradient compression garment, glove, padded, for nighttime use, custom, each
- ● A6522 Gradient compression garment, arm, padded, for nighttime use, each
- ● A6523 Gradient compression garment, arm, padded, for nighttime use, custom, each
- ● A6524 Gradient compression garment, lower leg and foot, padded, for nighttime use, each
- ● A6525 Gradient compression garment, lower leg and foot, padded, for nighttime use, custom, each
- ● A6526 Gradient compression garment, full leg and foot, padded, for nighttime use, each
- ● A6527 Gradient compression garment, full leg and foot, padded, for nighttime use, custom, each
- ● A6528 Gradient compression garment, bra, for nighttime use, each
- ● A6529 Gradient compression garment, bra, for nighttime use, custom, each

A6530 Gradient compression stocking, below knee, 18-30 mmHg, each

▲ A6531 Gradient compression stocking, below knee, 30-40 mmHg, used as a surgical dressing, each

▲ A6532 Gradient compression stocking, below knee, 40-50 mmHg, used as a surgical dressing, each

A6533 Gradient compression stocking, thigh length, 18-30 mmHg, each

A6534 Gradient compression stocking, thigh length, 30-40 mmHg, each

▲ A6535 Gradient compression stocking, thigh length, 40 mmHg or greater, each

A6536 Gradient compression stocking, full length/chap style, 18-30 mmHg, each

	A6537	Gradient compression stocking, full length/chap style, 30-40 mmHg, each
▲	A6538	Gradient compression stocking, full length/chap style, 40 mmHg or greater, each
	A6539	Gradient compression stocking, waist length, 18-30 mmHg, each
	A6540	Gradient compression stocking, waist length, 30-40 mmHg, each
▲	A6541	Gradient compression stocking, waist length, 40 mmHg or greater, each
	A6544	Gradient compression stocking, garter belt
▲	A6545	Gradient compression wrap, non-elastic, below knee, 30-50 mmHg, used as a surgical dressing, each
▲	A6549	Gradient compression garment, not otherwise specified
	A6550	Wound care set, for negative pressure wound therapy electrical pump, includes all supplies and accessories
•	A6552	Gradient compression stocking, below knee, 30-40 mmHg, each
•	A6553	Gradient compression stocking, below knee, 30-40 mmHg, custom, each
•	A6554	Gradient compression stocking, below knee, 40 mmHg or greater, each
•	A6555	Gradient compression stocking, below knee, 40 mmHg or greater, custom, each
•	A6556	Gradient compression stocking, thigh length, 18-30 mmHg, custom, each
•	A6557	Gradient compression stocking, thigh length, 30-40 mmHg, custom, each
•	A6558	Gradient compression stocking, thigh length, 40 mmHg or greater, custom, each
•	A6559	Gradient compression stocking, full length/chap style, 18-30 mmHg, custom, each
•	A6560	Gradient compression stocking, full length/chap style, 30-40 mmHg, custom, each
•	A6561	Gradient compression stocking, full length/chap style, 40 mmHg or greater, custom, each
•	A6562	Gradient compression stocking, waist length, 18-30 mmHg, custom, each
•	A6563	Gradient compression stocking, waist length, 30-40 mmHg, custom, each
•	A6564	Gradient compression stocking, waist length, 40 mmHg or greater, custom, each
•	A6565	Gradient compression gauntlet, custom, each
•	A6566	Gradient compression garment, neck/head, each
•	A6567	Gradient compression garment, neck/head, custom, each
•	A6568	Gradient compression garment, torso and shoulder, each
•	A6569	Gradient compression garment, torso/shoulder, custom, each
•	A6570	Gradient compression garment, genital region, each
•	A6571	Gradient compression garment, genital region, custom, each
•	A6572	Gradient compression garment, toe caps, each
•	A6573	Gradient compression garment, toe caps, custom, each
•	A6574	Gradient compression arm sleeve and glove combination, custom, each
•	A6575	Gradient compression arm sleeve and glove combination, each
•	A6576	Gradient compression arm sleeve, custom, medium weight, each
•	A6577	Gradient compression arm sleeve, custom, heavy weight, each
•	A6578	Gradient compression arm sleeve, each

- ● **A6579** Gradient compression glove, custom, medium weight, each
- ● **A6580** Gradient compression glove, custom, heavy weight, each
- ● **A6581** Gradient compression glove, each
- ● **A6582** Gradient compression gauntlet, each
- ● **A6583** Gradient compression wrap with adjustable straps, below knee, 30-50 mmHg, each
- ● **A6584** Gradient compression wrap with adjustable straps, not otherwise specified
- ● **A6585** Gradient pressure wrap with adjustable straps, above knee, each
- ● **A6586** Gradient pressure wrap with adjustable straps, full leg, each
- ● **A6587** Gradient pressure wrap with adjustable straps, foot, each
- ● **A6588** Gradient pressure wrap with adjustable straps, arm, each
- ● **A6589** Gradient pressure wrap with adjustable straps, bra, each
- ● **A6593** Accessory for gradient compression garment or wrap with adjustable straps, non-otherwise specified
- ● **A6594** Gradient compression bandaging supply, bandage liner, lower extremity, any size or length, each
- ● **A6595** Gradient compression bandaging supply, bandage liner, upper extremity, any size or length, each
- ● **A6596** Gradient compression bandaging supply, conforming gauze, per linear yard, any width, each
- ● **A6597** Gradient compression bandage roll, elastic long stretch, linear yard, any width, each
- ● **A6598** Gradient compression bandage roll, elastic medium stretch, per linear yard, any width, each
- ● **A6599** Gradient compression bandage roll, inelastic short stretch, per linear yard, any width, each
- ● **A6600** Gradient compression bandaging supply, high density foam sheet, per 250 square centimeters, each
- ● **A6601** Gradient compression bandaging supply, high density foam pad, any size or shape, each
- ● **A6602** Gradient compression bandaging supply, high density foam roll for bandage, per linear yard, any width, each
- ● **A6603** Gradient compression bandaging supply, low density channel foam sheet, per 250 square centimeters, each
- ● **A6604** Gradient compression bandaging supply, low density flat foam sheet, per 250 square centimeters, each
- ● **A6605** Gradient compression bandaging supply, padded foam, per linear yard, any width, each
- ● **A6606** Gradient compression bandaging supply, padded textile, per linear yard, any width, each
- ● **A6607** Gradient compression bandaging supply, tubular protective absorption layer, per linear yard, any width, each
- ● **A6608** Gradient compression bandaging supply, tubular protective absorption padded layer, per linear yard, any width, each
- ● **A6609** Gradient compression bandaging supply, not otherwise specified
- ● **A6610** Gradient compression stocking, below knee, 18-30 mmHg, custom, each
- **A7000** Canister, disposable, used with suction pump, each
- **A7001** Canister, non-disposable, used with suction pump, each
- **A7002** Tubing, used with suction pump, each
- **A7003** Administration set, with small volume nonfiltered pneumatic nebulizer, disposable
- **A7004** Small volume nonfiltered pneumatic nebulizer, disposable

A7005	Administration set, with small volume nonfiltered pneumatic nebulizer, non-disposable
A7006	Administration set, with small volume filtered pneumatic nebulizer
A7007	Large volume nebulizer, disposable, unfilled, used with aerosol compressor
A7008	Large volume nebulizer, disposable, prefilled, used with aerosol compressor
A7009	Reservoir bottle, non-disposable, used with large volume ultrasonic nebulizer
A7010	Corrugated tubing, disposable, used with large volume nebulizer, 100 feet
A7011	Corrugated tubing, non-disposable, used with large volume nebulizer, 10 feet
A7012	Water collection device, used with large volume nebulizer
A7013	Filter, disposable, used with aerosol compressor or ultrasonic generator
A7014	Filter, nondisposable, used with aerosol compressor or ultrasonic generator
A7015	Aerosol mask, used with DME nebulizer
A7016	Dome and mouthpiece, used with small volume ultrasonic nebulizer
A7017	Nebulizer, durable, glass or autoclavable plastic, bottle type, not used with oxygen
A7018	Water, distilled, used with large volume nebulizer, 1000 ml
A7020	Interface for cough stimulating device, includes all components, replacement only
• A7023	Mechanical allergen particle barrier/inhalation filter, cream, nasal, topical
A7025	High frequency chest wall oscillation system vest, replacement for use with patient owned equipment, each
A7026	High frequency chest wall oscillation system hose, replacement for use with patient owned equipment, each
A7027	Combination oral/nasal mask, used with continuous positive airway pressure device, each
A7028	Oral cushion for combination oral/nasal mask, replacement only, each
A7029	Nasal pillows for combination oral/nasal mask, replacement only, pair
A7030	Full face mask used with positive airway pressure device, each
A7031	Face mask interface, replacement for full face mask, each
A7032	Cushion for use on nasal mask interface, replacement only, each
A7033	Pillow for use on nasal cannula type interface, replacement only, pair
A7034	Nasal interface (mask or cannula type) used with positive airway pressure device, with or without head strap
A7035	Headgear used with positive airway pressure device
A7036	Chinstrap used with positive airway pressure device
A7037	Tubing used with positive airway pressure device
A7038	Filter, disposable, used with positive airway pressure device
A7039	Filter, non disposable, used with positive airway pressure device
A7040	One way chest drain valve
A7041	Water seal drainage container and tubing for use with implanted chest tube
A7042	Implanted pleural catheter, each
A7043	Vacuum drainage bottle and tubing for use with implanted catheter

A7044	Oral interface used with positive airway pressure device, each
A7045	Exhalation port with or without swivel used with accessories for positive airway devices, replacement only
A7046	Water chamber for humidifier, used with positive airway pressure device, replacement, each
A7047	Oral interface used with respiratory suction pump, each
A7048	Vacuum drainage collection unit and tubing kit, including all supplies needed for collection unit change, for use with implanted catheter, each
A7501	Tracheostoma valve, including diaphragm, each
A7502	Replacement diaphragm/faceplate for tracheostoma valve, each
A7503	Filter holder or filter cap, reusable, for use in a tracheostoma heat and moisture exchange system, each
A7504	Filter for use in a tracheostoma heat and moisture exchange system, each
A7505	Housing, reusable without adhesive, for use in a heat and moisture exchange system and/or with a tracheostoma valve, each
A7506	Adhesive disc for use in a heat and moisture exchange system and/or with tracheostoma valve, any type each
A7507	Filter holder and integrated filter without adhesive, for use in a tracheostoma heat and moisture exchange system, each
A7508	Housing and integrated adhesive, for use in a tracheostoma heat and moisture exchange system and/or with a tracheostoma valve, each
A7509	Filter holder and integrated filter housing, and adhesive, for use as a tracheostoma heat and moisture exchange system, each
A7520	Tracheostomy/laryngectomy tube, non-cuffed, polyvinylchloride (PVC), silicone or equal, each
A7521	Tracheostomy/laryngectomy tube, cuffed, polyvinylchloride (PVC), silicone or equal, each
A7522	Tracheostomy/laryngectomy tube, stainless steel or equal (sterilizable and reusable), each
A7523	Tracheostomy shower protector, each
A7524	Tracheostoma stent/stud/button, each
A7525	Tracheostomy mask, each
A7526	Tracheostomy tube collar/holder, each
A7527	Tracheostomy/laryngectomy tube plug/stop, each
A8000	Helmet, protective, soft, prefabricated, includes all components and accessories
A8001	Helmet, protective, hard, prefabricated, includes all components and accessories
A8002	Helmet, protective, soft, custom fabricated, includes all components and accessories
A8003	Helmet, protective, hard, custom fabricated, includes all components and accessories
A8004	Soft interface for helmet, replacement only

ADMINISTRATIVE, MISCELLANEOUS AND INVESTIGATIONAL

NOTE: The following codes do not imply that codes in other sections are necessarily covered.

Guidelines

In addition to the information presented in the INTRODUCTION, several other items unique to this section are defined or identified here:

1. **SPECIAL REPORT:** A service, material or supply that is rarely provided, unusual, variable or new may require a special report in determining medical appropriateness for reimbursement purposes. Pertinent information should include an adequate definition or description of the nature, extent, and need for the service, material or supply.

2. **CPT CODE CROSS-REFERENCE:** Unless specified otherwise, there is no equivalent CPT code for listings in this section.

Miscellaneous and Experimental

A9150	Non-prescription drugs
A9152	Single vitamin/mineral/trace element, oral, per dose, not otherwise specified
A9153	Multiple vitamins, with or without minerals and trace elements, oral, per dose, not otherwise specified
A9155	Artificial saliva, 30 ml
A9180	Pediculosis (lice infestation) treatment, topical, for administration by patient/caretaker
A9270	Non-covered item or service
A9272	Wound suction, disposable, includes dressing, all accessories and components, any type, each
A9273	Cold or hot fluid bottle, ice cap or collar, heat and/or cold wrap, any type
A9274	External ambulatory insulin delivery system, disposable, each, includes all supplies and accessories
A9275	Home glucose disposable monitor, includes test strips
A9276	Sensor; invasive (e.g., subcutaneous), disposable, for use with non-durable medical equipment interstitial continuous glucose monitoring system, one unit = 1 day supply
A9277	Transmitter; external, for use with non-durable medical equipment interstitial continuous glucose monitoring system
A9278	Receiver (monitor); external, for use with non-durable medical equipment interstitial continuous glucose monitoring system
A9279	Monitoring feature/device, stand-alone or integrated, any type, includes all accessories, components and electronics, not otherwise classified
A9280	Alert or alarm device, not otherwise classified
A9281	Reaching/grabbing device, any type, any length, each
A9282	Wig, any type, each
A9283	Foot pressure off loading/supportive device, any type, each
A9284	Spirometer, non-electronic, includes all accessories

A9285	Inversion/eversion correction device
A9286	Hygienic item or device, disposable or non-disposable, any type, each
A9291	Prescription digital cognitive and/or behavioral therapy, FDA cleared, per course of treatment
A9300	Exercise equipment
A9500	Technetium TC-99m sestamibi, diagnostic, per study dose
A9501	Technetium TC-99m teboroxime, diagnostic, per study dose
A9502	Technetium TC-99m tetrofosmin, diagnostic, per study dose
A9503	Technetium TC-99m medronate, diagnostic, per study dose, up to 30 millicuries
A9504	Technetium TC-99m apticide, diagnostic, per study dose, up to 20 millicuries
A9505	Thallium tl-201 thallous chloride, diagnostic, per millicurie
A9507	Indium in-111 capromab pendetide, diagnostic, per study dose, up to 10 millicuries
A9508	Iodine I-131 iobenguane sulfate, diagnostic, per 0.5 millicurie
A9509	Iodine i-123 sodium iodide, diagnostic, per millicurie
A9510	Technetium TC-99m disofenin, diagnostic, per study dose, up to 15 millicuries
A9512	Technetium TC-99m pertechnetate, diagnostic, per millicurie
A9513	Lutetium lu 177, dotatate, therapeutic, 1 millicurie
A9515	Choline c-11, diagnostic, per study dose up to 20 millicuries
A9516	Iodine i-123 sodium iodide, diagnostic, per 100 microcuries, up to 999 microcuries
A9517	Iodine I-131 sodium iodide capsule(s), therapeutic, per millicurie
A9520	Technetium TC-99m tilmanocept, diagnostic, up to 0.5 millicuries
A9521	Technetium TC-99m exametazime, diagnostic, per study dose, up to 25 millicuries
A9524	Iodine I-131 iodinated serum albumin, diagnostic, per 5 microcuries
A9526	Nitrogen n-13 ammonia, diagnostic, per study dose, up to 40 millicuries
A9527	Iodine I-125, sodium iodide solution, therapeutic, per millicurie
A9528	Iodine I-131 sodium iodide capsule(s), diagnostic, per millicurie
A9529	Iodine I-131 sodium iodide solution, diagnostic, per millicurie
A9530	Iodine I-131 sodium iodide solution, therapeutic, per millicurie
A9531	Iodine I-131 sodium iodide, diagnostic, per microcurie (up to 100 microcuries)
A9532	Iodine I-125 serum albumin, diagnostic, per 5 microcuries
A9536	Technetium TC-99m depreotide, diagnostic, per study dose, up to 35 millicuries
A9537	Technetium TC-99m mebrofenin, diagnostic, per study dose, up to 15 millicuries
A9538	Technetium TC-99m pyrophosphate, diagnostic, per study dose, up to 25 millicuries
A9539	Technetium TC-99m pentetate, diagnostic, per study dose, up to 25 millicuries
A9540	Technetium TC-99m macroaggregated albumin, diagnostic, per study dose, up to 10 millicuries
A9541	Technetium TC-99m sulfur colloid, diagnostic, per study dose, up to 20 millicuries
A9542	Indium in-111 ibritumomab tiuxetan, diagnostic, per study dose, up to 5 millicuries
A9543	Yttrium y-90 ibritumomab tiuxetan, therapeutic, per treatment dose, up to 40 millicuries

A9544 Iodine I-131 tositumomab, diagnostic, per study dose

A9545 Iodine I-131 tositumomab, therapeutic, per treatment dose

A9546 Cobalt co-57/58, cyanocobalamin, diagnostic, per study dose, up to 1 microcurie

A9547 Indium in-111 oxyquinoline, diagnostic, per 0.5 millicurie

A9548 Indium in-111 pentetate, diagnostic, per 0.5 millicurie

A9550 Technetium TC-99m sodium gluceptate, diagnostic, per study dose, up to 25 millicurie

A9551 Technetium TC-99m succimer, diagnostic, per study dose, up to 10 millicuries

A9552 Fluorodeoxyglucose f-18 FDG, diagnostic, per study dose, up to 45 millicuries

A9553 Chromium cr-51 sodium chromate, diagnostic, per study dose, up to 250 microcuries

A9554 Iodine I-125 sodium iothalamate, diagnostic, per study dose, up to 10 microcuries

A9555 Rubidium rb-82, diagnostic, per study dose, up to 60 millicuries

A9556 Gallium ga-67 citrate, diagnostic, per millicurie

A9557 Technetium TC-99m bicisate, diagnostic, per study dose, up to 25 millicuries

A9558 Xenon xe-133 gas, diagnostic, per 10 millicuries

A9559 Cobalt co-57 cyanocobalamin, oral, diagnostic, per study dose, up to 1 microcurie

A9560 Technetium TC-99m labeled red blood cells, diagnostic, per study dose, up to 30 millicuries

A9561 Technetium TC-99m oxidronate, diagnostic, per study dose, up to 30 millicuries

A9562 Technetium TC-99m mertiatide, diagnostic, per study dose, up to 15 millicuries

A9563 Sodium phosphate p-32, therapeutic, per millicurie

A9564 Chromic phosphate p-32 suspension, therapeutic, per millicurie

A9566 Technetium TC-99m fanolesomab, diagnostic, per study dose, up to 25 millicuries

A9567 Technetium TC-99m pentetate, diagnostic, aerosol, per study dose, up to 75 millicuries

A9568 Technetium TC-99m arcitumomab, diagnostic, per study dose, up to 45 millicuries

A9569 Technetium TC-99m exametazime labeled autologous white blood cells, diagnostic, per study dose

A9570 Indium in-111 labeled autologous white blood cells, diagnostic, per study dose

A9571 Indium in-111 labeled autologous platelets, diagnostic, per study dose

A9572 Indium in-111 pentetreotide, diagnostic, per study dose, up to 6 millicuries

A9575 Injection, gadoterate meglumine, 0.1 ml

A9576 Injection, gadoteridol, (ProHance multipack), per ml

A9577 Injection, gadobenate dimeglumine (MultiHance), per ml

A9578 Injection, gadobenate dimeglumine (MultiHance multipack), per ml

A9579 Injection, gadolinium-based magnetic resonance contrast agent, not otherwise specified (nos), per ml

A9580 Sodium fluoride f-18, diagnostic, per study dose, up to 30 millicuries

A9581 Injection, gadoxetate disodium, 1 ml

A9582 Iodine i-123 iobenguane, diagnostic, per study dose, up to 15 millicuries

A9583 Injection, gadofosveset trisodium, 1 ml

A9584 Iodine 1-123 ioflupane, diagnostic, per study dose, up to 5 millicuries
A9585 Injection, gadobutrol, 0.1 ml
A9586 Florbetapir f18, diagnostic, per study dose, up to 10 millicuries
A9587 Gallium ga-68, dotatate, diagnostic, 0.1 millicurie
A9588 Fluciclovine f-18, diagnostic, 1 millicurie
A9589 Instillation, hexaminolevulinate hydrochloride, 100 mg
A9590 Iodine I-131, iobenguane, 1 millicurie
A9591 Fluoroestradiol f 18, diagnostic, 1 millicurie
A9592 Copper cu-64, dotatate, diagnostic, 1 millicurie
A9593 Gallium ga-68 psma-11, diagnostic, (ucsf), 1 millicurie
A9594 Gallium ga-68 psma-11, diagnostic, (UCLA), 1 millicurie
A9595 Piflufolastat f-18, diagnostic, 1 millicurie
A9596 Gallium ga-68 gozetotide, diagnostic, (illuccix), 1 millicurie
A9597 Positron emission tomography radiopharmaceutical, diagnostic, for tumor identification, not otherwise classified
A9598 Positron emission tomography radiopharmaceutical, diagnostic, for non-tumor identification, not otherwise classified
A9599 Radiopharmaceutical, diagnostic, for beta-amyloid positron emission tomography (pet) imaging, per study dose, not otherwise specified
A9600 Strontium sr-89 chloride, therapeutic, per millicurie
A9601 Flortaucipir f 18 injection, diagnostic, 1 millicurie
A9602 Fluorodopa f-18, diagnostic, per millicurie
A9604 Samarium sm-153 lexidronam, therapeutic, per treatment dose, up to 150 millicuries
A9606 Radium ra-223 dichloride, therapeutic, per microcurie
A9607 Lutetium lu 177 vipivotide tetraxetan, therapeutic, 1 millicurie
● A9608 Flotufolastat f 18, diagnostic, 1 millicurie
● A9609 Fludeoxyglucose f18 up to 15 millicuries
A9698 Non-radioactive contrast imaging material, not otherwise classified, per study
A9699 Radiopharmaceutical, therapeutic, not otherwise classified
A9700 Supply of injectable contrast material for use in echocardiography, per study
A9800 Gallium ga-68 gozetotide, diagnostic, (locametz), 1 millicurie
A9900 Miscellaneous DME supply, accessory, and/or service component of another HCPCS code
A9901 DME delivery, set up, and/or dispensing service component of another HCPCS code
A9999 Miscellaneous DME supply or accessory, not otherwise specified

ENTERAL AND PARENTERAL THERAPY

Guidelines

In addition to the information presented in the INTRODUCTION, several other items unique to this section are defined or identified here:

1. **SUBSECTION INFORMATION:** Some of the listed subheadings or subsections have special needs or instructions unique to that section. Where these are indicated, special "notes" will be presented preceding or following the listings. Those subsections within the ENTERAL AND PARENTERAL THERAPY section that have "notes" are as follows:

SUBSECTION	CODE SERIES
Enteral formulae and enteral medical supplies	B4034-B5200

2. **UNLISTED SERVICE OR PROCEDURE:** A service or procedure may be provided that is not listed in this edition of HCPCS. When reporting such a service, the appropriate "unlisted procedure" code may be used to indicate the service, identifying it by "special report" as defined below. HCPCS terminology is inconsistent in defining unlisted procedures. The procedure definition may include the term(s) "unlisted", "not otherwise classified", "unspecified", "unclassified", "other" and "miscellaneous". Prior to using these codes, try to determine if a Local Level III code or CPT code is available. The "unlisted procedures" and accompanying codes for ENTERAL AND PARENTERAL THERAPY are as follows:

   B9998 NOC for enteral supplies
   B9999 NOC for parenteral supplies

3. **SPECIAL REPORT:** A service, material or supply that is rarely provided, unusual, variable or new may require a special report in determining medical appropriateness for reimbursement purposes. Pertinent information should include an adequate definition or description of the nature, extent, and need for the service, material or supply.

4. **MODIFIERS:** Listed services may be modified under certain circumstances. When appropriate, the modifying circumstance is identified by adding a modifier to the basic procedure code. CPT and HCPCS National Level II modifiers may be used with CPT and HCPCS National Level II procedure codes. Modifiers commonly used with ENTERAL AND PARENTERAL THERAPY are as follows:

   -CC Procedure code change (used when the procedure code submitted was changed either for administrative reasons or because an incorrect code was filed)

5. **CPT CODE CROSS-REFERENCE:** Unless specified otherwise, the equivalent CPT code for all listings in this section is 99070.

Enteral Formulae and Enteral Medical Supplies

B4034 Enteral feeding supply kit; syringe fed, per day, includes but not limited to feeding/flushing syringe, administration set tubing, dressings, tape

B4035 Enteral feeding supply kit; pump fed, per day, includes but not limited to feeding/flushing syringe, administration set tubing, dressings, tape

B4036 Enteral feeding supply kit; gravity fed, per day, includes but not limited to feeding/flushing syringe, administration set tubing, dressings, tape

B4081 Nasogastric tubing with stylet

B4082 Nasogastric tubing without stylet

B4083 Stomach tube - Levine type

B4087 Gastrostomy/jejunostomy tube, standard, any material, any type, each

B4088 Gastrostomy/jejunostomy tube, low-profile, any material, any type, each

B4100 Food thickener, administered orally, per ounce

B4102 Enteral formula, for adults, used to replace fluids and electrolytes (e.g., clear liquids), 500 ml = 1 unit

B4103 Enteral formula, for pediatrics, used to replace fluids and electrolytes (e.g., clear liquids), 500 ml = 1 unit

B4104 Additive for enteral formula (e.g., fiber)

B4105 In-line cartridge containing digestive enzyme(s) for enteral feeding, each

B4149 Enteral formula, manufactured blenderized natural foods with intact nutrients, includes proteins, fats, carbohydrates, vitamins and minerals, may include fiber, administered through an enteral feeding tube, 100 calories = 1 unit

B4150 Enteral formula, nutritionally complete with intact nutrients, includes proteins, fats, carbohydrates, vitamins and minerals, may include fiber, administered through an enteral feeding tube, 100 calories = 1 unit

B4152 Enteral formula, nutritionally complete, calorically dense (equal to or greater than 1.5 kcal/ml) with intact nutrients, includes proteins, fats, carbohydrates, vitamins and minerals, may include fiber, administered through an enteral feeding tube, 100 calories = 1 unit

B4153 Enteral formula, nutritionally complete, hydrolyzed proteins (amino acids and peptide chain), includes fats, carbohydrates, vitamins and minerals, may include fiber, administered through an enteral feeding tube, 100 calories = 1 unit

B4154 Enteral formula, nutritionally complete, for special metabolic needs, excludes inherited disease of metabolism, includes altered composition of proteins, fats, carbohydrates, vitamins and/or minerals, may include fiber, administered through an enteral feeding tube, 100 calories = 1 unit

B4155 Enteral formula, nutritionally incomplete/modular nutrients, includes specific nutrients, carbohydrates (e.g., glucose polymers), proteins/amino acids (e.g., glutamine, arginine), fat (e.g., medium chain triglycerides) or combination, administered through an enteral feeding tube, 100 calories = 1 unit

B4157 Enteral formula, nutritionally complete, for special metabolic needs for inherited disease of metabolism, includes proteins, fats, carbohydrates, vitamins and minerals, may include fiber, administered through an enteral feeding tube, 100 calories = 1 unit

B4158 Enteral formula, for pediatrics, nutritionally complete with intact nutrients, includes proteins, fats, carbohydrates, vitamins and minerals, may include fiber and/or iron, administered through an enteral feeding tube, 100 calories = 1 unit

B4159 Enteral formula, for pediatrics, nutritionally complete soy based with intact nutrients, includes proteins, fats, carbohydrates, vitamins and minerals, may include fiber and/or iron, administered through an enteral feeding tube, 100 calories = 1 unit

B4160 Enteral formula, for pediatrics, nutritionally complete calorically dense (equal to or greater than 0.7 kcal/ml) with intact nutrients, includes proteins, fats, carbohydrates, vitamins and minerals, may include fiber, administered through an enteral feeding tube, 100 calories = 1 unit

B4161 Enteral formula, for pediatrics, hydrolyzed/amino acids and peptide chain proteins, includes fats, carbohydrates, vitamins and minerals, may include fiber, administered through an enteral feeding tube, 100 calories = 1 unit

B4162 Enteral formula, for pediatrics, special metabolic needs for inherited disease of metabolism, includes proteins, fats, carbohydrates, vitamins and minerals, may include fiber, administered through an enteral feeding tube, 100 calories = 1 unit

Parenteral Nutrition

B4164 Parenteral nutrition solution: carbohydrates (dextrose), 50% or less (500 ml = 1 unit) - home mix

B4168 Parenteral nutrition solution; amino acid, 3.5%, (500 ml = 1 unit) - home mix

B4172 Parenteral nutrition solution; amino acid, 5.5% through 7%, (500 ml = 1 unit) - home mix

B4176 Parenteral nutrition solution; amino acid, 7% through 8.5%, (500 ml = 1 unit) - home mix

B4178 Parenteral nutrition solution: amino acid, greater than 8.5% (500 ml = 1 unit) - home mix

B4180 Parenteral nutrition solution; carbohydrates (dextrose), greater than 50% (500 ml = 1 unit) - home mix

B4185 Parenteral nutrition solution, not otherwise specified, 10 grams lipids

B4187 Omegaven, 10 grams lipids

B4189 Parenteral nutrition solution; compounded amino acid and carbohydrates with electrolytes, trace elements, and vitamins, including preparation, any strength, 10 to 51 grams of protein - premix

B4193 Parenteral nutrition solution; compounded amino acid and carbohydrates with electrolytes, trace elements, and vitamins, including preparation, any strength, 52 to 73 grams of protein - premix

B4197 Parenteral nutrition solution; compounded amino acid and carbohydrates with electrolytes, trace elements and vitamins, including preparation, any strength, 74 to 100 grams of protein - premix

B4199 Parenteral nutrition solution; compounded amino acid and carbohydrates with electrolytes, trace elements and vitamins, including preparation, any strength, over 100 grams of protein - premix

B4216 Parenteral nutrition; additives (vitamins, trace elements, heparin, electrolytes), home mix, per day

B4220 Parenteral nutrition supply kit; premix, per day

B4222 Parenteral nutrition supply kit; home mix, per day

B4224 Parenteral nutrition administration kit, per day

B5000 Parenteral nutrition solution compounded amino acid and carbohydrates with electrolytes, trace elements, and vitamins, including preparation, any strength, renal-Aminosyn-rf, nephramine, renamine-premix

B5100 Parenteral nutrition solution compounded amino acid and carbohydrates with electrolytes, trace elements, and vitamins, including preparation, any strength, hepatic, hepatamine-premix

B5200 Parenteral nutrition solution compounded amino acid and carbohydrates with electrolytes, trace elements, and vitamins, including preparation, any strength, stress-branch chain amino acids-freamine-HBc-premix

Enteral and Parenteral Pumps

B9000 Enteral nutrition infusion pump - without alarm

B9002 Enteral nutrition infusion pump, any type

B9004 Parenteral nutrition infusion pump, portable

B9006 Parenteral nutrition infusion pump, stationary

B9998 Noc for enteral supplies

B9999 Noc for parenteral supplies

B - C CODES

HOSPITAL OUTPATIENT PPS CODES

Guidelines

The "C" codes are unique temporary codes established by CMS for use under the Hospital Outpatient Prospective Payment System (OPPS). Non-OPPS use of these codes for Medicare is not valid.

The purpose of the "C" codes is to provide hospitals with a list of codes and long descriptors for drugs, biologicals and devices eligible for transitional pass-through payments, and for items classified in "new technology" ambulatory payment classifications (APCs) under the new Hospital Outpatient Prospective Payment System (OPPS).

The listing of HCPCS codes in this section does not assure coverage of the specific item or service in a given case. To be eligible for pass-through and new technology payments, the items reported with "C" codes must be considered reasonable and necessary.

All of the "C" codes are used exclusively for services paid under the Hospital Outpatient Prospective Payment System and may not be used to bill for services paid under other Medicare payment systems.

In addition to the information presented above, several other items unique to this section are defined here:

1. **SPECIAL REPORT:** A service, material or supply that is rarely provided, unusual, variable or new may require a special report in determining medical appropriateness for reimbursement purposes. Pertinent information should include an adequate definition or description of the nature, extent, and need for the service, material or supply.

2. **MODIFIERS:** Listed services may be modified under certain circumstances. When appropriate, the modifying circumstance is identified by adding a modifier to the basic procedure code. CPT and HCPCS National Level II modifiers may be used with CPT and HCPCS National Level II procedure codes.

Hospital Outpatient PPS Codes

C1052 Hemostatic agent, gastrointestinal, topical

C1062 Intravertebral body fracture augmentation with implant (e.g., metal, polymer)

C1300 Hyperbaric oxygen under pressure, full body chamber, per 30 minute interval

• **C1600** Catheter, transluminal intravascular lesion preparation device, bladed, sheathed (insertable)

• **C1601** Endoscope, single-use (i.e., disposable), pulmonary, imaging/illumination device (insertable)

• **C1602** Orthopedic/device/drug matrix/absorbable bone void filler, antimicrobial-eluting (implantable)

• **C1603** Retrieval device, insertable, laser (used to retrieve intravascular inferior vena cava filter)

• **C1604** Graft, transmural transvenous arterial bypass (implantable), with all delivery system components

C1713 Anchor/screw for opposing bone-to-bone or soft tissue-to-bone (implantable)

C1714 Catheter, transluminal atherectomy, directional

C1715 Brachytherapy needle

C1716 Brachytherapy source, non-stranded, gold-198, per source

C1717 Brachytherapy source, non-stranded, high dose rate iridium-192, per source

C1719 Brachytherapy source, non-stranded, non-high dose rate iridium-192, per source

C1721 Cardioverter-defibrillator, dual chamber (implantable)

C1722 Cardioverter-defibrillator, single chamber (implantable)

C1724 Catheter, transluminal atherectomy, rotational

C1725 Catheter, transluminal angioplasty, non-laser (may include guidance, infusion/perfusion capability)

C1726 Catheter, balloon dilatation, non-vascular

C1727 Catheter, balloon tissue dissector, non-vascular (insertable)

C1728 Catheter, brachytherapy seed administration

C1729 Catheter, drainage

C1730 Catheter, electrophysiology, diagnostic, other than 3d mapping (19 or fewer electrodes)

C1731 Catheter, electrophysiology, diagnostic, other than 3d mapping (20 or more electrodes)

C1732 Catheter, electrophysiology, diagnostic/ablation, 3d or vector mapping

C1733 Catheter, electrophysiology, diagnostic/ablation, other than 3d or vector mapping, other than cool-tip

C1734 Orthopedic/device/drug matrix for opposing bone-to-bone or soft tissue-to bone (implantable)

● **C1747** Endoscope, single-use (i.e., disposable), urinary tract, imaging/illumination device (insertable)

C1748 Endoscope, single-use (i.e., disposable), upper GI, imaging/illumination device (insertable)

C1749 Endoscope, retrograde imaging/illumination colonoscope device (implantable)

C1750 Catheter, hemodialysis/peritoneal, long-term

C1751 Catheter, infusion, inserted peripherally, centrally or midline (other than hemodialysis)

C1752 Catheter, hemodialysis/peritoneal, short-term

C1753 Catheter, intravascular ultrasound

C1754 Catheter, intradiscal

C1755 Catheter, intraspinal

C1756 Catheter, pacing, transesophageal

C1757 Catheter, thrombectomy/embolectomy

C1758 Catheter, ureteral

C1759 Catheter, intracardiac echocardiography

C1760 Closure device, vascular (implantable/insertable)

C1761 Catheter, transluminal intravascular lithotripsy, coronary

C1762 Connective tissue, human (includes fascia lata)

C1763 Connective tissue, non-human (includes synthetic)

C1764 Event recorder, cardiac (implantable)

C1765 Adhesion barrier

C1766 Introducer/sheath, guiding, intracardiac electrophysiological, steerable, other than peel-away

C1767 Generator, neurostimulator (implantable), non-rechargeable

C1768 Graft, vascular

C1769 Guide wire

C1770 Imaging coil, magnetic resonance (insertable)

C1771	Repair device, urinary, incontinence, with sling graft
C1772	Infusion pump, programmable (implantable)
C1773	Retrieval device, insertable (used to retrieve fractured medical devices)
C1776	Joint device (implantable)
C1777	Lead, cardioverter-defibrillator, endocardial single coil (implantable)
C1778	Lead, neurostimulator (implantable)
C1779	Lead, pacemaker, transvenous VDD single pass
C1780	Lens, intraocular (new technology)
C1781	Mesh (implantable)
C1782	Morcellator
C1783	Ocular implant, aqueous drainage assist device
C1784	Ocular device, intraoperative, detached retina
C1785	Pacemaker, dual chamber, rate-responsive (implantable)
C1786	Pacemaker, single chamber, rate-responsive (implantable)
C1787	Patient programmer, neurostimulator
C1788	Port, indwelling (implantable)
C1789	Prosthesis, breast (implantable)
C1813	Prosthesis, penile, inflatable
C1814	Retinal tamponade device, silicone oil
C1815	Prosthesis, urinary sphincter (implantable)
C1816	Receiver and/or transmitter, neurostimulator (implantable)
C1817	Septal defect implant system, intracardiac
C1818	Integrated keratoprosthesis
C1819	Surgical tissue localization and excision device (implantable)
C1820	Generator, neurostimulator (implantable), with rechargeable battery and charging system
C1821	Interspinous process distraction device (implantable)
C1822	Generator, neurostimulator (implantable), high frequency, with rechargeable battery and charging system
C1823	Generator, neurostimulator (implantable), non-rechargeable, with transvenous sensing and stimulation leads
C1824	Generator, cardiac contractility modulation (implantable)
C1825	Generator, neurostimulator (implantable), non-rechargeable with carotid sinus baroreceptor stimulation lead(s)
• **C1826**	Generator, neurostimulator (implantable), includes closed feedback loop leads and all implantable components, with rechargeable battery and charging system
• **C1827**	Generator, neurostimulator (implantable), non-rechargeable, with implantable stimulation lead and external paired stimulation controller
C1830	Powered bone marrow biopsy needle
C1831	Interbody cage, anterior, lateral or posterior, personalized (implantable)

C1832 Autograft suspension, including cell processing and application, and all system components

C1833 Monitor, cardiac, including intracardiac lead and all system components (implantable)

C1834 Pressure sensor system, includes all components (e.g., introducer, sensor), intramuscular (implantable), excludes mobile (wireless) software application

C1839 Iris prosthesis

C1840 Lens, intraocular (telescopic)

(**C1841** Retinal prosthesis, includes all internal and external components
Code deleted effective 12/31/2022, no HCPCS/CPT cross-reference provided.)

(**C1842** Retinal prosthesis, includes all internal and external components; add-on to c1841
Code deleted effective 12/31/2022, no HCPCS/CPT cross-reference provided.)

(**C1849** Skin substitute, synthetic, resorbable, per square centimeter
Code deleted effective 12/31/2022, no HCPCS/CPT cross-reference provided.)

C1874 Stent, coated/covered, with delivery system

C1875 Stent, coated/covered, without delivery system

C1876 Stent, non-coated/non-covered, with delivery system

C1877 Stent, non-coated/non-covered, without delivery system

C1878 Material for vocal cord medialization, synthetic (implantable)

C1880 Vena cava filter

C1881 Dialysis access system (implantable)

C1882 Cardioverter-defibrillator, other than single or dual chamber (implantable)

C1883 Adapter/extension, pacing lead or neurostimulator lead (implantable)

C1884 Embolization protective system

C1885 Catheter, transluminal angioplasty, laser

C1886 Catheter, extravascular tissue ablation, any modality (insertable)

C1887 Catheter, guiding (may include infusion/perfusion capability)

C1888 Catheter, ablation, non-cardiac, endovascular (implantable)

C1889 Implantable/insertable device, not otherwise classified

C1890 No implantable/insertable device used with device-intensive procedures

C1891 Infusion pump, non-programmable, permanent (implantable)

C1892 Introducer/sheath, guiding, intracardiac electrophysiological, fixed-curve, peel-away

C1893 Introducer/sheath, guiding, intracardiac electrophysiological, fixed-curve, other than peel-away

C1894 Introducer/sheath, other than guiding, other than intracardiac electrophysiological, non-laser

C1895 Lead, cardioverter-defibrillator, endocardial dual coil (implantable)

C1896 Lead, cardioverter-defibrillator, other than endocardial single or dual coil (implantable)

C1897 Lead, neurostimulator test kit (implantable)

C1898 Lead, pacemaker, other than transvenous VDD single pass

C1899 Lead, pacemaker/cardioverter-defibrillator combination (implantable)

C1900 Lead, left ventricular coronary venous system

C1982	Catheter, pressure-generating, one-way valve, intermittently occlusive
C2596	Probe, image-guided, robotic, waterjet ablation
C2613	Lung biopsy plug with delivery system
C2614	Probe, percutaneous lumbar discectomy
C2615	Sealant, pulmonary, liquid
C2616	Brachytherapy source, non-stranded, yttrium-90, per source
C2617	Stent, non-coronary, temporary, without delivery system
C2618	Probe/needle, cryoablation
C2619	Pacemaker, dual chamber, non rate-responsive (implantable)
C2620	Pacemaker, single chamber, non rate-responsive (implantable)
C2621	Pacemaker, other than single or dual chamber (implantable)
C2622	Prosthesis, penile, non-inflatable
C2623	Catheter, transluminal angioplasty, drug-coated, non-laser
C2624	Implantable wireless pulmonary artery pressure sensor with delivery catheter, including all system components
C2625	Stent, non-coronary, temporary, with delivery system
C2626	Infusion pump, non-programmable, temporary (implantable)
C2627	Catheter, suprapubic/cystoscopic
C2628	Catheter, occlusion
C2629	Introducer/sheath, other than guiding, other than intracardiac electrophysiological, laser
C2630	Catheter, electrophysiology, diagnostic/ablation, other than 3d or vector mapping, cool-tip
C2631	Repair device, urinary, incontinence, without sling graft
C2634	Brachytherapy source, non-stranded, high activity, iodine-125, greater than 1.01 mci (nist), per source
C2635	Brachytherapy source, non-stranded, high activity, palladium-103, greater than 2.2 mci (nist), per source
C2636	Brachytherapy linear source, non-stranded, palladium-103, per 1 mm
C2637	Brachytherapy source, non-stranded, ytterbium-169, per source
C2638	Brachytherapy source, stranded, iodine-125, per source
C2639	Brachytherapy source, non-stranded, iodine-125, per source
C2640	Brachytherapy source, stranded, palladium-103, per source
C2641	Brachytherapy source, non-stranded, palladium-103, per source
C2642	Brachytherapy source, stranded, cesium-131, per source
C2643	Brachytherapy source, non-stranded, cesium-131, per source
C2644	Brachytherapy source, cesium-131 chloride solution, per millicurie
C2645	Brachytherapy planar source, palladium-103, per square millimeter
C2698	Brachytherapy source, stranded, not otherwise specified, per source
C2699	Brachytherapy source, non-stranded, not otherwise specified, per source

C5271 Application of low cost skin substitute graft to trunk, arms, legs, total wound surface area up to 100 sq cm; first 25 sq cm or less wound surface area

C5272 Application of low cost skin substitute graft to trunk, arms, legs, total wound surface area up to 100 sq cm; each additional 25 sq cm wound surface area, or part thereof (list separately in addition to code for primary procedure)

C5273 Application of low cost skin substitute graft to trunk, arms, legs, total wound surface area greater than or equal to 100 sq cm; first 100 sq cm wound surface area, or 1% of body area of infants and children

C5274 Application of low cost skin substitute graft to trunk, arms, legs, total wound surface area greater than or equal to 100 sq cm; each additional 100 sq cm wound surface area, or part thereof, or each additional 1% of body area of infants and children, or part thereof (list separately in addition to code for primary procedure)

C5275 Application of low cost skin substitute graft to face, scalp, eyelids, mouth, neck, ears, orbits, genitalia, hands, feet, and/or multiple digits, total wound surface area up to 100 sq cm; first 25 sq cm or less wound surface area

C5276 Application of low cost skin substitute graft to face, scalp, eyelids, mouth, neck, ears, orbits, genitalia, hands, feet, and/or multiple digits, total wound surface area up to 100 sq cm; each additional 25 sq cm wound surface area, or part thereof (list separately in addition to code for primary procedure)

C5277 Application of low cost skin substitute graft to face, scalp, eyelids, mouth, neck, ears, orbits, genitalia, hands, feet, and/or multiple digits, total wound surface area greater than or equal to 100 sq cm; first 100 sq cm wound surface area, or 1% of body area of infants and children

C5278 Application of low cost skin substitute graft to face, scalp, eyelids, mouth, neck, ears, orbits, genitalia, hands, feet, and/or multiple digits, total wound surface area greater than or equal to 100 sq cm; each additional 100 sq cm wound surface area, or part thereof, or each additional 1% of body area of infants and children, or part thereof (list separately in addition to code for primary procedure)

• **C7500** Debridement, bone including epidermis, dermis, subcutaneous tissue, muscle and/or fascia, if performed, first 20 sq cm or less with manual preparation and insertion of deep (e.g., subfacial) drug-delivery device(s)

• **C7501** Percutaneous breast biopsies using stereotactic guidance, with placement of breast localization device(s) (e.g., clip, metallic pellet), when performed, and imaging of the biopsy specimen, when performed, all lesions unilateral and bilateral (for single lesion biopsy, use appropriate code)

• **C7502** Percutaneous breast biopsies using magnetic resonance guidance, with placement of breast localization device(s) (e.g., clip, metallic pellet), when performed, and imaging of the biopsy specimen, when performed, all lesions unilateral or bilateral (for single lesion biopsy, use appropriate code)

• **C7503** Open biopsy or excision of deep cervical node(s) with intraoperative identification (e.g., mapping) of sentinel lymph node(s) including injection of non-radioactive dye when performed

• **C7504** Percutaneous vertebroplasties (bone biopsies included when performed), first cervicothoracic and any additional cervicothoracic or lumbosacral vertebral bodies, unilateral or bilateral injection, inclusive of all imaging guidance

• **C7505** Percutaneous vertebroplasties (bone biopsies included when performed), first lumbosacral and any additional cervicothoracic or lumbosacral vertebral bodies, unilateral or bilateral injection, inclusive of all imaging guidance

• **C7506** Arthrodesis, interphalangeal joints, with or without internal fixation

• **C7507** Percutaneous vertebral augmentations, first thoracic and any additional thoracic or lumbar vertebral bodies, including cavity creations (fracture reductions and bone biopsies included when performed) using mechanical device (e.g., kyphoplasty), unilateral or bilateral cannulations, inclusive of all imaging guidance

- **C7509** Bronchoscopy, rigid or flexible, diagnostic with cell washing(s) when performed, with computer-assisted image-guided navigation, including fluoroscopic guidance when performed
- **C7510** Bronchoscopy, rigid or flexible, with bronchial alveolar lavage(s), with computer-assisted image-guided navigation, including fluoroscopic guidance when performed
- **C7511** Bronchoscopy, rigid or flexible, with single or multiple bronchial or endobronchial biopsy(ies), single or multiple sites, with computer-assisted image-guided navigation, including fluoroscopic guidance when performed
- **C7512** Bronchoscopy, rigid or flexible, with single or multiple bronchial or endobronchial biopsy(ies), single or multiple sites, with transendoscopic endobronchial ultrasound (ebus) during bronchoscopic diagnostic or therapeutic intervention(s) for peripheral lesion(s), including fluoroscopic guidance when performed
- **C7513** Dialysis circuit, introduction of needle(s) and/or catheter(s), with diagnostic angiography of the dialysis circuit, including all direct puncture(s) and catheter placement(s), injection(s) of contrast, all necessary imaging from the arterial anastomosis and adjacent artery through entire venous outflow including the inferior or superior vena cava, fluoroscopic guidance, with transluminal balloon angioplasty of central dialysis segment, performed through dialysis circuit, including all required imaging, radiological supervision and interpretation, image documentation and report
- **C7514** Dialysis circuit, introduction of needle(s) and/or catheter(s), with diagnostic angiography of the dialysis circuit, including all direct puncture(s) and catheter placement(s), injection(s) of contrast, all necessary imaging from the arterial anastomosis and adjacent artery through entire venous outflow including the inferior or superior vena cava, fluoroscopic guidance, with all angioplasty in the central dialysis segment, and transcatheter placement of intravascular stent(s), central dialysis segment, performed through dialysis circuit, including all required imaging, radiological supervision and interpretation, image documentation and report
- **C7515** Dialysis circuit, introduction of needle(s) and/or catheter(s), with diagnostic angiography of the dialysis circuit, including all direct puncture(s) and catheter placement(s), injection(s) of contrast, all necessary imaging from the arterial anastomosis and adjacent artery through entire venous outflow including the inferior or superior vena cava, fluoroscopic guidance, with dialysis circuit permanent endovascular embolization or occlusion of main circuit or any accessory veins, including all required imaging, radiological supervision and interpretation, image documentation and report
- **C7516** Catheter placement in coronary artery(s) for coronary angiography, including intraprocedural injection(s) for coronary angiography, with endoluminal imaging of initial coronary vessel or graft using intravascular ultrasound (IVUS) or optical coherence tomography (oct) during diagnostic evaluation and/or therapeutic intervention including imaging supervision, interpretation and report
- **C7517** Catheter placement in coronary artery(s) for coronary angiography, including intraprocedural injection(s) for coronary angiography, with iliac and/or femoral artery angiography, non-selective, bilateral or ipsilateral to catheter insertion, performed at the same time as cardiac catheterization and/or coronary angiography, includes positioning or placement of the catheter in the distal aorta or ipsilateral femoral or iliac artery, injection of dye, production of permanent images, and radiologic supervision and interpretation
- **C7518** Catheter placement in coronary artery(ies) for coronary angiography, including intraprocedural injection(s) for coronary angiography, imaging supervision and interpretation, with catheter placement(s) in bypass graft(s) (internal mammary, free arterial, venous grafts) including intraprocedural injection(s) for bypass graft angiography with endoluminal imaging of initial coronary vessel or graft using intravascular ultrasound (IVUS) or optical coherence tomography (oct) during diagnostic evaluation and/or therapeutic intervention including imaging, supervision, interpretation and report
- **C7519** Catheter placement in coronary artery(ies) for coronary angiography, including intraprocedural injection(s) for coronary angiography, imaging supervision and interpretation, with catheter placement(s) in bypass graft(s) (internal mammary, free arterial, venous grafts) including intraprocedural injection(s) for bypass graft angiography with intravascular doppler velocity

and/or pressure derived coronary flow reserve measurement (initial coronary vessel or graft) during coronary angiography including pharmacologically induced stress

- **C7520** Catheter placement in coronary artery(ies) for coronary angiography, including intraprocedural injection(s) for coronary angiography, imaging supervision and interpretation, with catheter placement(s) in bypass graft(s) (internal mammary, free arterial, venous grafts) includes intraprocedural injection(s) for bypass graft angiography with iliac and/or femoral artery angiography, non-selective, bilateral or ipsilateral to catheter insertion, performed at the same time as cardiac catheterization and/or coronary angiography, includes positioning or placement of the catheter in the distal aorta or ipsilateral femoral or iliac artery, injection of dye, production of permanent images, and radiologic supervision and interpretation
- **C7521** Catheter placement in coronary artery(ies) for coronary angiography, including intraprocedural injection(s) for coronary angiography with right heart catheterization with endoluminal imaging of initial coronary vessel or graft using intravascular ultrasound (IVUS) or optical coherence tomography (oct) during diagnostic evaluation and/or therapeutic intervention including imaging supervision, interpretation and report
- **C7522** Catheter placement in coronary artery(ies) for coronary angiography, including intraprocedural injection(s) for coronary angiography, imaging supervision and interpretation with right heart catheterization, with intravascular doppler velocity and/or pressure derived coronary flow reserve measurement (initial coronary vessel or graft) during coronary angiography including pharmacologically induced stress
- **C7523** Catheter placement in coronary artery(ies) for coronary angiography, including intraprocedural injection(s) for coronary angiography, imaging supervision and interpretation, with left heart catheterization including intraprocedural injection(s) for left ventriculography, when performed, with endoluminal imaging of initial coronary vessel or graft using intravascular ultrasound (IVUS) or optical coherence tomography (oct) during diagnostic evaluation and/or therapeutic intervention including imaging supervision, interpretation and report
- **C7524** Catheter placement in coronary artery(ies) for coronary angiography, including intraprocedural injection(s) for coronary angiography, imaging supervision and interpretation, with left heart catheterization including intraprocedural injection(s) for left ventriculography, when performed, with intravascular doppler velocity and/or pressure derived coronary flow reserve measurement (initial coronary vessel or graft) during coronary angiography including pharmacologically induced stress
- **C7525** Catheter placement in coronary artery(ies) for coronary angiography, including intraprocedural injection(s) for coronary angiography, imaging supervision and interpretation, with left heart catheterization including intraprocedural injection(s) for left ventriculography, when performed, catheter placement(s) in bypass graft(s) (internal mammary, free arterial, venous grafts) with bypass graft angiography with endoluminal imaging of initial coronary vessel or graft using intravascular ultrasound (IVUS) or optical coherence tomography (oct) during diagnostic evaluation and/or therapeutic intervention including imaging supervision, interpretation and report
- **C7526** Catheter placement in coronary artery(ies) for coronary angiography, including intraprocedural injection(s) for coronary angiography, imaging supervision and interpretation, with left heart catheterization including intraprocedural injection(s) for left ventriculography, when performed, catheter placement(s) in bypass graft(s) (internal mammary, free arterial, venous grafts) with bypass graft angiography with intravascular doppler velocity and/or pressure derived coronary flow reserve measurement (initial coronary vessel or graft) during coronary angiography including pharmacologically induced stress
- **C7527** Catheter placement in coronary artery(ies) for coronary angiography, including intraprocedural injection(s) for coronary angiography, imaging supervision and interpretation, with right and left heart catheterization including intraprocedural injection(s) for left ventriculography, when performed, with endoluminal imaging of initial coronary vessel or graft using intravascular ultrasound (IVUS) or optical coherence tomography (oct) during diagnostic evaluation and/or therapeutic intervention including imaging supervision, interpretation and report
- **C7528** Catheter placement in coronary artery(ies) for coronary angiography, including intraprocedural

B - C CODES

injection(s) for coronary angiography, imaging supervision and interpretation, with right and left heart catheterization including intraprocedural injection(s) for left ventriculography, when performed, with intravascular doppler velocity and/or pressure derived coronary flow reserve measurement (initial coronary vessel or graft) during coronary angiography including pharmacologically induced stress

- **C7529** Catheter placement in coronary artery(ies) for coronary angiography, including intraprocedural injection(s) for coronary angiography, imaging supervision and interpretation, with right and left heart catheterization including intraprocedural injection(s) for left ventriculography, when performed, catheter placement(s) in bypass graft(s) (internal mammary, free arterial, venous grafts) with bypass graft angiography with intravascular doppler velocity and/or pressure derived coronary flow reserve measurement (initial coronary vessel or graft) during coronary angiography including pharmacologically induced stress
- **C7530** Dialysis circuit, introduction of needle(s) and/or catheter(s), with diagnostic angiography of the dialysis circuit, including all direct puncture(s) and catheter placement(s), injection(s) of contrast, all necessary imaging from the arterial anastomosis and adjacent artery through entire venous outflow including the inferior or superior vena cava, fluoroscopic guidance, with transluminal balloon angioplasty, peripheral dialysis segment, including all imaging and radiological supervision and interpretation necessary to perform the angioplasty and all angioplasty in the central dialysis segment, with transcatheter placement of intravascular stent(s), central dialysis segment, performed through dialysis circuit, including all imaging, radiological supervision and interpretation, documentation and report
- **C7531** Revascularization, endovascular, open or percutaneous, femoral, popliteal artery(ies), unilateral, with transluminal angioplasty with intravascular ultrasound (initial noncoronary vessel) during diagnostic evaluation and/or therapeutic intervention, including radiological supervision and interpretation
- **C7532** Transluminal balloon angioplasty (except lower extremity artery(ies) for occlusive disease, intracranial, coronary, pulmonary, or dialysis circuit), initial artery, open or percutaneous, including all imaging and radiological supervision and interpretation necessary to perform the angioplasty within the same artery, with intravascular ultrasound (initial noncoronary vessel) during diagnostic evaluation and/or therapeutic intervention, including radiological supervision and interpretation
- **C7533** Percutaneous transluminal coronary angioplasty, single major coronary artery or branch with transcatheter placement of radiation delivery device for subsequent coronary intravascular brachytherapy
- **C7534** Revascularization, endovascular, open or percutaneous, femoral, popliteal artery(ies), unilateral, with atherectomy, includes angioplasty within the same vessel, when performed with intravascular ultrasound (initial noncoronary vessel) during diagnostic evaluation and/or therapeutic intervention, including radiological supervision and interpretation
- **C7535** Revascularization, endovascular, open or percutaneous, femoral, popliteal artery(ies), unilateral, with transluminal stent placement(s), includes angioplasty within the same vessel, when performed, with intravascular ultrasound (initial noncoronary vessel) during diagnostic evaluation and/or therapeutic intervention, including radiological supervision and interpretation
- **C7537** Insertion of new or replacement of permanent pacemaker with atrial transvenous electrode(s), with insertion of pacing electrode, cardiac venous system, for left ventricular pacing, at time of insertion of implantable defibrillator or pacemaker pulse generator (e.g., for upgrade to dual chamber system)
- **C7538** Insertion of new or replacement of permanent pacemaker with ventricular transvenous electrode(s), with insertion of pacing electrode, cardiac venous system, for left ventricular pacing, at time of insertion of implantable defibrillator or pacemaker pulse generator (e.g., for upgrade to dual chamber system)
- **C7539** Insertion of new or replacement of permanent pacemaker with atrial and ventricular transvenous

electrode(s), with insertion of pacing electrode, cardiac venous system, for left ventricular pacing, at time of insertion of implantable defibrillator or pacemaker pulse generator (e.g., for upgrade to dual chamber system)

- • **C7540** Removal of permanent pacemaker pulse generator with replacement of pacemaker pulse generator, dual lead system, with insertion of pacing electrode, cardiac venous system, for left ventricular pacing, at time of insertion of implantable defibrillator or pacemaker pulse generator (e.g., for upgrade to dual chamber system)
- • **C7541** Diagnostic endoscopic retrograde cholangiopancreatography (ERCP), including collection of specimen(s) by brushing or washing, when performed, with endoscopic cannulation of papilla with direct visualization of pancreatic/common bile ducts(s)
- • **C7542** Endoscopic retrograde cholangiopancreatography (ERCP) with biopsy, single or multiple, with endoscopic cannulation of papilla with direct visualization of pancreatic/common bile ducts(s)
- • **C7543** Endoscopic retrograde cholangiopancreatography (ERCP) with sphincterotomy/papillotomy, with endoscopic cannulation of papilla with direct visualization of pancreatic/common bile ducts(s)
- • **C7544** Endoscopic retrograde cholangiopancreatography (ERCP) with removal of calculi/debris from biliary/pancreatic duct(s), with endoscopic cannulation of papilla with direct visualization of pancreatic/common bile ducts(s)
- • **C7545** Percutaneous exchange of biliary drainage catheter (e.g., external, internal-external, or conversion of internal-external to external only), with removal of calculi/debris from biliary duct(s) and/or gallbladder, including destruction of calculi by any method (e.g., mechanical, electrohydraulic, lithotripsy) when performed, including diagnostic cholangiography(ies) when performed, imaging guidance (e.g., fluoroscopy), and all associated radiological supervision and interpretation
- • **C7546** Removal and replacement of externally accessible nephroureteral catheter (e.g., external/internal stent) requiring fluoroscopic guidance, with ureteral stricture balloon dilation, including imaging guidance and all associated radiological supervision and interpretation
- • **C7547** Convert nephrostomy catheter to nephroureteral catheter, percutaneous via pre-existing nephrostomy tract, with ureteral stricture balloon dilation, including diagnostic nephrostogram and/or ureterogram when performed, imaging guidance (e.g., ultrasound and/or fluoroscopy) and all associated radiological supervision and interpretation
- • **C7548** Exchange nephrostomy catheter, percutaneous, with ureteral stricture balloon dilation, including diagnostic nephrostogram and/or ureterogram when performed, imaging guidance (e.g., ultrasound and/or fluoroscopy) and all associated radiological supervision and interpretation
- • **C7549** Change of ureterostomy tube or externally accessible ureteral stent via ileal conduit with ureteral stricture balloon dilation, including imaging guidance (e.g., ultrasound and/or fluoroscopy) and all associated radiological supervision and interpretation
- • **C7550** Cystourethroscopy, with biopsy(ies) with adjunctive blue light cystoscopy with fluorescent imaging agent
- • **C7551** Excision of major peripheral nerve neuroma, except sciatic, with implantation of nerve end into bone or muscle
- • **C7552** Catheter placement in coronary artery(s) for coronary angiography, including intraprocedural injection(s) for coronary angiography, imaging supervision and interpretation; with catheter placement(s) in bypass graft(s) (internal mammary, free arterial, venous grafts) including intraprocedural injection(s) for bypass graft angiography and right heart catheterization with intravascular doppler velocity and/or pressure derived coronary flow reserve measurement (coronary vessel or graft) during coronary angiography including pharmacologically induced stress, initial vessel
- • **C7553** Catheter placement in coronary artery(s) for coronary angiography, including intraprocedural injection(s) for coronary angiography, imaging supervision and interpretation; with right and left heart catheterization including intraprocedural injection(s) for left ventriculography, when performed, catheter placement(s) in bypass graft(s) (internal mammary, free arterial, venous grafts) with bypass graft angiography with pharmacologic agent administration (e.g., inhaled nitric

oxide, intravenous infusion of nitroprusside, dobutamine, milrinone, or other agent) including assessing hemodynamic measurements before, during, after and repeat pharmacologic agent administration, when performed

- **C7554** Cystourethroscopy with adjunctive blue light cystoscopy with fluorescent imaging agent
- **C7555** Thyroidectomy, total or complete with parathyroid autotransplantation
- **C7556** Bronchoscopy, rigid or flexible, with bronchial alveolar lavage and transendoscopic endobronchial ultrasound (ebus) during bronchoscopic diagnostic or therapeutic intervention(s) for peripheral lesion(s), including fluoroscopic guidance, when performed
- **C7557** Catheter placement in coronary artery(s) for coronary angiography, including intraprocedural injection(s) for coronary angiography, imaging supervision and interpretation with left heart catheterization including intraprocedural injection(s) for left ventriculography, when performed and intraprocedural coronary fractional flow reserve (FFR) with 3d functional mapping of color-coded FFR values for the coronary tree, derived from coronary angiogram data, for real-time review and interpretation of possible atherosclerotic stenosis(es) intervention
- **C7558** Catheter placement in coronary artery(s) for coronary angiography, including intraprocedural injection(s) for coronary angiography, imaging supervision and interpretation with right and left heart catheterization including intraprocedural injection(s) for left ventriculography, when performed, catheter placement(s) in bypass graft(s) (internal mammary, free arterial, venous grafts) with bypass graft angiography with pharmacologic agent administration (eg, inhaled nitric oxide, intravenous infusion of nitroprusside, dobutamine, milrinone, or other agent) including assessing hemodynamic measurements before, during, after and repeat pharmacologic agent administration, when performed
- **C7560** Endoscopic retrograde cholangiopancreatography (ERCP) with removal of foreign body(s) or stent(s) from biliary/pancreatic duct(s) and endoscopic cannulation of papilla with direct visualization of pancreatic/common bile duct(s)
- **C7561** Debridement, bone (includes epidermis, dermis, subcutaneous tissue, muscle and/or fascia, if performed); first 20 sq cm or less with manual preparation and insertion of drug-delivery device(s), deep (e.g., subfascial)
- **C7556** Bronchoscopy, rigid or flexible, with bronchial alveolar lavage and transendoscopic endobronchial ultrasound (ebus) during bronchoscopic diagnostic or therapeutic intervention(s) for peripheral lesion(s), including fluoroscopic guidance, when performed
- **C7900** Service for diagnosis, evaluation, or treatment of a mental health or substance use disorder, initial 15-29 minutes, provided remotely by hospital staff who are licensed to provide mental health services under applicable state law(s), when the patient is in their home, and there is no associated professional service
- **C7901** Service for diagnosis, evaluation, or treatment of a mental health or substance use disorder, initial 30-60 minutes, provided remotely by hospital staff who are licensed to provided mental health services under applicable state law(s), when the patient is in their home, and there is no associated professional service
- **C7902** Service for diagnosis, evaluation, or treatment of a mental health or substance use disorder, each additional 15 minutes, provided remotely by hospital staff who are licensed to provide mental health services under applicable state law(s), when the patient is in their home, and there is no associated professional service (list separately in addition to code for primary service)
- **C7903** Group psychotherapy service for diagnosis, evaluation, or treatment of a mental health or substance use disorder provided remotely by hospital staff who are licensed to provide mental health services under applicable state law(s), when the patient is in their home, and there is no associated professional service

C8900 Magnetic resonance angiography with contrast, abdomen

C8901 Magnetic resonance angiography without contrast, abdomen

C8902 Magnetic resonance angiography without contrast followed by with contrast, abdomen

C8903 Magnetic resonance imaging with contrast, breast; unilateral

C8904 Magnetic resonance imaging without contrast, breast; unilateral

C8905 Magnetic resonance imaging without contrast followed by with contrast, breast; unilateral

C8906 Magnetic resonance imaging with contrast, breast; bilateral

C8907 Magnetic resonance imaging without contrast, breast; bilateral

C8908 Magnetic resonance imaging without contrast followed by with contrast, breast; bilateral

C8909 Magnetic resonance angiography with contrast, chest (excluding myocardium)

C8910 Magnetic resonance angiography without contrast, chest (excluding myocardium)

C8911 Magnetic resonance angiography without contrast followed by with contrast, chest (excluding myocardium)

C8912 Magnetic resonance angiography with contrast, lower extremity

C8913 Magnetic resonance angiography without contrast, lower extremity

C8914 Magnetic resonance angiography without contrast followed by with contrast, lower extremity

C8918 Magnetic resonance angiography with contrast, pelvis

C8919 Magnetic resonance angiography without contrast, pelvis

C8920 Magnetic resonance angiography without contrast followed by with contrast, pelvis

C8921 Transthoracic echocardiography with contrast, or without contrast followed by with contrast, for congenital cardiac anomalies; complete

C8922 Transthoracic echocardiography with contrast, or without contrast followed by with contrast, for congenital cardiac anomalies; follow-up or limited study

C8923 Transthoracic echocardiography with contrast, or without contrast followed by with contrast, real-time with image documentation (2d), includes m-mode recording, when performed, complete, without spectral or color doppler echocardiography

C8924 Transthoracic echocardiography with contrast, or without contrast followed by with contrast, real-time with image documentation (2d), includes m-mode recording, when performed, follow-up or limited study

C8925 Transesophageal echocardiography (tee) with contrast, or without contrast followed by with contrast, real time with image documentation (2d) (with or without m-mode recording); including probe placement, image acquisition, interpretation and report

C8926 Transesophageal echocardiography (tee) with contrast, or without contrast followed by with contrast, for congenital cardiac anomalies; including probe placement, image acquisition, interpretation and report

C8927 Transesophageal echocardiography (tee) with contrast, or without contrast followed by with contrast, for monitoring purposes, including probe placement, real time 2-dimensional image acquisition and interpretation leading to ongoing (continuous) assessment of (dynamically changing) cardiac pumping function and to therapeutic measures on an immediate time basis

C8928 Transthoracic echocardiography with contrast, or without contrast followed by with contrast, real-time with image documentation (2d), includes m-mode recording, when performed, during rest

and cardiovascular stress test using treadmill, bicycle exercise and/or pharmacologically induced stress, with interpretation and report

C8929 Transthoracic echocardiography with contrast, or without contrast followed by with contrast, real-time with image documentation (2d), includes m-mode recording, when performed, complete, with spectral doppler echocardiography, and with color flow doppler echocardiography

C8930	Transthoracic echocardiography, with contrast, or without contrast followed by with contrast, real-time with image documentation (2d), includes m-mode recording, when performed, during rest and cardiovascular stress test using treadmill, bicycle exercise and/or pharmacologically induced stress, with interpretation and report; including performance of continuous electrocardiographic monitoring, with physician supervision
C8931	Magnetic resonance angiography with contrast, spinal canal and contents
C8932	Magnetic resonance angiography without contrast, spinal canal and contents
C8933	Magnetic resonance angiography without contrast followed by with contrast, spinal canal and contents
C8934	Magnetic resonance angiography with contrast, upper extremity
C8935	Magnetic resonance angiography without contrast, upper extremity
C8936	Magnetic resonance angiography without contrast followed by with contrast, upper extremity
C8937	Computer-aided detection, including computer algorithm analysis of breast MRI image data for lesion detection/characterization, pharmacokinetic analysis, with further physician review for interpretation (list separately in addition to code for primary procedure)
C8957	Intravenous infusion for therapy/diagnosis; initiation of prolonged infusion (more than 8 hours), requiring use of portable or implantable pump
C9014	Injection, cerliponase alfa, 1 mg
C9015	Injection, c-1 esterase inhibitor (human), haegarda, 10 units
C9016	Injection, triptorelin extended release, 3.75 mg
C9021	Injection, obinutuzumab, 10 mg
C9022	Injection, elosulfase alfa, 1mg
C9023	Injection, testosterone undecanoate, 1 mg
C9024	Injection, liposomal, 1 mg daunorubicin and 2.27 mg cytarabine
C9025	Injection, ramucirumab, 5 mg
C9026	Injection, vedolizumab, 1 mg
C9027	Injection, pembrolizumab, 1 mg
C9028	Injection, inotuzumab ozogamicin, 0.1 mg
C9029	Injection, guselkumab, 1 mg
C9030	Injection, copanlisib, 1 mg
C9031	Lutetium lu 177, dotatate, therapeutic, 1 mci
C9032	Injection, voretigene neparvovec-rzyl, 1 billion vector genome
C9033	Injection, fosnetupitant 235 mg and palonosetron 0.25 mg
C9034	Injection, dexamethasone 9%, intraocular, 1 mcg
C9035	Injection, aripiprazole lauroxil (aristada initio), 1 mg
C9036	Injection, patisiran, 0.1 mg
C9037	Injection, risperidone (perseris), 0.5 mg
C9038	Injection, mogamulizumab-kpkc, 1 mg
C9039	Injection, plazomicin, 5 mg
C9040	Injection, fremanezumab-vfrm, 1mg

C9041	Injection, coagulation factor xa (recombinant), inactivated (andexxa), 10 mg
C9042	Injection, bendamustine HCl (belrapzo), 1 mg
C9043	Injection, levoleucovorin, 1 mg
C9044	Injection, cemiplimab-rwlc, 1 mg
C9045	Injection, moxetumomab pasudotox-tdfk, 0.01 mg
C9046	Cocaine hydrochloride nasal solution (goprelto), 1 mg
C9047	Injection, caplacizumab-yhdp, 1 mg
C9048	Dexamethasone, lacrimal ophthalmic insert, 0.1 mg
C9049	Injection, tagraxofusp-erzs, 10 mcg
C9050	Injection, emapalumab-lzsg, 1 mg
C9051	Injection, omadacycline, 1 mg
C9052	Injection, ravulizumab-cwvz, 10 mg
C9053	Injection, crizanlizumab-tmca, 1 mg
C9054	Injection, lefamulin (xenleta), 1 mg
C9055	Injection, brexanolone, 1mg
C9056	Injection, givosiran, 0.5 mg
C9057	Injection, cetirizine hydrochloride, 1 mg
C9058	Injection, pegfilgrastim-bmez, biosimilar, (ziextenzo) 0.5 mg
C9059	Injection, meloxicam, 1 mg
C9060	Fluoroestradiol f18, diagnostic, 1 mci
C9061	Injection, teprotumumab-trbw, 10 mg
C9062	Injection, daratumumab 10 mg and hyaluronidase-fihj
C9063	Injection, eptinezumab-jjmr, 1 mg
C9064	Mitomycin pyelocalyceal instillation, 1 mg
C9065	Injection, romidepsin, non-lyophilized (e.g., liquid), 1mg
C9066	Injection, sacituzumab govitecan-hziy, 2.5 mg
C9067	Gallium ga-68, dotatoc, diagnostic, 0.01 mci
C9068	Copper cu-64, dotatate, diagnostic, 1 millicurie
C9069	Injection, belantamab mafodontin-blmf, 0.5 mg
C9070	Injection, tafasitamab-cxix, 2 mg
C9071	Injection, viltolarsen, 10 mg
C9072	Injection, immune globulin (asceniv), 500 mg
C9073	Brexucabtagene autoleucel, up to 200 million autologous anti-cd19 car positive viable t cells, including leukapheresis and dose preparation procedures, per therapeutic dose
C9074	Injection, lumasiran, 0.5 mg
C9075	Injection, casimersen, 10 mg

C9076	Lisocabtagene maraleucel, up to 110 million autologous anti-cd19 car-positive viable t cells, including leukapheresis and dose preparation procedures, per therapeutic dose
C9077	Injection, cabotegravir and rilpivirine, 2mg/3mg
C9078	Injection, trilaciclib, 1 mg
C9079	Injection, evinacumab-dgnb, 5 mg
C9080	Injection, melphalan flufenamide hydrochloride, 1 mg
C9081	Idecabtagene vicleucel, up to 460 million autologous anti-bcma car-positive viable t cells, including leukapheresis and dose preparation procedures, per therapeutic dose
C9082	Injection, dostarlimab-gxly, 100 mg
C9083	Injection, amivantamab-vmjw, 10 mg
C9084	Injection, loncastuximab tesirine-lpyl, 0.1 mg
C9085	Injection, avalglucosidase alfa-ngpt, 4 mg
C9086	Injection, anifrolumab-fnia, 1 mg
C9087	Injection, cyclophosphamide, (auromedics), 10 mg
C9088	Instillation, bupivacaine and meloxicam, 1 mg/0.03 mg
C9089	Bupivacaine, collagen-matrix implant, 1 mg
C9090	Injection, plasminogen, human-tvmh, 1 mg
C9091	Injection, sirolimus protein-bound particles, 1 mg
C9092	Injection, triamcinolone acetonide, suprachoroidal (xipere), 1 mg
C9093	Injection, ranibizumab, via sustained release intravitreal implant (susvimo), 0.1 mg
C9094	Injection, sutimlimab-jome, 10 mg
C9095	Injection, tebentafusp-tebn, 1 mcg
C9096	Injection, filgrastim-ayow, biosimilar, (releuko), 1 microgram
C9097	Injection, faricimab-svoa, 0.1 mg
C9098	Ciltacabtagene autoleucel, up to 100 million autologous b-cell maturation antigen (bcma) directed car-positive t cells, including leukapheresis and dose preparation procedures, per therapeutic dose
C9101	Injection, oliceridine, 0.1 mg
C9113	Injection, pantoprazole sodium, per vial
C9121	Injection, argatroban, per 5 mg
C9122	Mometasone furoate sinus implant, 10 micrograms (sinuva)
C9132	Prothrombin complex concentrate (human), kcentra, per i.u. of factor ix activity
C9133	Factor ix (antihemophilic factor, recombinant), rixubis, per i.u.
C9134	Factor xiii (antihemophilic factor, recombinant), tretten, per 10 i.u.
C9135	Factor ix (antihemophilic factor, recombinant), alprolix, per i.u.
C9136	Injection, factor viii, fc fusion protein, (recombinant), per i.u.
C9137	Injection, factor viii (antihemophilic factor, recombinant) pegylated, 1 i.u.
C9138	Injection, factor viii (antihemophilic factor, recombinant) (nuwiq), 1 i.u.
C9139	Injection, factor ix, albumin fusion protein (recombinant), idelvion, 1 i.u.

C9140 Injection, factor viii (antihemophilic factor, recombinant) (afstyla), 1 i.u.

C9141 Injection, factor viii, (antihemophilic factor, recombinant), pegylated-aucl (jivi), 1 i.u.

(C9142 Injection, bevacizumab-maly, biosimilar, (alymsys), 10 mg
Code deleted effective 12/31/2022, no HCPCS/CPT cross-reference provided.)

• C9143 Cocaine hydrochloride nasal solution (numbrino), 1 mg

• C9144 Injection, bupivacaine (posimir), 1 mg

(C9152 Injection, aripiprazole, (abilify asimtufii), 1 mg

(C9153 Injection, amisulpride, 1 mg

(C9154 Injection, buprenorphine extended-release (brixadi), 1 mg

(C9155 Injection, epcoritamab-bysp, 0.16 mg

(C9156 Flotufolastat f 18, diagnostic, 1 millicurie

(C9157 Injection, tofersen, 1 mg

(C9158 Injection, risperidone, (uzedy), 1 mg

• C9159 Injection, prothrombin complex concentrate (human), balfaxar, per i.u. of factor ix activity

• C9160 Injection, daxibotulinumtoxina-lanm, 1 unit

• C9161 Injection, aflibercept hd, 1 mg

• C9162 Injection, avacincaptad pegol, 0.1 mg

• C9163 Injection, talquetamab-tgvs, 0.25 mg

• C9164 Cantharidin for topical administration, 0.7%, single unit dose applicator (3.2 mg)

• C9165 Injection, elranatamab-bcmm, 1 mg

C9248 Injection, clevidipine butyrate, 1 mg

C9250 Human plasma fibrin sealant, vapor-heated, solvent-detergent (artiss), 2 ml

C9254 Injection, lacosamide, 1 mg

C9257 Injection, bevacizumab, 0.25 mg

C9275 Injection, hexaminolevulinate hydrochloride, 100 mg, per study dose

C9285 Lidocaine 70 mg/tetracaine 70 mg, per patch

C9290 Injection, bupivacaine liposome, 1 mg

C9293 Injection, glucarpidase, 10 units

C9349 PuraPly, and PuraPly antimicrobial, any type, per square centimeter

C9352 Microporous collagen implantable tube (neuragen nerve guide), per centimeter length

C9353 Microporous collagen implantable slit tube (neurawrap nerve protector), per centimeter length

C9354 Acellular pericardial tissue matrix of non-human origin (veritas), per square centimeter

C9355 Collagen nerve cuff (neuromatrix), per 0.5 centimeter length

C9356 Tendon, porous matrix of cross-linked collagen and glycosaminoglycan matrix (tenoglide tendon protector sheet), per square centimeter

C9358 Dermal substitute, native, non-denatured collagen, fetal bovine origin (surgimend collagen matrix), per 0.5 square centimeters

C9359 Porous purified collagen matrix bone void filler (integra mozaik osteoconductive scaffold putty, integra os osteoconductive scaffold putty), per 0.5 cc

C9360	Dermal substitute, native, non-denatured collagen, neonatal bovine origin (surgimend collagen matrix), per 0.5 square centimeters
C9361	Collagen matrix nerve wrap (neuromend collagen nerve wrap), per 0.5 centimeter length
C9362	Porous purified collagen matrix bone void filler (integra mozaik osteoconductive scaffold strip), per 0.5 cc
C9363	Skin substitute, integra meshed bilayer wound matrix, per square centimeter
C9364	Porcine implant, permacol, per square centimeter
C9399	Unclassified drugs or biologicals
C9407	Iodine I-131 iobenguane, diagnostic, 1 millicurie
C9408	Iodine I-131 iobenguane, therapeutic, 1 millicurie
C9441	Injection, ferric carboxymaltose, 1 mg
C9442	Injection, belinostat, 10 mg
C9443	Injection, dalbavancin, 10 mg
C9444	Injection, oritavancin, 10 mg
C9445	Injection, c-1 esterase inhibitor (recombinant), ruconest, 10 units
C9446	Injection, tedizolid phosphate, 1 mg
C9447	Injection, phenylephrine and ketorolac, 4 ml vial
C9448	Netupitant 300 mg and palonosetron 0.5 mg, oral
C9449	Injection, blinatumomab, 1 mcg
C9450	Injection, fluocinolone acetonide intravitreal implant, 0.01 mg
C9451	Injection, peramivir, 1 mg
C9452	Injection, ceftolozane 50 mg and tazobactam 25 mg
C9453	Injection, nivolumab, 1 mg
C9454	Injection, pasireotide long acting, 1 mg
C9455	Injection, siltuximab, 10 mg
C9456	Injection, isavuconazonium sulfate, 1 mg
C9457	Injection, sulfur hexafluoride lipid microsphere, per ml
C9458	Florbetaben f18, diagnostic, per study dose, up to 8.1 millicuries
C9459	Flutemetamol f18, diagnostic, per study dose, up to 5 millicuries
C9460	Injection, cangrelor, 1 mg
C9461	Choline c 11, diagnostic, per study dose
C9462	Injection, delafloxacin, 1 mg
C9463	Injection, aprepitant, 1 mg
C9464	Injection, rolapitant, 0.5 mg
C9465	Hyaluronan or derivative, durolane, for intra-articular injection, per dose
C9466	Injection, benralizumab, 1 mg
C9467	Injection, rituximab and hyaluronidase, 10 mg
C9468	Injection, factor ix (antihemophilic factor, recombinant), glycopegylated, rebinyn, 1 i.u.

C9469 Injection, triamcinolone acetonide, preservative-free, extended-release, microsphere formulation, 1 mg

C9470 Injection, aripiprazole lauroxil, 1 mg

C9471 Hyaluronan or derivative, hymovis, for intra-articular injection, 1 mg

C9472 Injection, talimogene laherparepvec, 1 million plaque forming units (pfu)

C9473 Injection, mepolizumab, 1 mg

C9474 Injection, irinotecan liposome, 1 mg

C9475 Injection, necitumumab, 1 mg

C9476 Injection, daratumumab, 10 mg

C9477 Injection, elotuzumab, 1 mg

C9478 Injection, sebelipase alfa, 1 mg

C9479 Instillation, ciprofloxacin otic suspension, 6 mg

C9480 Injection, trabectedin, 0.1 mg

C9481 Injection, reslizumab, 1 mg

C9482 Injection, sotalol hydrochloride, 1 mg

C9483 Injection, atezolizumab, 10 mg

C9484 Injection, eteplirsen, 10 mg

C9485 Injection, olaratumab, 10 mg

C9486 Injection, granisetron extended release, 0.1 mg

C9487 Ustekinumab, for intravenous injection, 1 mg

C9488 Injection, conivaptan hydrochloride, 1 mg

C9489 Injection, nusinersen, 0.1 mg

C9490 Injection, bezlotoxumab, 10 mg

C9491 Injection, avelumab, 10 mg

C9492 Injection, durvalumab, 10 mg

C9493 Injection, edaravone, 1 mg

C9494 Injection, ocrelizumab, 1 mg

C9497 Loxapine, inhalation powder, 10 mg

C9507 Plasma, high titer covid-19 convalescent, each unit

C9600 Percutaneous transcatheter placement of drug eluting intracoronary stent(s), with coronary angioplasty when performed; single major coronary artery or branch

C9601 Percutaneous transcatheter placement of drug-eluting intracoronary stent(s), with coronary angioplasty when performed; each additional branch of a major coronary artery (list separately in addition to code for primary procedure)

C9602 Percutaneous transluminal coronary atherectomy, with drug eluting intracoronary stent, with coronary angioplasty when performed; single major coronary artery or branch

C9603 Percutaneous transluminal coronary atherectomy, with drug-eluting intracoronary stent, with coronary angioplasty when performed; each additional branch of a major coronary artery (list separately in addition to code for primary procedure)

C9604 Percutaneous transluminal revascularization of or through coronary artery bypass graft (internal mammary, free arterial, venous), any combination of drug-eluting intracoronary stent, atherectomy and angioplasty, including distal protection when performed; single vessel

C9605 Percutaneous transluminal revascularization of or through coronary artery bypass graft (internal mammary, free arterial, venous), any combination of drug-eluting intracoronary stent, atherectomy and angioplasty, including distal protection when performed; each additional branch subtended by the bypass graft (list separately in addition to code for primary procedure)

C9606 Percutaneous transluminal revascularization of acute total/subtotal occlusion during acute myocardial infarction, coronary artery or coronary artery bypass graft, any combination of drug-eluting intracoronary stent, atherectomy and angioplasty, including aspiration thrombectomy when performed, single vessel

C9607 Percutaneous transluminal revascularization of chronic total occlusion, coronary artery, coronary artery branch, or coronary artery bypass graft, any combination of drug-eluting intracoronary stent, atherectomy and angioplasty; single vessel

C9608 Percutaneous transluminal revascularization of chronic total occlusion, coronary artery, coronary artery branch, or coronary artery bypass graft, any combination of drug-eluting intracoronary stent, atherectomy and angioplasty; each additional coronary artery, coronary artery branch, or bypass graft (list separately in addition to code for primary procedure)

C9724 Endoscopic full-thickness plication of the stomach using endoscopic plication system (eps); includes endoscopy

C9725 Placement of endorectal intracavitary applicator for high intensity brachytherapy

C9726 Placement and removal (if performed) of applicator into breast for intraoperative radiation therapy, add-on to primary breast procedure

C9727 Insertion of implants into the soft palate; minimum of three implants

C9728 Placement of interstitial device(s) for radiation therapy/surgery guidance (e.g., fiducial markers, dosimeter), for other than the following sites (any approach): abdomen, pelvis, prostate, retroperitoneum, thorax, single or multiple

C9733 Non-ophthalmic fluorescent vascular angiography

C9734 Focused ultrasound ablation/therapeutic intervention, other than uterine leiomyomata, with magnetic resonance (MR) guidance

C9735 Anoscopy; with directed submucosal injection(s), any substance

C9737 Laparoscopy, surgical, esophageal sphincter augmentation with device (e.g., magnetic band)

C9738 Adjunctive blue light cystoscopy with fluorescent imaging agent (list separately in addition to code for primary procedure)

C9739 Cystourethroscopy, with insertion of transprostatic implant; 1 to 3 implants

C9740 Cystourethroscopy, with insertion of transprostatic implant; 4 or more implants

C9741 Right heart catheterization with implantation of wireless pressure sensor in the pulmonary artery, including any type of measurement, angiography, imaging supervision, interpretation, and report

C9742 Laryngoscopy, flexible fiberoptic, with injection into vocal cord(s), therapeutic, including diagnostic laryngoscopy, if performed

C9743 Injection/implantation of bulking or spacer material (any type) with or without image guidance (not to be used if a more specific code applies)

C9744 Ultrasound, abdominal, with contrast

C9745 Nasal endoscopy, surgical; balloon dilation of eustachian tube

C9746 Transperineal implantation of permanent adjustable balloon continence device, with cystourethroscopy, when performed and/or fluoroscopy, when performed

C9747 Ablation of prostate, transrectal, high intensity focused ultrasound (HIFU), including imaging guidance

C9748 Transurethral destruction of prostate tissue; by radiofrequency water vapor (steam) thermal therapy

C9749 Repair of nasal vestibular lateral wall stenosis with implant(s)

C9750 Insertion or removal and replacement of intracardiac ischemia monitoring system including imaging supervision and interpretation and peri-operative interrogation and programming; complete system (includes device and electrode)

C9751 Bronchoscopy, rigid or flexible, transbronchial ablation of lesion(s) by microwave energy, including fluoroscopic guidance, when performed, with computed tomography acquisition(s) and 3-d rendering, computer-assisted, image-guided navigation, and endobronchial ultrasound (ebus) guided transtracheal and/or transbronchial sampling (e.g., aspiration[s]/biopsy[ies]) and all mediastinal and/or hilar lymph node stations or structures and therapeutic intervention(s)

C9752 Destruction of intraosseous basivertebral nerve, first two vertebral bodies, including imaging guidance (e.g., fluoroscopy), lumbar/sacrum

C9753 Destruction of intraosseous basivertebral nerve, each additional vertebral body, including imaging guidance (e.g., fluoroscopy), lumbar/sacrum (list separately in addition to code for primary procedure)

C9754 Creation of arteriovenous fistula, percutaneous; direct, any site, including all imaging and radiologic supervision and interpretation, when performed and secondary procedures to redirect blood flow (e.g., transluminal balloon angioplasty, coil embolization, when performed)

C9755 Creation of arteriovenous fistula, percutaneous using magnetic-guided arterial and venous catheters and radiofrequency energy, including flow-directing procedures (e.g., vascular coil embolization with radiologic supervision and interpretation, when performed) and fistulogram(s), angiography, venography, and/or ultrasound, with radiologic supervision and interpretation, when performed

C9756 Intraoperative near-infrared fluorescence lymphatic mapping of lymph node(s) (sentinel or tumor draining) with administration of indocyanine green (ICG) (list separately in addition to code for primary procedure)

C9757 Laminotomy (hemilaminectomy), with decompression of nerve root(s), including partial facetectomy, foraminotomy and excision of herniated intervertebral disc, and repair of annular defect with implantation of bone anchored annular closure device, including annular defect measurement, alignment and sizing assessment, and image guidance; 1 interspace, lumbar

C9758 Blinded procedure for NYHA class iii/iv heart failure; transcatheter implantation of interatrial shunt or placebo control, including right heart catheterization, trans-esophageal echocardiography (tee)/intracardiac echocardiography (ice), and all imaging with or without guidance (e.g., ultrasound, fluoroscopy), performed in an approved investigational device exemption (ide) study

C9759 Transcatheter intraoperative blood vessel microinfusion(s) (e.g., intraluminal, vascular wall and/or perivascular) therapy, any vessel, including radiological supervision and interpretation, when performed

C9760 Non-randomized, non-blinded procedure for NYHA class ii, iii, iv heart failure; transcatheter implantation of interatrial shunt, including right and left heart catheterization, transeptal puncture, trans-esophageal echocardiography (tee)/intracardiac echocardiography (ice), and all imaging with or without guidance (e.g., ultrasound, fluoroscopy), performed in an approved investigational device exemption (ide) study

C9761 Cystourethroscopy, with ureteroscopy and/or pyeloscopy, with lithotripsy, and ureteral catheterization for steerable vacuum aspiration of the kidney, collecting system, ureter, bladder, and urethra if applicable (must use a steerable ureteral catheter)

C9762 Cardiac magnetic resonance imaging for morphology and function, quantification of segmental dysfunction; with strain imaging

C9763 Cardiac magnetic resonance imaging for morphology and function, quantification of segmental dysfunction; with stress imaging

C9764 Revascularization, endovascular, open or percutaneous, lower extremity artery(ies), except tibial/peroneal; with intravascular lithotripsy, includes angioplasty within the same vessel(s), when performed

C9765 Revascularization, endovascular, open or percutaneous, lower extremity artery(ies), except tibial/peroneal; with intravascular lithotripsy, and transluminal stent placement(s), includes angioplasty within the same vessel(s), when performed

C9766 Revascularization, endovascular, open or percutaneous, lower extremity artery(ies), except tibial/peroneal; with intravascular lithotripsy and atherectomy, includes angioplasty within the same vessel(s), when performed

C9767 Revascularization, endovascular, open or percutaneous, lower extremity artery(ies), except tibial/peroneal; with intravascular lithotripsy and transluminal stent placement(s), and atherectomy, includes angioplasty within the same vessel(s), when performed

C9768 Endoscopic ultrasound-guided direct measurement of hepatic portosystemic pressure gradient by any method (list separately in addition to code for primary procedure)

C9769 Cystourethroscopy, with insertion of temporary prostatic implant/stent with fixation/anchor and incisional struts

(**C9770** Vitrectomy, mechanical, pars plana approach, with subretinal injection of pharmacologic/biologic agent

(**C9771** Nasal/sinus endoscopy, cryoablation nasal tissue(s) and/or nerve(s), unilateral or bilateral

C9772 Revascularization, endovascular, open or percutaneous, tibial/peroneal artery(ies), with intravascular lithotripsy, includes angioplasty within the same vessel (s), when performed

C9773 Revascularization, endovascular, open or percutaneous, tibial/peroneal artery(ies); with intravascular lithotripsy, and transluminal stent placement(s), includes angioplasty within the same vessel(s), when performed

C9774 Revascularization, endovascular, open or percutaneous, tibial/peroneal artery(ies); with intravascular lithotripsy and atherectomy, includes angioplasty within the same vessel (s), when performed

C9775 Revascularization, endovascular, open or percutaneous, tibial/peroneal artery(ies); with intravascular lithotripsy and transluminal stent placement(s), and atherectomy, includes angioplasty within the same vessel (s), when performed

C9776 Intraoperative near-infrared fluorescence imaging of major extra-hepatic bile duct(s) (e.g., cystic duct, common bile duct and common hepatic duct) with intravenous administration of indocyanine green (ICG) (list separately in addition to code for primary procedure)

C9777 Esophageal mucosal integrity testing by electrical impedance, transoral, includes esophagoscopy or esophagogastroduodenoscopy

C9778 Colpopexy, vaginal; minimally invasive extra-peritoneal approach (sacrospinous)

C9779 Endoscopic submucosal dissection (ESD), including endoscopy or colonoscopy, mucosal closure, when performed

C9780 Insertion of central venous catheter through central venous occlusion via inferior and superior approaches (e.g., inside-out technique), including imaging guidance

C9781 Arthroscopy, shoulder, surgical; with implantation of subacromial spacer (e.g., balloon), includes debridement (e.g., limited or extensive), subacromial decompression, acromioplasty, and biceps tenodesis when performed

C9782 Blinded procedure for New York Heart Association (NYHA) class ii or iii heart failure, or Canadian cardiovascular society (ccs) class iii or iv chronic refractory angina; transcatheter intramyocardial transplantation of autologous bone marrow cells (e.g., mononuclear) or placebo control, autologous bone marrow harvesting and preparation for transplantation, left heart catheterization including ventriculography, all laboratory services, and all imaging with or without

B - C CODES

B - C CODES

guidance (e.g., transthoracic echocardiography, ultrasound, fluoroscopy), performed in an approved investigational device exemption (ide) study

C9783 Blinded procedure for transcatheter implantation of coronary sinus reduction device or placebo control, including vascular access and closure, right heart catheterization, venous and coronary sinus angiography, imaging guidance and supervision and interpretation when performed in an approved investigational device exemption (ide) study

(**C9788** Opto-acoustic imaging, breast (including axilla when performed), unilateral, with image documentation, analysis and report, obtained with ultrasound examination

• **C9793** 3d predictive model generation for pre-planning of a cardiac procedure, using data from cardiac computed tomographic angiography with report

• **C9794** Therapeutic radiology simulation-aided field setting; complex, including acquisition of pet and CT imaging data required for radiopharmaceutical-directed radiation therapy treatment planning (i.e., modeling)

• **C9795** Stereotactic body radiation therapy, treatment delivery, per fraction to 1 or more lesions, including image guidance and real-time positron emissions-based delivery adjustments to 1 or more lesions, entire course not to exceed 5 fractions

C9800 Dermal injection procedure(s) for facial lipodystrophy syndrome (LDS) and provision of Radiesse or Sculptra dermal filler, including all items and supplies

(**C9803** Hospital outpatient clinic visit specimen collection for severe acute respiratory syndrome coronavirus 2 (sars-cov-2) (coronavirus disease [covid-19]), any specimen source
Code deleted effective 12/31/2023, no HCPCS/CPT cross-reference provided.)

C9898 Radiolabeled product provided during a hospital inpatient stay

C9899 Implanted prosthetic device, payable only for inpatients who do not have inpatient coverage

DURABLE MEDICAL EQUIPMENT

Guidelines

In addition to the information presented in the INTRODUCTION, several other items unique to this section are defined or identified here:

1. **DEFINITION OF DURABLE MEDICAL EQUIPMENT:** Durable medical equipment (DME) can withstand repeated use and is used primarily to serve a medical purpose. It generally is not useful in the absence of an illness or injury and is appropriate for use in the home. Expendable medical supplies, such as incontinent pads, lamb's wool pads, catheters, ace bandages, elastic stockings, surgical face masks, irrigating kits, sheets and bags, are not considered to be DME.

2. **REASONABLE AND NECESSARY:** DME may not be covered in every instance. The equipment must be reasonable and necessary for the illness or injury being treated or for improving the functioning of a malformed body part. A physician's prescription is normally sufficient to establish that the equipment is necessary. To determine reasonableness, the following conditions must be met: the expense must be proportionate to the therapeutic benefits of using the equipment; the cost must not substantially exceed a medically appropriate care plan; and the item must not serve the same purpose as equipment already available to the patient. Claims for items that are not reasonable will be denied except when it is determined that no alternative plan of care is available for which payment could be made.

3. **SUBSECTION INFORMATION:** Some of the listed subheadings or subsections have special needs or instructions unique to that section. Where these are indicated, special "notes" will be presented preceding or following the listings. Those subsections within the DURABLE MEDICAL EQUIPMENT section that have "notes" are as follows:

SUBSECTION	CODE SERIES
Artificial kidney machines and accessories	E1510–E1699

4. **UNLISTED SERVICE OR PROCEDURE:** A service or procedure may be provided that is not listed in this edition of HCPCS. When reporting such a service, the appropriate "unlisted procedure" code may be used to indicate the service, identifying it by "special report" as defined below. HCPCS terminology is inconsistent in defining unlisted procedures. The procedure definition may include the term(s) "unlisted", "not otherwise classified", "unspecified", "unclassified", "other" and "miscellaneous". Prior to using these codes, try to determine if a Local Level III code or CPT code is available. The "unlisted procedures" and accompanying codes for DURABLE MEDICAL EQUIPMENT are as follows:

   E1399 Durable medical equipment, miscellaneous
   E1699 Dialysis equipment, not otherwise specified

5. **SPECIAL REPORT:** A service, material or supply that is rarely provided, unusual, variable or new may require a special report in determining medical appropriateness for reimbursement purposes. Pertinent information should include an adequate definition or description of the nature, extent, and need for the service, material or supply.

6. **MODIFIERS:** Listed services may be modified under certain circumstances. When appropriate, the modifying circumstance is identified by adding a modifier to the basic procedure code. CPT and HCPCS National Level II modifiers may be used with CPT and HCPCS National Level II procedure codes. Modifiers commonly used with DURABLE MEDICAL EQUIPMENT are as follows:

   -CC Procedure code change (use "CC" when the procedure code submitted was changed either for administrative reasons or because an incorrect code was filed)

E CODES

-LL Lease/rental (used the "LL" modifier when DME rental is to be applied against the purchase price)

-LT Left side (used to identify procedures performed on the left side of the body)

-MS Six-month maintenance and servicing fee for reasonable and necessary parts and labor which are not covered under any manufacturer or supplier warranty

-NR New when rented (use the "NR" modifier when DME which was new at the time of rental is subsequently purchased)

-NU New equipment

-QE Prescribed amount of oxygen is less than 1 liter per minute (LPM)

-QF Prescribed amount of oxygen exceeds 4 liters per minute (LPM) and portable oxygen is prescribed

-QG Prescribed amount of oxygen is greater than 4 liters per minute (LPM)

-QH Oxygen conserving device is being used with an oxygen delivery system

-QT Recording and storage on tape by an analog tape recorder

-RP Replacement and repair (may be used to indicate replacement of DME, orthotic and prosthetic devices which have been in use for some time. The claim shows the code for the part, followed by the "RP" modifier and the charge for the part.)

-RR Rental (used when DME is to be rented)

-RT Right side (used to identify procedures performed on the right side of the body)

-TC Technical component.

Under certain circumstances, a charge may be made for the technical component alone. Under those circumstances, the technical component charge is identified by adding modifier -TC to the usual procedure code. Technical component charges are institutional charges and are not billed separately by physicians. However, portable x-ray suppliers bill only for technical component and should utilize modifier -TC. The charge data from portable x-ray suppliers will then be used to build customary and prevailing profiles.

-UE Used durable medical equipment

7. **CPT CODE CROSS-REFERENCE:** Unless otherwise specified, the equivalent CPT code for all listings in this section is 99070.

8. **DURABLE MEDICAL EQUIPMENT REGIONAL CARRIERS (DMERCS):** Effective October 1, 1993 claims for durable medical equipment (DME) must be billed to one of four regional carriers depending upon the residence of the beneficiary. The transition dates for DMERC claims is from November 1, 1993 to March 1, 1994 depending upon the state you practice in. See the Introduction for a complete discussion of DMERCs.

Durable Medical Equipment Canes

E0100 Cane, includes canes of all materials, adjustable or fixed, with tip

E0105 Cane, quad or three prong, includes canes of all materials, adjustable or fixed, with tips

Crutches

E0110 Crutches, forearm, includes crutches of various materials, adjustable or fixed, pair, complete with tips and handgrips

E0111 Crutch forearm, includes crutches of various materials, adjustable or fixed, each, with tip and handgrips

E0112 Crutches underarm, wood, adjustable or fixed, pair, with pads, tips and handgrips

E0113 Crutch underarm, wood, adjustable or fixed, each, with pad, tip and handgrip

E0114 Crutches underarm, other than wood, adjustable or fixed, pair, with pads, tips and handgrips

E0116 Crutch, underarm, other than wood, adjustable or fixed, with pad, tip, handgrip, with or without shock absorber, each

E0117 Crutch, underarm, articulating, spring assisted, each

E0118 Crutch substitute, lower leg platform, with or without wheels, each

Walkers

E0130 Walker, rigid (pickup), adjustable or fixed height

E0135 Walker, folding (pickup), adjustable or fixed height

E0140 Walker, with trunk support, adjustable or fixed height, any type

E0141 Walker, rigid, wheeled, adjustable or fixed height

E0143 Walker, folding, wheeled, adjustable or fixed height

E0144 Walker, enclosed, four sided framed, rigid or folding, wheeled with posterior seat

E0147 Walker, heavy duty, multiple braking system, variable wheel resistance

E0148 Walker, heavy duty, without wheels, rigid or folding, any type, each

E0149 Walker, heavy duty, wheeled, rigid or folding, any type

Attachments

E0153 Platform attachment, forearm crutch, each

E0154 Platform attachment, walker, each

E0155 Wheel attachment, rigid pick-up walker, per pair

E0156 Seat attachment, walker

E0157 Crutch attachment, walker, each

E0158 Leg extensions for walker, per set of four (4)

E0159 Brake attachment for wheeled walker, replacement, each

Commodes

E0160 Sitz type bath or equipment, portable, used with or without commode

E0161 Sitz type bath or equipment, portable, used with or without commode, with faucet attachment/s

E0162 Sitz bath chair

E0163 Commode chair, mobile or stationary, with fixed arms

E0165 Commode chair, mobile or stationary, with detachable arms

E0167 Pail or pan for use with commode chair, replacement only

E CODES

E0168 Commode chair, extra wide and/or heavy duty, stationary or mobile, with or without arms, any type, each

E0170 Commode chair with integrated seat lift mechanism, electric, any type

E0171 Commode chair with integrated seat lift mechanism, non-electric, any type

E0172 Seat lift mechanism placed over or on top of toilet, any type

E0175 Foot rest, for use with commode chair, each

Decubitus Care Equipment

E0181 Powered pressure reducing mattress overlay/pad, alternating, with pump, includes heavy duty

E0182 Pump for alternating pressure pad, for replacement only

E0183 Powered pressure reducing underlay/pad, alternating, with pump, includes heavy duty

E0184 Dry pressure mattress

E0185 Gel or gel-like pressure pad for mattress, standard mattress length and width

E0186 Air pressure mattress

E0187 Water pressure mattress

E0188 Synthetic sheepskin pad

E0189 Lambswool sheepskin pad, any size

E0190 Positioning cushion/pillow/wedge, any shape or size, includes all components and accessories

E0191 Heel or elbow protector, each

E0193 Powered air flotation bed (low air loss therapy)

E0194 Air fluidized bed

E0196 Gel pressure mattress

E0197 Air pressure pad for mattress, standard mattress length and width

E0198 Water pressure pad for mattress, standard mattress length and width

E0199 Dry pressure pad for mattress, standard mattress length and width

Heat/Cold Application

E0200 Heat lamp, without stand (table model), includes bulb, or infrared element

E0202 Phototherapy (bilirubin) light with photometer

E0203 Therapeutic lightbox, minimum 10,000 lux, table top model

E0205 Heat lamp, with stand, includes bulb, or infrared element

E0210 Electric heat pad, standard

E0215 Electric heat pad, moist

E0217 Water circulating heat pad with pump

E0218 Fluid circulating cold pad with pump, any type

E0221 Infrared heating pad system

E0225 Hydrocollator unit, includes pads

E0231 Non-contact wound warming device (temperature control unit, ac adapter and power cord) for use with warming card and wound cover

E0232 Warming card for use with the non contact wound warming device and non contact wound warming wound cover

E0235 Paraffin bath unit, portable (see medical supply code a4265 for paraffin)

E0236 Pump for water circulating pad

E0239 Hydrocollator unit, portable

Bath and Toilet Aids

E0240 Bath/shower chair, with or without wheels, any size

E0241 Bath tub wall rail, each

E0242 Bath tub rail, floor base

E0243 Toilet rail, each

E0244 Raised toilet seat

E0245 Tub stool or bench

E0246 Transfer tub rail attachment

E0247 Transfer bench for tub or toilet with or without commode opening

E0248 Transfer bench, heavy duty, for tub or toilet with or without commode opening

E0249 Pad for water circulating heat unit, for replacement only

Hospital Beds and Accessories

E0250 Hospital bed, fixed height, with any type of side rails, with mattress

E0251 Hospital bed, fixed height, with any type of side rails, without mattress

E0255 Hospital bed, variable height, hi-lo, with any type of side rails, with mattress

E0256 Hospital bed, variable height, hi-lo, with any type of side rails, without mattress

E0260 Hospital bed, semi-electric (head and foot adjustment), with any type of side rails, with mattress

E0261 Hospital bed, semi-electric (head and foot adjustment), with any type of side rails, without mattress

E0265 Hospital bed, total electric (head, foot and height adjustments), with any type of side rails, with mattress

E0266 Hospital bed, total electric (head, foot and height adjustments), with any type of side rails, without mattress

E0270 Hospital bed, institutional type includes oscillating, circulating and Stryker frame, with mattress

E0271 Mattress, innerspring

E0272 Mattress, foam rubber

E0273 Bed board

E0274 Over-bed table

E0275 Bed pan, standard, metal or plastic

E0276 Bed pan, fracture, metal or plastic

E0277 Powered pressure-reducing air mattress

E0280 Bed cradle, any type

E0290 Hospital bed, fixed height, without side rails, with mattress

E0291 Hospital bed, fixed height, without side rails, without mattress

E0292 Hospital bed, variable height, hi-lo, without side rails, with mattress

E0293 Hospital bed, variable height, hi-lo, without side rails, without mattress

E0294 Hospital bed, semi-electric (head and foot adjustment), without side rails, with mattress

E0295 Hospital bed, semi-electric (head and foot adjustment), without side rails, without mattress

E0296 Hospital bed, total electric (head, foot and height adjustments), without side rails, with mattress

E0297 Hospital bed, total electric (head, foot and height adjustments), without side rails, without mattress

E0300 Pediatric crib, hospital grade, fully enclosed, with or without top enclosure

E0301 Hospital bed, heavy duty, extra wide, with weight capacity greater than 350 pounds, but less than or equal to 600 pounds, with any type of side rails, without mattress

E0302 Hospital bed, extra heavy duty, extra wide, with weight capacity greater than 600 pounds, with any type of side rails, without mattress

E0303 Hospital bed, heavy duty, extra wide, with weight capacity greater than 350 pounds, but less than or equal to 600 pounds, with any type of side rails, with mattress

E0304 Hospital bed, extra heavy duty, extra wide, with weight capacity greater than 600 pounds, with any type of side rails, with mattress

E0305 Bed side rails, half length

E0310 Bed side rails, full length

E0315 Bed accessory: board, table, or support device, any type

E0316 Safety enclosure frame/canopy for use with hospital bed, any type

E0325 Urinal; male, jug-type, any material

E0326 Urinal; female, jug-type, any material

E0328 Hospital bed, pediatric, manual, 360 degree side enclosures, top of headboard, footboard and side rails up to 24 inches above the spring, includes mattress

E0329 Hospital bed, pediatric, electric or semi-electric, 360 degree side enclosures, top of headboard, footboard and side rails up to 24 inches above the spring, includes mattress

E0350 Control unit for electronic bowel irrigation/evacuation system

E0352 Disposable pack (water reservoir bag, speculum, valving mechanism and collection bag/box) for use with the electronic bowel irrigation/evacuation system

E0370 Air pressure elevator for heel

E0371 Nonpowered advanced pressure reducing overlay for mattress, standard mattress length and width

E0372 Powered air overlay for mattress, standard mattress length and width

E0373 Nonpowered advanced pressure reducing mattress

Oxygen and Related Respiratory Equipment

E0424 Stationary compressed gaseous oxygen system, rental; includes container, contents, regulator, flowmeter, humidifier, nebulizer, cannula or mask, and tubing

E0430 Portable gaseous oxygen system, purchase; includes regulator, flowmeter, humidifier, cannula or mask, and tubing

E0431 Portable gaseous oxygen system, rental; includes portable container, regulator, flowmeter, humidifier, cannula or mask, and tubing

E0433 Portable liquid oxygen system, rental; home liquefier used to fill portable liquid oxygen containers, includes portable containers, regulator, flowmeter, humidifier, cannula or mask and tubing, with or without supply reservoir and contents gauge

E0434 Portable liquid oxygen system, rental; includes portable container, supply reservoir, humidifier, flowmeter, refill adaptor, contents gauge, cannula or mask, and tubing

E0435 Portable liquid oxygen system, purchase; includes portable container, supply reservoir, flowmeter, humidifier, contents gauge, cannula or mask, tubing and refill adaptor

E0439 Stationary liquid oxygen system, rental; includes container, contents, regulator, flowmeter, humidifier, nebulizer, cannula or mask, & tubing

E0440 Stationary liquid oxygen system, purchase; includes use of reservoir, contents indicator, regulator, flowmeter, humidifier, nebulizer, cannula or mask, and tubing

E0441 Stationary oxygen contents, gaseous, 1 month's supply = 1 unit

E0442 Stationary oxygen contents, liquid, 1 month's supply = 1 unit

E0443 Portable oxygen contents, gaseous, 1 month's supply = 1 unit

E0444 Portable oxygen contents, liquid, 1 month's supply = 1 unit

E0445 Oximeter device for measuring blood oxygen levels non-invasively

E0446 Topical oxygen delivery system, not otherwise specified, includes all supplies and accessories

E0447 Portable oxygen contents, liquid, 1 month's supply = 1 unit, prescribed amount at rest or nighttime exceeds 4 liters per minute (lpm)

E0450 Volume control ventilator, without pressure support mode, may include pressure control mode, used with invasive interface (e.g., tracheostomy tube)

E0455 Oxygen tent, excluding croup or pediatric tents

E0457 Chest shell (cuirass)

E0459 Chest wrap

E0460 Negative pressure ventilator; portable or stationary

E0461 Volume control ventilator, without pressure support mode, may include pressure control mode, used with non-invasive interface (e.g., mask)

E0462 Rocking bed with or without side rails

E0463 Pressure support ventilator with volume control mode, may include pressure control mode, used with invasive interface (e.g., tracheostomy tube)

E0464 Pressure support ventilator with volume control mode, may include pressure control mode, used with non-invasive interface (e.g., mask)

E0465 Home ventilator, any type, used with invasive interface, (e.g., tracheostomy tube)

E0466 Home ventilator, any type, used with non-invasive interface, (e.g., mask, chest shell)

E0467 Home ventilator, multi-function respiratory device, also performs any or all of the additional functions of oxygen concentration, drug nebulization, aspiration, and cough stimulation, includes all accessories, components and supplies for all functions

E0470 Respiratory assist device, bi-level pressure capability, without backup rate feature, used with noninvasive interface, e.g., nasal or facial mask (intermittent assist device with continuous positive airway pressure device)

E0471 Respiratory assist device, bi-level pressure capability, with back-up rate feature, used with noninvasive interface, e.g., nasal or facial mask (intermittent assist device with continuous positive airway pressure device)

E0472 Respiratory assist device, bi-level pressure capability, with backup rate feature, used with invasive interface, e.g., tracheostomy tube (intermittent assist device with continuous positive airway pressure device)

E0480 Percussor, electric or pneumatic, home model

E0481 Intrapulmonary percussive ventilation system and related accessories

E0482 Cough stimulating device, alternating positive and negative airway pressure

E0483 High frequency chest wall oscillation system, with full anterior and/or posterior thoracic region receiving simultaneous external oscillation, includes all accessories and supplies, each

E0484 Oscillatory positive expiratory pressure device, non-electric, any type, each

E0485 Oral device/appliance used to reduce upper airway collapsibility, adjustable or non-adjustable, prefabricated, includes fitting and adjustment

E0486 Oral device/appliance used to reduce upper airway collapsibility, adjustable or non-adjustable, custom fabricated, includes fitting and adjustment

E0487 Spirometer, electronic, includes all accessories

● **E0492** Power source and control electronics unit for oral device/appliance for neuromuscular electrical stimulation of the tongue muscle, controlled by phone application

● **E0493** Oral device/appliance for neuromuscular electrical stimulation of the tongue muscle, used in conjunction with the power source and control electronics unit, controlled by phone application, 90-day supply

IPPB Machines

E0500 IPPB machine, all types, with built-in nebulization; manual or automatic valves; internal or external power source

Humidifiers/Nebulizers for Use With Oxygen IPPB Equipment

● **E0530** Electronic positional obstructive sleep apnea treatment, with sensor, includes all components and accessories, any type

E0550 Humidifier, durable for extensive supplemental humidification during IPPB treatments or oxygen delivery

E0550 Humidifier, durable for extensive supplemental humidification during IPPB treatments or oxygen delivery

E0555 Humidifier, durable, glass or autoclavable plastic bottle type, for use with regulator or flowmeter

E0560 Humidifier, durable for supplemental humidification during IPPB treatment or oxygen delivery

E0561 Humidifier, non-heated, used with positive airway pressure device

E0562 Humidifier, heated, used with positive airway pressure device

E0565 Compressor, air power source for equipment which is not self-contained, or cylinder driven

E0570 Nebulizer, with compressor

E0572 Aerosol compressor, adjustable pressure, light duty for intermittent use

E0574 Ultrasonic/electronic aerosol generator with small volume nebulizer

E0575 Nebulizer, ultrasonic, large volume

E0580 Nebulizer, durable, glass or autoclavable plastic, bottle type, for use with regulator or flowmeter

E0585 Nebulizer, with compressor and heater

Suction Pump/Room Vaporizers

E0600 Respiratory suction pump, home model, portable or stationary, electric

E0601 Continuous positive airway pressure (CPAP) device

E0602 Breast pump, manual, any type

E0603 Breast pump, electric (ac and/or dc), any type

E0604 Breast pump, hospital grade, electric (ac and / or dc), any type

E0605 Vaporizer, room type

E0606 Postural drainage board

Monitoring Equipment

E0607 Home blood glucose monitor

Pacemaker Monitor

E0610 Pacemaker monitor, self-contained, (checks battery depletion, includes audible and visible check systems)

E0615 Pacemaker monitor, self contained, checks battery depletion and other pacemaker components, includes digital/visible check systems

E0616 Implantable cardiac event recorder with memory, activator and programmer

E0617 External defibrillator with integrated electrocardiogram analysis

E0618 Apnea monitor, without recording feature

E0619 Apnea monitor, with recording feature

E0620 Skin piercing device for collection of capillary blood, laser, each

Patient Lifts

E0621 Sling or seat, patient lift, canvas or nylon

E0625 Patient lift, bathroom or toilet, not otherwise classified

E0627 Seat lift mechanism, electric, any type

E0628 Separate seat lift mechanism for use with patient owned furniture-electric

E0629 Seat lift mechanism, non-electric, any type

E0630 Patient lift, hydraulic or mechanical, includes any seat, sling, strap(s) or pad(s)

E0635 Patient lift, electric with seat or sling

E0636 Multipositional patient support system, with integrated lift, patient accessible controls

E0637 Combination sit to stand frame/table system, any size including pediatric, with seat lift feature, with or without wheels

E0638 Standing frame/table system, one position (e.g., upright, supine or prone stander), any size including pediatric, with or without wheels

E0639 Patient lift, moveable from room to room with disassembly and reassembly, includes all components/accessories

E0640 Patient lift, fixed system, includes all components/accessories

E0641 Standing frame/table system, multi-position (e.g., three-way stander), any size including pediatric, with or without wheels

E0642 Standing frame/table system, mobile (dynamic stander), any size including pediatric

Pneumatic Compressor and Appliances (Lymphedema Pump)

E0651 Pneumatic compressor, segmental home model without calibrated gradient pressure

E0652 Pneumatic compressor, segmental home model with calibrated gradient pressure

E0655 Non-segmental pneumatic appliance for use with pneumatic compressor, half arm

E0656 Segmental pneumatic appliance for use with pneumatic compressor, trunk

E0657 Segmental pneumatic appliance for use with pneumatic compressor, chest

E0660 Non-segmental pneumatic appliance for use with pneumatic compressor, full leg

E0665 Non-segmental pneumatic appliance for use with pneumatic compressor, full arm

E0666 Non-segmental pneumatic appliance for use with pneumatic compressor, half leg

E0667 Segmental pneumatic appliance for use with pneumatic compressor, full leg

E0668 Segmental pneumatic appliance for use with pneumatic compressor, full arm

E0669 Segmental pneumatic appliance for use with pneumatic compressor, half leg

E0670 Segmental pneumatic appliance for use with pneumatic compressor, integrated, 2 full legs and trunk

E0671 Segmental gradient pressure pneumatic appliance, full leg

E0672 Segmental gradient pressure pneumatic appliance, full arm

E0673 Segmental gradient pressure pneumatic appliance, half leg

E0675 Pneumatic compression device, high pressure, rapid inflation/deflation cycle, for arterial insufficiency (unilateral or bilateral system)

E0676 Intermittent limb compression device (includes all accessories), not otherwise specified

• E0678 Non-pneumatic sequential compression garment, full leg

• E0679 Non-pneumatic sequential compression garment, half leg

• E0680 Non-pneumatic compression controller with sequential calibrated gradient pressure

• E0681 Non-pneumatic compression controller without calibrated gradient pressure

• E0682 Non-pneumatic sequential compression garment, full arm

Ultraviolet Cabinet

E0691 Ultraviolet light therapy system, includes bulbs/lamps, timer and eye protection; treatment area 2 square feet or less

E0692 Ultraviolet light therapy system panel, includes bulbs/lamps, timer and eye protection, 4 foot panel

E0693 Ultraviolet light therapy system panel, includes bulbs/lamps, timer and eye protection, 6 foot panel

E0694 Ultraviolet multidirectional light therapy system in 6 foot cabinet, includes bulbs/lamps, timer and eye protection

Safety Equipment

E0700 Safety equipment, device or accessory, any type

Restraints

E0705 Transfer device, any type, each

E0710 Restraints, any type (body, chest, wrist or ankle)

Transcutaneous and/or Neuromuscular Electrical Nerve Stimulators - TENS

E0720 Transcutaneous electrical nerve stimulation (tens) device, two lead, localized stimulation

E0730 Transcutaneous electrical nerve stimulation (tens) device, four or more leads, for multiple nerve stimulation

E0731 Form fitting conductive garment for delivery of tens or NMES (with conductive fibers separated from the patient's skin by layers of fabric)

• **E0732** Cranial electrotherapy stimulation (CES) system, any type

• **E0733** Transcutaneous electrical nerve stimulator for electrical stimulation of the trigeminal nerve

• **E0734** External upper limb tremor stimulator of the peripheral nerves of the wrist

• **E0735** Non-invasive vagus nerve stimulator

E0740 Non-implanted pelvic floor electrical stimulator, complete system

E0744 Neuromuscular stimulator for scoliosis

E0745 Neuromuscular stimulator, electronic shock unit

E0746 Electromyography (EMG), biofeedback device

E0747 Osteogenesis stimulator, electrical, non-invasive, other than spinal applications

E0748 Osteogenesis stimulator, electrical, non-invasive, spinal applications

E0749 Osteogenesis stimulator, electrical, surgically implanted

E0755 Electronic salivary reflex stimulator (intra-oral/non-invasive)

E0760 Osteogenesis stimulator, low intensity ultrasound, non-invasive

E0761 Non-thermal pulsed high frequency radio waves, high peak power electromagnetic energy treatment device

E0762 Transcutaneous electrical joint stimulation device system, includes all accessories

E0764 Functional neuromuscular stimulation, transcutaneous stimulation of sequential muscle groups of ambulation with computer control, used for walking by spinal cord injured, entire system, after completion of training program

E0765 FDA approved nerve stimulator, with replaceable batteries, for treatment of nausea and vomiting

E0766 Electrical stimulation device used for cancer treatment, includes all accessories, any type

E0769 Electrical stimulation or electromagnetic wound treatment device, not otherwise classified

E0770 Functional electrical stimulator, transcutaneous stimulation of nerve and/or muscle groups, any type, complete system, not otherwise specified

Infusion Pumps

E0776 IV pole

E0779 Ambulatory infusion pump, mechanical, reusable, for infusion 8 hours or greater

E0780 Ambulatory infusion pump, mechanical, reusable, for infusion less than 8 hours

E0781 Ambulatory infusion pump, single or multiple channels, electric or battery operated, with administrative equipment, worn by patient

E0782 Infusion pump, implantable, non-programmable (includes all components, e.g., pump, catheter, connectors, etc.)

E0783 Infusion pump system, implantable, programmable (includes all components, e.g., pump, catheter, connectors, etc.)

E0784 External ambulatory infusion pump, insulin

E0785 Implantable intraspinal (epidural/intrathecal) catheter used with implantable infusion pump, replacement

E0786 Implantable programmable infusion pump, replacement (excludes implantable intraspinal catheter)

E0787 External ambulatory infusion pump, insulin, dosage rate adjustment using therapeutic continuous glucose sensing

E0791 Parenteral infusion pump, stationary, single or multi-channel

Traction Equipment

E0830 Ambulatory traction device, all types, each

E0840 Traction frame, attached to headboard, cervical traction

E0849 Traction equipment, cervical, free-standing stand/frame, pneumatic, applying traction force to other than mandible

E0850 Traction stand, free standing, cervical traction

E0855 Cervical traction equipment not requiring additional stand or frame

E0856 Cervical traction device, with inflatable air bladder(s)

E0860 Traction equipment, overdoor, cervical

E0870 Traction frame, attached to footboard, extremity traction, (e.g., buck's)

E0880 Traction stand, free standing, extremity traction

E0890 Traction frame, attached to footboard, pelvic traction

E0900 Traction stand, free standing, pelvic traction, (e.g., buck's)

Trapeze Equipment, Fracture Frame, and Other Orthopedic Devices

E0910 Trapeze bars, a/k/a patient helper, attached to bed, with grab bar

E0911 Trapeze bar, heavy duty, for patient weight capacity greater than 250 pounds, attached to bed, with grab bar

E0912 Trapeze bar, heavy duty, for patient weight capacity greater than 250 pounds, free standing, complete with grab bar

E0920 Fracture frame, attached to bed, includes weights

E0930 Fracture frame, free standing, includes weights

E0935 Continuous passive motion exercise device for use on knee only

E0936 Continuous passive motion exercise device for use other than knee

E0940 Trapeze bar, free standing, complete with grab bar

E0941 Gravity assisted traction device, any type

E0942 Cervical head harness/halter

E0944 Pelvic belt/harness/boot

E0945 Extremity belt/harness

E0946 Fracture, frame, dual with cross bars, attached to bed, (e.g., balken, 4 poster)

E0947 Fracture frame, attachments for complex pelvic traction

E0948 Fracture frame, attachments for complex cervical traction

Wheelchair Accessories

E0950	Wheelchair accessory, tray, each
E0951	Heel loop/holder, any type, with or without ankle strap, each
E0952	Toe loop/holder, any type, each
E0953	Wheelchair accessory, lateral thigh or knee support, any type including fixed mounting hardware, each
E0954	Wheelchair accessory, foot box, any type, includes attachment and mounting hardware, each foot
E0955	Wheelchair accessory, headrest, cushioned, any type, including fixed mounting hardware, each
E0956	Wheelchair accessory, lateral trunk or hip support, any type, including fixed mounting hardware, each
E0957	Wheelchair accessory, medial thigh support, any type, including fixed mounting hardware, each
E0958	Manual wheelchair accessory, one-arm drive attachment, each
E0959	Manual wheelchair accessory, adapter for amputee, each
E0960	Wheelchair accessory, shoulder harness/straps or chest strap, including any type mounting hardware
E0961	Manual wheelchair accessory, wheel lock brake extension (handle), each
E0966	Manual wheelchair accessory, headrest extension, each
E0967	Manual wheelchair accessory, hand rim with projections, any type, replacement only, each
E0968	Commode seat, wheelchair
E0969	Narrowing device, wheelchair
E0970	No. 2 footplates, except for elevating leg rest
E0971	Manual wheelchair accessory, anti-tipping device, each
E0973	Wheelchair accessory, adjustable height, detachable armrest, complete assembly, each
E0974	Manual wheelchair accessory, anti-rollback device, each
E0978	Wheelchair accessory, positioning belt/safety belt/pelvic strap, each
E0980	Safety vest, wheelchair
E0981	Wheelchair accessory, seat upholstery, replacement only, each
E0982	Wheelchair accessory, back upholstery, replacement only, each
E0983	Manual wheelchair accessory, power add-on to convert manual wheelchair to motorized wheelchair, joystick control
E0984	Manual wheelchair accessory, power add-on to convert manual wheelchair to motorized wheelchair, tiller control
E0985	Wheelchair accessory, seat lift mechanism
E0986	Manual wheelchair accessory, push-rim activated power assist system
E0988	Manual wheelchair accessory, lever-activated, wheel drive, pair
E0990	Wheelchair accessory, elevating leg rest, complete assembly, each
E0992	Manual wheelchair accessory, solid seat insert
E0994	Arm rest, each
E0995	Wheelchair accessory, calf rest/pad, replacement only, each
E1002	Wheelchair accessory, power seating system, tilt only

E CODES

E1003 Wheelchair accessory, power seating system, recline only, without shear reduction

E1004 Wheelchair accessory, power seating system, recline only, with mechanical shear reduction

E1005 Wheelchair accessory, power seating system, recline only, with power shear reduction

E1006 Wheelchair accessory, power seating system, combination tilt and recline, without shear reduction

E1007 Wheelchair accessory, power seating system, combination tilt and recline, with mechanical shear reduction

E1008 Wheelchair accessory, power seating system, combination tilt and recline, with power shear reduction

E1009 Wheelchair accessory, addition to power seating system, mechanically linked leg elevation system, including pushrod and leg rest, each

E1010 Wheelchair accessory, addition to power seating system, power leg elevation system, including leg rest, pair

E1011 Modification to pediatric size wheelchair, width adjustment package (not to be dispensed with initial chair)

E1012 Wheelchair accessory, addition to power seating system, center mount power elevating leg rest/platform, complete system, any type, each

E1014 Reclining back, addition to pediatric size wheelchair

E1015 Shock absorber for manual wheelchair, each

E1016 Shock absorber for power wheelchair, each

E1017 Heavy duty shock absorber for heavy duty or extra heavy duty manual wheelchair, each

E1018 Heavy duty shock absorber for heavy duty or extra heavy duty power wheelchair, each

E1020 Residual limb support system for wheelchair, any type

E1028 Wheelchair accessory, manual swing away, retractable or removable mounting hardware for joystick, other control interface or positioning accessory

E1029 Wheelchair accessory, ventilator tray, fixed

E1030 Wheelchair accessory, ventilator tray, gimbaled

Rollabout Chair

E1031 Rollabout chair, any and all types with casters 5" or greater

E1035 Multi-positional patient transfer system, with integrated seat, operated by care giver, patient weight capacity up to and including 300 lbs

E1036 Multi-positional patient transfer system, extra-wide, with integrated seat, operated by caregiver, patient weight capacity greater than 300 lbs

E1037 Transport chair, pediatric size

E1038 Transport chair, adult size, patient weight capacity up to and including 300 pounds

E1039 Transport chair, adult size, heavy duty, patient weight capacity greater than 300 pounds

Wheelchairs; Fully-Reclining, Semi-Reclining, Standard, Amputee, and Special Size

E1050 Fully-reclining wheelchair, fixed full length arms, swing away detachable elevating leg rests

E1060 Fully-reclining wheelchair, detachable arms, desk or full length, swing away detachable elevating leg rests

E1070 Fully-reclining wheelchair, detachable arms (desk or full length) swing away detachable footrest

E1083	Hemi-wheelchair, fixed full length arms, swing away detachable elevating leg rest
E1084	Hemi-wheelchair, detachable arms desk or full length arms, swing away detachable elevating leg rests
E1085	Hemi-wheelchair, fixed full length arms, swing away detachable foot rests
E1086	Hemi-wheelchair detachable arms desk or full length, swing away detachable footrests
E1087	High strength lightweight wheelchair, fixed full length arms, swing away detachable elevating leg rests
E1088	High strength lightweight wheelchair, detachable arms desk or full length, swing away detachable elevating leg rests
E1089	High strength lightweight wheelchair, fixed length arms, swing away detachable footrest
E1090	High strength lightweight wheelchair, detachable arms desk or full length, swing away detachable foot rests
E1092	Wide heavy duty wheel chair, detachable arms (desk or full length), swing away detachable elevating leg rests
E1093	Wide heavy duty wheelchair, detachable arms desk or full length arms, swing away detachable footrests
E1100	Semi-reclining wheelchair, fixed full length arms, swing away detachable elevating leg rests
E1110	Semi-reclining wheelchair, detachable arms (desk or full length) elevating leg rest
E1130	Standard wheelchair, fixed full length arms, fixed or swing away detachable footrests
E1140	Wheelchair, detachable arms, desk or full length, swing away detachable footrests
E1150	Wheelchair, detachable arms, desk or full length swing away detachable elevating leg rests
E1160	Wheelchair, fixed full length arms, swing away detachable elevating leg rests
E1161	Manual adult size wheelchair, includes tilt in space
E1170	Amputee wheelchair, fixed full length arms, swing away detachable elevating leg rests
E1171	Amputee wheelchair, fixed full length arms, without footrests or leg rest
E1172	Amputee wheelchair, detachable arms (desk or full length) without footrests or leg rest
E1180	Amputee wheelchair, detachable arms (desk or full length) swing away detachable footrests
E1190	Amputee wheelchair, detachable arms (desk or full length) swing away detachable elevating leg rests
E1195	Heavy duty wheelchair, fixed full length arms, swing away detachable elevating leg rests
E1200	Amputee wheelchair, fixed full length arms, swing away detachable footrest
E1220	Wheelchair; specially sized or constructed, (indicate brand name, model number, if any) and justification
E1221	Wheelchair with fixed arm, footrests
E1222	Wheelchair with fixed arm, elevating leg rests
E1223	Wheelchair with detachable arms, footrests
E1224	Wheelchair with detachable arms, elevating leg rests
E1225	Wheelchair accessory, manual semi-reclining back, (recline greater than 15 degrees, but less than 80 degrees), each
E1226	Wheelchair accessory, manual fully reclining back, (recline greater than 80 degrees), each
E1227	Special height arms for wheelchair

E CODES

Not payable by Medicare | Non-covered by Medicare | Special coverage instructions | Carrier judgement

E1228 Special back height for wheelchair

E1229 Wheelchair, pediatric size, not otherwise specified

Power Operated Vehicle

E1230 Power operated vehicle (three or four wheel nonhighway) specify brand name and model number

Wheelchairs; Lightweight and Heavy Duty

E1231 Wheelchair, pediatric size, tilt-in-space, rigid, adjustable, with seating system

E1232 Wheelchair, pediatric size, tilt-in-space, folding, adjustable, with seating system

E1233 Wheelchair, pediatric size, tilt-in-space, rigid, adjustable, without seating system

E1234 Wheelchair, pediatric size, tilt-in-space, folding, adjustable, without seating system

E1235 Wheelchair, pediatric size, rigid, adjustable, with seating system

E1236 Wheelchair, pediatric size, folding, adjustable, with seating system

E1237 Wheelchair, pediatric size, rigid, adjustable, without seating system

E1238 Wheelchair, pediatric size, folding, adjustable, without seating system

E1239 Power wheelchair, pediatric size, not otherwise specified

E1240 Lightweight wheelchair, detachable arms, (desk or full length) swing away detachable, elevating leg rest

E1250 Lightweight wheelchair, fixed full length arms, swing away detachable footrest

E1260 Lightweight wheelchair, detachable arms (desk or full length) swing away detachable footrest

E1270 Lightweight wheelchair, fixed full length arms, swing away detachable elevating leg rests

E1280 Heavy duty wheelchair, detachable arms (desk or full length) elevating leg rests

E1285 Heavy duty wheelchair, fixed full length arms, swing away detachable footrest

E1290 Heavy duty wheelchair, detachable arms (desk or full length) swing away detachable footrest

E1295 Heavy duty wheelchair, fixed full length arms, elevating leg rest

E1296 Special wheelchair seat height from floor

E1297 Special wheelchair seat depth, by upholstery

E1298 Special wheelchair seat depth and/or width, by construction

Whirlpool Equipment

E1300 Whirlpool, portable (overtub type)

• **E1301** Whirlpool tub, walk-in, portable

E1310 Whirlpool, non-portable (built-in type)

Additional Oxygen Related Supplies and Equipment

E1352 Oxygen accessory, flow regulator capable of positive inspiratory pressure

E1353 Regulator

E1354 Oxygen accessory, wheeled cart for portable cylinder or portable concentrator, any type, replacement only, each

E1355 Stand/rack

E1356 Oxygen accessory, battery pack/cartridge for portable concentrator, any type, replacement only, each

E1357 Oxygen accessory, battery charger for portable concentrator, any type, replacement only, each

E1358 Oxygen accessory, dc power adapter for portable concentrator, any type, replacement only, each

E1372 Immersion external heater for nebulizer

E1390 Oxygen concentrator, single delivery port, capable of delivering 85 percent or greater oxygen concentration at the prescribed flow rate

E1391 Oxygen concentrator, dual delivery port, capable of delivering 85 percent or greater oxygen concentration at the prescribed flow rate, each

E1392 Portable oxygen concentrator, rental

E1399 Durable medical equipment, miscellaneous

E1405 Oxygen and water vapor enriching system with heated delivery

E1406 Oxygen and water vapor enriching system without heated delivery

Artificial Kidney Machines and Accessories

E1500 Centrifuge, for dialysis

E1510 Kidney, dialysate delivery syst kidney machine, pump recirculating, air removal syst, flowrate meter, power off, heater and temperature control with alarm, I.V. poles, pressure gauge, concentrate container

E1520 Heparin infusion pump for hemodialysis

E1530 Air bubble detector for hemodialysis, each, replacement

E1540 Pressure alarm for hemodialysis, each, replacement

E1550 Bath conductivity meter for hemodialysis, each

E1560 Blood leak detector for hemodialysis, each, replacement

E1570 Adjustable chair, for ESRD patients

E1575 Transducer protectors/fluid barriers, for hemodialysis, any size, per 10

E1580 Unipuncture control system for hemodialysis

E1590 Hemodialysis machine

E1592 Automatic intermittent peritoneal dialysis system

E1594 Cycler dialysis machine for peritoneal dialysis

E1600 Delivery and/or installation charges for hemodialysis equipment

E1610 Reverse osmosis water purification system, for hemodialysis

E1615 Deionizer water purification system, for hemodialysis

E1620 Blood pump for hemodialysis, replacement

E1625 Water softening system, for hemodialysis

E1629 Tablo hemodialysis system for the billable dialysis service

E1630 Reciprocating peritoneal dialysis system

E1632 Wearable artificial kidney, each

E1634 Peritoneal dialysis clamps, each

E1635 Compact (portable) travel hemodialyzer system

E CODES

E1636	Sorbent cartridges, for hemodialysis, per 10
E1637	Hemostats, each
E1639	Scale, each
E1699	Dialysis equipment, not otherwise specified
E1700	Jaw motion rehabilitation system
E1701	Replacement cushions for jaw motion rehabilitation system, pkg. of 6
E1702	Replacement measuring scales for jaw motion rehabilitation system, pkg. of 200
E1800	Dynamic adjustable elbow extension/flexion device, includes soft interface material
E1801	Static progressive stretch elbow device, extension and/or flexion, with or without range of motion adjustment, includes all components and accessories
E1802	Dynamic adjustable forearm pronation/supination device, includes soft interface material
E1805	Dynamic adjustable wrist extension / flexion device, includes soft interface material
E1806	Static progressive stretch wrist device, flexion and/or extension, with or without range of motion adjustment, includes all components and accessories
E1810	Dynamic adjustable knee extension / flexion device, includes soft interface material
E1811	Static progressive stretch knee device, extension and/or flexion, with or without range of motion adjustment, includes all components and accessories
E1812	Dynamic knee, extension/flexion device with active resistance control
E1815	Dynamic adjustable ankle extension/flexion device, includes soft interface material
E1816	Static progressive stretch ankle device, flexion and/or extension, with or without range of motion adjustment, includes all components and accessories
E1818	Static progressive stretch forearm pronation / supination device, with or without range of motion adjustment, includes all components and accessories
E1820	Replacement soft interface material, dynamic adjustable extension/flexion device
E1821	Replacement soft interface material/cuffs for bi-directional static progressive stretch device
E1825	Dynamic adjustable finger extension/flexion device, includes soft interface material
E1830	Dynamic adjustable toe extension/flexion device, includes soft interface material
E1831	Static progressive stretch toe device, extension and/or flexion, with or without range of motion adjustment, includes all components and accessories
E1840	Dynamic adjustable shoulder flexion / abduction / rotation device, includes soft interface material
E1841	Static progressive stretch shoulder device, with or without range of motion adjustment, includes all components and accessories
E1902	Communication board, non-electronic augmentative or alternative communication device
E2000	Gastric suction pump, home model, portable or stationary, electric
• E2001	Suction pump, home model, portable or stationary, electric, any type, for use with external urine management system
E2100	Blood glucose monitor with integrated voice synthesizer
E2101	Blood glucose monitor with integrated lancing/blood sample
E2102	Adjunctive, non-implanted continuous glucose monitor or receiver
E2103	Non-adjunctive, non-implanted continuous glucose monitor or receiver

E CODES

E2120 Pulse generator system for tympanic treatment of inner ear endolymphatic fluid

Extension/Flexion Devices

E1700 Jaw motion rehabilitation system

Manual Wheelchair Accessories

E2201 Manual wheelchair accessory, nonstandard seat frame, width greater than or equal to 20 inches and less than 24 inches

E2202 Manual wheelchair accessory, nonstandard seat frame width, 24-27 inches

E2203 Manual wheelchair accessory, nonstandard seat frame depth, 20 to less than 22 inches

E2204 Manual wheelchair accessory, nonstandard seat frame depth, 22 to 25 inches

E2205 Manual wheelchair accessory, hand rim without projections (includes ergonomic or contoured), any type, replacement only, each

E2206 Manual wheelchair accessory, wheel lock assembly, complete, replacement only, each

E2207 Wheelchair accessory, crutch and cane holder, each

E2208 Wheelchair accessory, cylinder tank carrier, each

E2209 Accessory, arm trough, with or without hand support, each

E2210 Wheelchair accessory, bearings, any type, replacement only, each

E2211 Manual wheelchair accessory, pneumatic propulsion tire, any size, each

E2212 Manual wheelchair accessory, tube for pneumatic propulsion tire, any size, each

E2213 Manual wheelchair accessory, insert for pneumatic propulsion tire (removable), any type, any size, each

E2214 Manual wheelchair accessory, pneumatic caster tire, any size, each

E2215 Manual wheelchair accessory, tube for pneumatic caster tire, any size, each

E2216 Manual wheelchair accessory, foam filled propulsion tire, any size, each

E2217 Manual wheelchair accessory, foam filled caster tire, any size, each

E2218 Manual wheelchair accessory, foam propulsion tire, any size, each

E2219 Manual wheelchair accessory, foam caster tire, any size, each

E2220 Manual wheelchair accessory, solid (rubber/plastic) propulsion tire, any size, replacement only, each

E2221 Manual wheelchair accessory, solid (rubber/plastic) caster tire (removable), any size, replacement only, each

E2222 Manual wheelchair accessory, solid (rubber/plastic) caster tire with integrated wheel, any size, replacement only, each

E2224 Manual wheelchair accessory, propulsion wheel excludes tire, any size, replacement only, each

E2225 Manual wheelchair accessory, caster wheel excludes tire, any size, replacement only, each

E2226 Manual wheelchair accessory, caster fork, any size, replacement only, each

E2227 Manual wheelchair accessory, gear reduction drive wheel, each

E2228 Manual wheelchair accessory, wheel braking system and lock, complete, each

E2230 Manual wheelchair accessory, manual standing system

E2231 Manual wheelchair accessory, solid seat support base (replaces sling seat), includes any type mounting hardware

E2291 Back, planar, for pediatric size wheelchair including fixed attaching hardware

E2292 Seat, planar, for pediatric size wheelchair including fixed attaching hardware

E2293 Back, contoured, for pediatric size wheelchair including fixed attaching hardware

E2294 Seat, contoured, for pediatric size wheelchair including fixed attaching hardware

E2295 Manual wheelchair accessory, for pediatric size wheelchair, dynamic seating frame, allows coordinated movement of multiple positioning features

E2300 Wheelchair accessory, power seat elevation system, any type

E2301 Wheelchair accessory, power standing system, any type

Power Wheelchair Accessories

E2310 Power wheelchair accessory, electronic connection between wheelchair controller and one power seating system motor, including all related electronics, indicator feature, mechanical function selection switch, and fixed mounting hardware

E2311 Power wheelchair accessory, electronic connection between wheelchair controller and two or more power seating system motors, including all related electronics, indicator feature, mechanical function selection switch, and fixed mounting hardware

E2312 Power wheelchair accessory, hand or chin control interface, mini-proportional remote joystick, proportional, including fixed mounting hardware

E2313 Power wheelchair accessory, harness for upgrade to expandable controller, including all fasteners, connectors and mounting hardware, each

E2321 Power wheelchair accessory, hand control interface, remote joystick, nonproportional, including all related electronics, mechanical stop switch, and fixed mounting hardware

E2322 Power wheelchair accessory, hand control interface, multiple mechanical switches, nonproportional, including all related electronics, mechanical stop switch, and fixed mounting hardware

E2323 Power wheelchair accessory, specialty joystick handle for hand control interface, prefabricated

E2324 Power wheelchair accessory, chin cup for chin control interface

E2325 Power wheelchair accessory, sip and puff interface, nonproportional, including all related electronics, mechanical stop switch, and manual swing away mounting hardware

E2326 Power wheelchair accessory, breath tube kit for sip and puff interface

E2327 Power wheelchair accessory, head control interface, mechanical, proportional, including all related electronics, mechanical direction change switch, and fixed mounting hardware

E2328 Power wheelchair accessory, head control or extremity control interface, electronic, proportional, including all related electronics and fixed mounting hardware

E2329 Power wheelchair accessory, head control interface, contact switch mechanism, nonproportional, including all related electronics, mechanical stop switch, mechanical direction change switch, head array, and fixed mounting hardware

E2330 Power wheelchair accessory, head control interface, proximity switch mechanism, nonproportional, including all related electronics, mechanical stop switch, mechanical direction change switch, head array, and fixed mounting hardware

E2331 Power wheelchair accessory, attendant control, proportional, including all related electronics and fixed mounting hardware

E2340 Power wheelchair accessory, nonstandard seat frame width, 20-23 inches

E2341 Power wheelchair accessory, nonstandard seat frame width, 24-27 inches

E2342	Power wheelchair accessory, nonstandard seat frame depth, 20 or 21 inches
E2343	Power wheelchair accessory, nonstandard seat frame depth, 22-25 inches
E2351	Power wheelchair accessory, electronic interface to operate speech generating device using power wheelchair control interface
E2358	Power wheelchair accessory, group 34 non-sealed lead acid battery, each
E2359	Power wheelchair accessory, group 34 sealed lead acid battery, each (e.g., gel cell, absorbed glass mat)
E2360	Power wheelchair accessory, 22nf non-sealed lead acid battery, each
E2361	Power wheelchair accessory, 22nf sealed lead acid battery, each, (e.g., gel cell, absorbed glass mat)
E2362	Power wheelchair accessory, group 24 non-sealed lead acid battery, each
E2363	Power wheelchair accessory, group 24 sealed lead acid battery, each (e.g., gel cell, absorbed glass mat)
E2364	Power wheelchair accessory, u-1 non-sealed lead acid battery, each
E2365	Power wheelchair accessory, u-1 sealed lead acid battery, each (e.g., gel cell, absorbed glass mat)
E2366	Power wheelchair accessory, battery charger, single mode, for use with only one battery type, sealed or non-sealed, each
E2367	Power wheelchair accessory, battery charger, dual mode, for use with either battery type, sealed or non-sealed, each
E2368	Power wheelchair component, drive wheel motor, replacement only
E2369	Power wheelchair component, drive wheel gear box, replacement only
E2370	Power wheelchair component, integrated drive wheel motor and gear box combination, replacement only
E2371	Power wheelchair accessory, group 27 sealed lead acid battery, (e.g., gel cell, absorbed glass mat), each
E2372	Power wheelchair accessory, group 27 non-sealed lead acid battery, each
E2373	Power wheelchair accessory, hand or chin control interface, compact remote joystick, proportional, including fixed mounting hardware
E2374	Power wheelchair accessory, hand or chin control interface, standard remote joystick (not including controller), proportional, including all related electronics and fixed mounting hardware, replacement only
E2375	Power wheelchair accessory, non-expandable controller, including all related electronics and mounting hardware, replacement only
E2376	Power wheelchair accessory, expandable controller, including all related electronics and mounting hardware, replacement only
E2377	Power wheelchair accessory, expandable controller, including all related electronics and mounting hardware, upgrade provided at initial issue
E2378	Power wheelchair component, actuator, replacement only
E2381	Power wheelchair accessory, pneumatic drive wheel tire, any size, replacement only, each
E2382	Power wheelchair accessory, tube for pneumatic drive wheel tire, any size, replacement only, each
E2383	Power wheelchair accessory, insert for pneumatic drive wheel tire (removable), any type, any size, replacement only, each
E2384	Power wheelchair accessory, pneumatic caster tire, any size, replacement only, each
E2385	Power wheelchair accessory, tube for pneumatic caster tire, any size, replacement only, each

E2386 Power wheelchair accessory, foam filled drive wheel tire, any size, replacement only, each

E2387 Power wheelchair accessory, foam filled caster tire, any size, replacement only, each

E2388 Power wheelchair accessory, foam drive wheel tire, any size, replacement only, each

E2389 Power wheelchair accessory, foam caster tire, any size, replacement only, each

E2390 Power wheelchair accessory, solid (rubber/plastic) drive wheel tire, any size, replacement only, each

E2391 Power wheelchair accessory, solid (rubber/plastic) caster tire (removable), any size, replacement only, each

E2392 Power wheelchair accessory, solid (rubber/plastic) caster tire with integrated wheel, any size, replacement only, each

E2394 Power wheelchair accessory, drive wheel excludes tire, any size, replacement only, each

E2395 Power wheelchair accessory, caster wheel excludes tire, any size, replacement only, each

E2396 Power wheelchair accessory, caster fork, any size, replacement only, each

E2397 Power wheelchair accessory, lithium-based battery, each

E2398 Wheelchair accessory, dynamic positioning hardware for back

E2402 Negative pressure wound therapy electrical pump, stationary or portable

Speech Generating Device and Accessories

E2500 Speech generating device, digitized speech, using pre-recorded messages, less than or equal to 8 minutes recording time

E2502 Speech generating device, digitized speech, using pre-recorded messages, greater than 8 minutes but less than or equal to 20 minutes recording time

E2504 Speech generating device, digitized speech, using pre-recorded messages, greater than 20 minutes but less than or equal to 40 minutes recording time

E2506 Speech generating device, digitized speech, using pre-recorded messages, greater than 40 minutes recording time

E2508 Speech generating device, synthesized speech, requiring message formulation by spelling and access by physical contact with the device

E2510 Speech generating device, synthesized speech, permitting multiple methods of message formulation and multiple methods of device access

E2511 Speech generating software program, for personal computer or personal digital assistant

E2512 Accessory for speech generating device, mounting system

E2599 Accessory for speech generating device, not otherwise classified

Wheelchair Cushions and Support Devices

E2601 General use wheelchair seat cushion, width less than 22 inches, any depth

E2602 General use wheelchair seat cushion, width 22 inches or greater, any depth

E2603 Skin protection wheelchair seat cushion, width less than 22 inches, any depth

E2604 Skin protection wheelchair seat cushion, width 22 inches or greater, any depth

E2605 Positioning wheelchair seat cushion, width less than 22 inches, any depth

E2606 Positioning wheelchair seat cushion, width 22 inches or greater, any depth

E2607 Skin protection and positioning wheelchair seat cushion, width less than 22 inches, any depth

E2608 Skin protection and positioning wheelchair seat cushion, width 22 inches or greater, any depth

E2609 Custom fabricated wheelchair seat cushion, any size

E2610 Wheelchair seat cushion, powered

E2611 General use wheelchair back cushion, width less than 22 inches, any height, including any type mounting hardware

E2612 General use wheelchair back cushion, width 22 inches or greater, any height, including any type mounting hardware

E2613 Positioning wheelchair back cushion, posterior, width less than 22 inches, any height, including any type mounting hardware

E2614 Positioning wheelchair back cushion, posterior, width 22 inches or greater, any height, including any type mounting hardware

E2615 Positioning wheelchair back cushion, posterior-lateral, width less than 22 inches, any height, including any type mounting hardware

E2616 Positioning wheelchair back cushion, posterior-lateral, width 22 inches or greater, any height, including any type mounting hardware

E2617 Custom fabricated wheelchair back cushion, any size, including any type mounting hardware

E2619 Replacement cover for wheelchair seat cushion or back cushion, each

E2620 Positioning wheelchair back cushion, planar back with lateral supports, width less than 22 inches, any height, including any type mounting hardware

E2621 Positioning wheelchair back cushion, planar back with lateral supports, width 22 inches or greater, any height, including any type mounting hardware

E2622 Skin protection wheelchair seat cushion, adjustable, width less than 22 inches, any depth

E2623 Skin protection wheelchair seat cushion, adjustable, width 22 inches or greater, any depth

E2624 Skin protection and positioning wheelchair seat cushion, adjustable, width less than 22 inches, any depth

E2625 Skin protection and positioning wheelchair seat cushion, adjustable, width 22 inches or greater, any depth

E2626 Wheelchair accessory, shoulder elbow, mobile arm support attached to wheelchair, balanced, adjustable

E2627 Wheelchair accessory, shoulder elbow, mobile arm support attached to wheelchair, balanced, adjustable rancho type

E2628 Wheelchair accessory, shoulder elbow, mobile arm support attached to wheelchair, balanced, reclining

E2629 Wheelchair accessory, shoulder elbow, mobile arm support attached to wheelchair, balanced, friction arm support (friction dampening to proximal and distal joints)

E2630 Wheelchair accessory, shoulder elbow, mobile arm support, monosuspension arm and hand support, overhead elbow forearm hand sling support, yoke type suspension support

E2631 Wheelchair accessory, addition to mobile arm support, elevating proximal arm

E2632 Wheelchair accessory, addition to mobile arm support, offset or lateral rocker arm with elastic balance control

E2633 Wheelchair accessory, addition to mobile arm support, supinator

• **E3000** Speech volume modulation system, any type, including all components and accessories

Gait Trainer

E8000 Gait trainer, pediatric size, posterior support, includes all accessories and components

E8001 Gait trainer, pediatric size, upright support, includes all accessories and components

E8002 Gait trainer, pediatric size, anterior support, includes all accessories and components

PROCEDURES AND PROFESSIONAL SERVICES

Guidelines

In addition to the information presented in the INTRODUCTION, several other items unique to this section are defined or identified here:

1. **TEMPORARY CODES**: The codes listed in this section are assigned by CMS on a temporary basis to identify procedures/services.

Procedures/Professional Services

G0008 Administration of influenza virus vaccine

G0009 Administration of pneumococcal vaccine

G0010 Administration of hepatitis b vaccine

• **G0011** Individual counseling for pre-exposure prophylaxis (prep) by physician or qualified health care professional (qhp)to prevent human immunodeficiency virus (HIV), includes HIV risk assessment (initial or continued assessment of risk), HIV risk reduction and medication adherence, 15-30 minutes

• **G0012** Injection of pre-exposure prophylaxis (prep) drug for HIV prevention, under skin or into muscle

• **G0013** Individual counseling for pre-exposure prophylaxis (prep) by clinical staff to prevent human immunodeficiency virus (HIV), includes HIV risk assessment (initial or continued assessment of risk), HIV risk reduction and medication adherence

• **G0017** Psychotherapy for crisis furnished in an applicable site of service (any place of service at which the non-facility rate for psychotherapy for crisis services applies, other than the office setting); first 60 minutes

• **G0018** Psychotherapy for crisis furnished in an applicable site of service (any place of service at which the non-facility rate for psychotherapy for crisis services applies, other than the office setting); each additional 30 minutes (list separately in addition to code for primary service)

• **G0019** Community health integration services performed by certified or trained auxiliary personnel, including a community health worker, under the direction of a physician or other practitioner; 60 minutes per calendar month, in the following activities to address social determinants of health (sdoh) need(s) that are significantly limiting the ability to diagnose or treat problem(s) addressed in an initiating visit: person-centered assessment, performed to better understand the individualized context of the intersection between the sdoh need(s) and the problem(s) addressed in the initiating visit. ++ conducting a person-centered assessment to understand patient's life story, strengths, needs, goals, preferences and desired outcomes, including understanding cultural and linguistic factors and including unmet sdoh needs (that are not separately billed). ++ facilitating patient-driven goal-setting and establishing an action plan. ++ providing tailored support to the patient as needed to accomplish the practitioner's treatment plan. practitioner, home-, and community-based care coordination. ++ coordinating receipt of needed services from healthcare practitioners, providers, and facilities; and from home- and community-based service providers, social service providers, and caregiver (if applicable). ++ communication with practitioners, home- and community-based service providers, hospitals, and skilled nursing facilities (or other health care facilities) regarding the patient's psychosocial strengths and needs, functional deficits, goals, preferences, and desired outcomes, including cultural and linguistic factors. ++ coordination of care transitions between and among health care practitioners and settings, including transitions involving referral to other clinicians; follow-up after an emergency department visit; or follow-up after discharges from hospitals, skilled nursing facilities or other health care facilities. ++ facilitating access to community-based social services (e.g., housing, utilities, transportation, food assistance) to address the sdoh need(s). health education- helping the patient contextualize health education provided by the patient's treatment team with the patient's individual needs, goals, and preferences, in the context of the sdoh need(s) and educating the patient on how to best participate in medical decision-making. building patient self-advocacy skills, so that the patient can interact with members of the health care team and related community-based services addressing the sdoh need(s), in ways that are more likely to promote personalized and effective diagnosis or treatment. health care access / health system navigation. ++ helping the patient access healthcare, including identifying appropriate practitioners or providers for clinical care and helping secure appointments with them. facilitating behavioral change as necessary for meeting diagnosis and treatment goals, including promoting patient motivation to participate in care and reach person-centered diagnosis or treatment goals. facilitating and providing social and emotional support to help the patient cope with the problem(s) addressed in the initiating visit, the sdoh need(s), and adjust daily routines to better meet diagnosis and treatment goals. leveraging lived experience when applicable to provide support, mentorship, or inspiration to meet treatment goals

● **G0022** Community health integration services, each additional 30 minutes per calendar month (list separately in addition to G0019)

● **G0023** Principal illness navigation services by certified or trained auxiliary personnel under the direction of a physician or other practitioner, including a patient navigator; 60 minutes per calendar month, in the following activities: person-centered assessment, performed to better understand the individual context of the serious, high-risk condition. ++ conducting a person-centered assessment to understand the patient's life story, strengths, needs, goals, preferences, and desired outcomes, including understanding cultural and linguistic factors and including unmet sdoh needs (that are not separately billed). ++ facilitating patient-driven goal setting and establishing an action plan. ++ providing tailored support as needed to accomplish the practitioner's treatment plan. identifying or referring patient (and caregiver or family, if applicable) to appropriate supportive services. practitioner, home, and community-based care coordination. ++ coordinating receipt of needed services from healthcare practitioners, providers, and facilities; home- and community-based service providers; and caregiver (if applicable). ++ communication with practitioners, home-, and community-based service providers, hospitals, and skilled nursing facilities (or other health care facilities) regarding the patient's psychosocial strengths and needs, functional deficits, goals, preferences, and desired outcomes, including cultural and linguistic factors. ++ coordination of care transitions between and among health care practitioners and settings, including transitions involving referral to other clinicians; follow-up after an emergency department visit; or follow-up after discharges from hospitals, skilled nursing facilities or other health care facilities. ++ facilitating access to community-based social services (e.g., housing, utilities, transportation, likely to promote personalized and effective treatment of their condition. health care access / health system navigation. ++ helping the patient access healthcare, including identifying appropriate practitioners or providers for clinical care, and helping secure appointments with them. ++ providing the patient with information/resources to consider participation in clinical trials or clinical research as applicable. facilitating behavioral change as necessary for meeting diagnosis and treatment goals, including promoting patient motivation to participate in care and reach person-centered diagnosis or treatment goals. facilitating and providing social and emotional support to help the patient cope with the condition, sdoh need(s), and adjust daily routines to better meet diagnosis and treatment goals. leverage knowledge of the serious, high-risk condition and/or lived experience when applicable to provide support, mentorship, or inspiration to meet treatment goals

● **G0024** Principal illness navigation services, additional 30 minutes per calendar month (list separately in addition to G0023)

G0027 Semen analysis; presence and/or motility of sperm excluding Huhner

(**G0028** Documentation of medical reason(s) for not screening for tobacco use (e.g., limited life expectancy, other medical reason)

Code deleted effective 12/31/2022, no HCPCS/CPT cross-reference provided.)

G0029 Tobacco screening not performed, or tobacco cessation intervention not provided during the

G - H CODES

measurement period or in the six months prior to the measurement period

G0030 Patient screened for tobacco use and received tobacco cessation intervention during the measurement period or in the six months prior to the measurement period (counseling, pharmacotherapy, or both), if identified as a tobacco user

G0031 Palliative care services given to patient any time during the measurement period

G0032 Two or more antipsychotic prescriptions ordered for patients who had a diagnosis of schizophrenia, schizoaffective disorder, or bipolar disorder on or between January 1 of the year prior to the measurement period and the index prescription start date (ipsd) for antipsychotics

G0033 Two or more benzodiazepine prescriptions ordered for patients who had a diagnosis of seizure disorders, rapid eye movement sleep behavior disorder, benzodiazepine withdrawal, ethanol withdrawal, or severe generalized anxiety disorder on or between January 1 of the year prior to the measurement period and the ipsd for benzodiazepines

G0034 Patients receiving palliative care during the measurement period

G0035 Patient has any emergency department encounter during the performance period with place of service indicator 23

G0036 Patient or care partner decline assessment

G0037 On date of encounter, patient is not able to participate in assessment or screening, including non-verbal patients, delirious, severely aphasic, severely developmentally delayed, severe visual or hearing impairment and for those patients, no knowledgeable informant available

G0038 Clinician determines patient does not require referral

G0039 Patient not referred; reason not otherwise specified

G0040 Patient already receiving physical/occupational/speech/recreational therapy during the measurement period

G0041 Patient and/or care partner decline referral

G0042 Referral to physical, occupational, speech, or recreational therapy

G0043 Patients with mechanical prosthetic heart valve

G0044 Patients with moderate or severe mitral stenosis

G0045 Clinical follow-up and MRS score assessed at 90 days following endovascular stroke intervention

G0046 Clinical follow-up and MRS score not assessed at 90 days following endovascular stroke intervention

G0047 Pediatric patient with minor blunt head trauma and pecarn prediction criteria are not assessed

G0048 Patients who receive palliative care services any time during the intake period through the end of the measurement year

G0049 With maintenance hemodialysis (in-center and home hd) for the complete reporting month

G0050 Patients with a catheter that have limited life expectancy

G0051 Patients under hospice care in the current reporting month

G0052 Patients on peritoneal dialysis for any portion of the reporting month

G0053 Advancing rheumatology patient care MIPS value pathways

G0054 Coordinating stroke care to promote prevention and cultivate positive outcomes MIPS value pathways

G0055 Advancing care for heart disease MIPS value pathways

(**G0056** Optimizing chronic disease management MIPS value pathways

G0057 Proposed adopting best practices and promoting patient safety within emergency medicine MIPS value pathways

G - H CODES

G0058 Improving care for lower extremity joint repair MIPS value pathways

G0059 Patient safety and support of positive experiences with anesthesia MIPS value pathways

G0060 Allergy/immunology MIPS specialty set

G0061 Anesthesiology MIPS specialty set

G0062 Audiology MIPS specialty set

G0063 Cardiology MIPS specialty set

G0064 Certified nurse midwife MIPS specialty set

G0065 Chiropractic medicine MIPS specialty set

G0066 Clinical social work MIPS specialty set

G0067 Dentistry MIPS specialty set

G0068 Professional services for the administration of anti-infective, pain management, chelation, pulmonary hypertension, inotropic, or other intravenous infusion drug or biological (excluding chemotherapy or other highly complex drug or biological) for each infusion drug administration calendar day in the individual's home, each 15 minutes

G0069 Professional services for the administration of subcutaneous immunotherapy or other subcutaneous infusion drug or biological for each infusion drug administration calendar day in the individual's home, each 15 minutes

G0070 Professional services for the administration of intravenous chemotherapy or other intravenous highly complex drug or biological infusion for each infusion drug administration calendar day in the individual's home, each 15 minutes

G0071 Payment for communication technology-based services for 5 minutes or more of a virtual (non-face-to-face) communication between an rural health clinic (rhc) or federally qualified health center (fqhc) practitioner and rhc or fqhc patient, or 5 minutes or more of remote evaluation of recorded video and/or images by an rhc or fqhc practitioner, occurring in lieu of an office visit; rhc or fqhc only

G0076 Brief (20 minutes) care management home visit for a new patient. for use only in a Medicare-approved cmmi model. (services must be furnished within a beneficiary's home, domiciliary, rest home, assisted living and/or nursing facility)

G0077 Limited (30 minutes) care management home visit for a new patient. for use only in a Medicare-approved cmmi model. (services must be furnished within a beneficiary's home, domiciliary, rest home, assisted living and/or nursing facility)

G0078 Moderate (45 minutes) care management home visit for a new patient. for use only in a Medicare-approved cmmi model. (services must be furnished within a beneficiary's home, domiciliary, rest home, assisted living and/or nursing facility)

G0079 Comprehensive (60 minutes) care management home visit for a new patient. for use only in a Medicare-approved cmmi model. (services must be furnished within a beneficiary's home, domiciliary, rest home, assisted living and/or nursing facility)

G0080 Extensive (75 minutes) care management home visit for a new patient. for use only in a Medicare-approved cmmi model. (services must be furnished within a beneficiary's home, domiciliary, rest home, assisted living and/or nursing facility)

G0081 Brief (20 minutes) care management home visit for an existing patient. for use only in a Medicare-approved cmmi model. (services must be furnished within a beneficiary's home, domiciliary, rest home, assisted living and/or nursing facility)

G0082 Limited (30 minutes) care management home visit for an existing patient. for use only in a Medicare-approved cmmi model. (services must be furnished within a beneficiary's home, domiciliary, rest home, assisted living and/or nursing facility)

G0083 Moderate (45 minutes) care management home visit for an existing patient. for use only in a Medicare-approved cmmi model. (services must be furnished within a beneficiary's home, domiciliary, rest home, assisted living and/or nursing facility)

G0084 Comprehensive (60 minutes) care management home visit for an existing patient. for use only in a Medicare-approved cmmi model. (services must be furnished within a beneficiary's home, domiciliary, rest home, assisted living and/or nursing facility)

G0085 Extensive (75 minutes) care management home visit for an existing patient. for use only in a Medicare-approved cmmi model. (services must be furnished within a beneficiary's home, domiciliary, rest home, assisted living and/or nursing facility)

G0086 Limited (30 minutes) care management home care plan oversight. for use only in a Medicare-approved cmmi model. (services must be furnished within a beneficiary's home, domiciliary, rest home, assisted living and/or nursing facility)

G0087 Comprehensive (60 minutes) care management home care plan oversight. for use only in a Medicare-approved cmmi model. (services must be furnished within a beneficiary's home, domiciliary, rest home, assisted living and/or nursing facility)

G0088 Professional services, initial visit, for the administration of anti-infective, pain management, chelation, pulmonary hypertension, inotropic, or other intravenous infusion drug or biological (excluding chemotherapy or other highly complex drug or biological) for each infusion drug administration calendar day in the individual's home, each 15 minutes

G0089 Professional services, initial visit, for the administration of subcutaneous immunotherapy or other subcutaneous infusion drug or biological for each infusion drug administration calendar day in the individual's home, each 15 minutes

G0090 Professional services, initial visit, for the administration of intravenous chemotherapy or other highly complex infusion drug or biological for each infusion drug administration calendar day in the individual's home, each 15 minutes

G0101 Cervical or vaginal cancer screening; pelvic and clinical breast examination

G0102 Prostate cancer screening; digital rectal examination

G0103 Prostate cancer screening; prostate specific antigen test (PSA)

G0104 Colorectal cancer screening; flexible sigmoidoscopy

G0105 Colorectal cancer screening; colonoscopy on individual at high risk

G0106 Colorectal cancer screening; alternative to G0104, screening sigmoidoscopy, barium enema

G0108 Diabetes outpatient self-management training services, individual, per 30 minutes

G0109 Diabetes outpatient self-management training services, group session (2 or more), per 30 minutes

G0117 Glaucoma screening for high risk patients furnished by an optometrist or ophthalmologist

G0118 Glaucoma screening for high risk patient furnished under the direct supervision of an optometrist or ophthalmologist

G0120 Colorectal cancer screening; alternative to G0105, screening colonoscopy, barium enema.

G0121 Colorectal cancer screening; colonoscopy on individual not meeting criteria for high risk

G0122 Colorectal cancer screening; barium enema

G0123 Screening cytopathology, cervical or vaginal (any reporting system), collected in preservative fluid, automated thin layer preparation, screening by cytotechnologist under physician supervision

G0124 Screening cytopathology, cervical or vaginal (any reporting system), collected in preservative fluid, automated thin layer preparation, requiring interpretation by physician

G0127 Trimming of dystrophic nails, any number

G0128 Direct (face-to-face with patient) skilled nursing services of a registered nurse provided in a comprehensive outpatient rehabilitation facility, each 10 minutes beyond the first 5 minutes

▲ **G0129** Occupational therapy services requiring the skills of a qualified occupational therapist, furnished as a component of a partial hospitalization or intensive outpatient treatment program, per session (45 minutes or more)

G0130 Single energy x-ray absorptiometry (sexa) bone density study, one or more sites; appendicular skeleton (peripheral) (e.g., radius, wrist, heel)

• **G0136** Administration of a standardized, evidence-based social determinants of health risk assessment tool, 5-15 minutes

• **G0137** Intensive outpatient services; weekly bundle, minimum of 9 services over a 7 contiguous day period, which can include individual and group therapy with physicians or psychologists (or other mental health professionals to the extent authorized under state law); occupational therapy requiring the skills of a qualified occupational therapist; services of social workers, trained psychiatric nurses, and other staff trained to work with psychiatric patients; individualized activity therapies that are not primarily recreational or diversionary; family counseling (the primary purpose of which is treatment of the individual's condition); patient training and education (to the extent that training and educational activities are closely and clearly related to individual's care and treatment); diagnostic services; and such other items and services (excluding meals and transportation) that are reasonable and necessary for the diagnosis or active treatment of the individual's condition, reasonably expected to improve or maintain the individual's condition and functional level and to prevent relapse or hospitalization, and furnished pursuant to such guidelines relating to frequency and duration of services in accordance with a physician certification and plan of treatment (provision of the services by a Medicare-enrolled opioid treatment program); list separately in addition to code for primary procedure

• **G0140** Principal illness navigation - peer support by certified or trained auxiliary personnel under the direction of a physician or other practitioner, including a certified peer specialist; 60 minutes per calendar month, in the following activities: person-centered interview, performed to better understand the individual context of the serious, high-risk condition. ++ conducting a person-centered interview to understand the patient's life story, strengths, needs, goals, preferences, and desired outcomes, including understanding cultural and linguistic factors, and including unmet sdoh needs (that are not billed separately). ++ facilitating patient-driven goal setting and establishing an action plan. ++ providing tailored support as needed to accomplish the person-centered goals in the practitioner's treatment plan. identifying or referring patient (and caregiver or family, if applicable) to appropriate supportive services. practitioner, home, and community-based care communication. ++ assist the patient in communicating with their practitioners, home-, and community-based service providers, hospitals, and skilled nursing facilities (or other health care facilities) regarding the patient's psychosocial strengths and needs, goals, preferences, and desired outcomes, including cultural and linguistic factors. ++ facilitating access to community-based social services (e.g., housing, utilities, transportation, food assistance) as needed to address sdoh need(s). health education. helping the patient contextualize health education provided by the patient's treatment team with the patient's individual needs, goals, preferences, and sdoh need(s), and educating the patient (and caregiver if applicable) on how to best participate in medical decision-making. building patient self-advocacy skills, so that the patient can interact with members of the health care team and related community-based services (as needed), in ways that are more likely to promote personalized and effective treatment of their condition. developing and proposing strategies to help meet person-centered treatment goals and supporting the patient in using chosen strategies to reach person-centered treatment goals. facilitating and providing social and emotional support to help the patient cope with the condition, sdoh need(s), and adjust daily routines to better meet person-centered diagnosis and treatment goals. leverage knowledge of the serious, high-risk condition and/or lived experience when applicable to provide support, mentorship, or inspiration to meet treatment goals

G0141 Screening cytopathology smears, cervical or vaginal, performed by automated system, with manual rescreening, requiring interpretation by physician

G0143 Screening cytopathology, cervical or vaginal (any reporting system), collected in preservative fluid, automated thin layer preparation, with manual screening and rescreening by cytotechnologist under physician supervision

G0144 Screening cytopathology, cervical or vaginal (any reporting system), collected in preservative

G - H CODES

fluid, automated thin layer preparation, with screening by automated system, under physician supervision

G0145 Screening cytopathology, cervical or vaginal (any reporting system), collected in preservative fluid, automated thin layer preparation, with screening by automated system and manual rescreening under physician supervision

• **G0146** Principal illness navigation - peer support, additional 30 minutes per calendar month (list separately in addition to G0140)

G0147 Screening cytopathology smears, cervical or vaginal, performed by automated system under physician supervision

G0148 Screening cytopathology smears, cervical or vaginal, performed by automated system with manual rescreening

G0151 Services performed by a qualified physical therapist in the home health or hospice setting, each 15 minutes

G0152 Services performed by a qualified occupational therapist in the home health or hospice setting, each 15 minutes

G0153 Services performed by a qualified speech-language pathologist in the home health or hospice setting, each 15 minutes

G0154 Direct skilled nursing services of a licensed nurse (LPN or RN) in the home health or hospice setting, each 15 minutes

G0155 Services of clinical social worker in home health or hospice settings, each 15 minutes

G0156 Services of home health/hospice aide in home health or hospice settings, each 15 minutes

G0157 Services performed by a qualified physical therapist assistant in the home health or hospice setting, each 15 minutes

G0158 Services performed by a qualified occupational therapist assistant in the home health or hospice setting, each 15 minutes

G0159 Services performed by a qualified physical therapist, in the home health setting, in the establishment or delivery of a safe and effective physical therapy maintenance program, each 15 minutes

G0160 Services performed by a qualified occupational therapist, in the home health setting, in the establishment or delivery of a safe and effective occupational therapy maintenance program, each 15 minutes

G0161 Services performed by a qualified speech-language pathologist, in the home health setting, in the establishment or delivery of a safe and effective speech-language pathology maintenance program, each 15 minutes

G0162 Skilled services by a registered nurse (RN) for management and evaluation of the plan of care; each 15 minutes (the patient's underlying condition or complication requires an RN to ensure that essential non-skilled care achieves its purpose in the home health or hospice setting)

G0163 Skilled services of a licensed nurse (LPN or RN) for the observation and assessment of the patient's condition, each 15 minutes (the change in the patient's condition requires skilled nursing personnel to identify and evaluate the patient's need for possible modification of treatment in the home health or hospice setting)

G0164 Skilled services of a licensed nurse (LPN or RN), in the training and/or education of a patient or family member, in the home health or hospice setting, each 15 minutes

G0166 External counterpulsation, per treatment session

G0168 Wound closure utilizing tissue adhesive(s) only

G0173 Linear accelerator based stereotactic radiosurgery, complete course of therapy in one session

G0175 Scheduled interdisciplinary team conference (minimum of three exclusive of patient care nursing staff) with patient present

G0176 Activity therapy, such as music, dance, art or play therapies not for recreation, related to the care and treatment of patient's disabling mental health problems, per session (45 minutes or more)

G0177 Training and educational services related to the care and treatment of patient's disabling mental health problems per session (45 minutes or more)

G0179 Physician or allowed practitioner re-certification for Medicare-covered home health services under a home health plan of care (patient not present), including contacts with home health agency and review of reports of patient status required by physicians and allowed practitioners to affirm the initial implementation of the plan of care

G0180 Physician or allowed practitioner certification for Medicare-covered home health services under a home health plan of care (patient not present), including contacts with home health agency and review of reports of patient status required by physicians and allowed practitioners to affirm the initial implementation of the plan of care

G0181 Physician or allowed practitioner supervision of a patient receiving Medicare-covered services provided by a participating home health agency (patient not present) requiring complex and multidisciplinary care modalities involving regular physician or allowed practitioner development and/or revision of care plans

G0182 Physician supervision of a patient under a Medicare-approved hospice (patient not present) requiring complex and multidisciplinary care modalities involving regular physician development and/or revision of care plans, review of subsequent reports of patient status, review of laboratory and other studies, communication (including telephone calls) with other health care professionals involved in the patient's care, integration of new information into the medical treatment plan and/or adjustment of medical therapy, within a calendar month, 30 minutes or more

G0186 Destruction of localized lesion of choroid (for example, choroidal neovascularization); photocoagulation, feeder vessel technique (one or more sessions)

G0202 Screening mammography, bilateral (2-view study of each breast), including computer-aided detection (cad) when performed

G0204 Diagnostic mammography, including computer-aided detection (cad) when performed; bilateral

G0206 Diagnostic mammography, including computer-aided detection (cad) when performed; unilateral

G0219 Pet imaging whole body; melanoma for non-covered indications

G0235 Pet imaging, any site, not otherwise specified

G0237 Therapeutic procedures to increase strength or endurance of respiratory muscles, face to face, one on one, each 15 minutes (includes monitoring)

G0238 Therapeutic procedures to improve respiratory function, other than described by G0237, one on one, face to face, per 15 minutes (includes monitoring)

G0239 Therapeutic procedures to improve respiratory function or increase strength or endurance of respiratory muscles, two or more individuals (includes monitoring)

G0245 Initial physician evaluation and management of a diabetic patient with diabetic sensory neuropathy resulting in a loss of protective sensation (lops) which must include: (1) the diagnosis of lops, (2) a patient history, (3) a physical examination that consists of at least the following elements: (a) visual inspection of the forefoot, hindfoot and toe web spaces, (b) evaluation of a protective sensation, (c) evaluation of foot structure and biomechanics, (d) evaluation of vascular status and skin integrity, and (e) evaluation and recommendation of footwear and (4) patient education

G0246 Follow-up physician evaluation and management of a diabetic patient with diabetic sensory neuropathy resulting in a loss of protective sensation (lops) to include at least the following: (1) a patient history, (2) a physical examination that includes: (a) visual inspection of the forefoot, hindfoot and toe web spaces, (b) evaluation of protective sensation, (c) evaluation of foot structure and biomechanics, (d) evaluation of vascular status and skin integrity, and (e) evaluation and recommendation of footwear, and (3) patient education

G0247 Routine foot care by a physician of a diabetic patient with diabetic sensory neuropathy resulting in a loss of protective sensation (lops) to include the local care of superficial wounds (i.e., superficial to muscle and fascia) and at least the following if present: (1) local care of superficial wounds, (2) debridement of corns and calluses, and (3) trimming and debridement of nails

G0248 Demonstration, prior to initiation of home INR monitoring, for patient with either mechanical heart valve(s), chronic atrial fibrillation, or venous thromboembolism who meets Medicare coverage criteria, under the direction of a physician; includes: face-to-face demonstration of use and care of the INR monitor, obtaining at least one blood sample, provision of instructions for reporting home INR test results, and documentation of patient's ability to perform testing and report results

G0249 Provision of test materials and equipment for home INR monitoring of patient with either mechanical heart valve(s), chronic atrial fibrillation, or venous thromboembolism who meets Medicare coverage criteria; includes provision of materials for use in the home and reporting of test results to physician; testing not occurring more frequently than once a week; testing materials, billing units of service include 4 tests

G0250 Physician review, interpretation, and patient management of home INR testing for patient with either mechanical heart valve(s), chronic atrial fibrillation, or venous thromboembolism who meets Medicare coverage criteria; testing not occurring more frequently than once a week; billing units of service include 4 tests

G0251 Linear accelerator based stereotactic radiosurgery, delivery including collimator changes and custom plugging, fractionated treatment, all lesions, per session, maximum five sessions per course of treatment

G0252 Pet imaging, full and partial-ring pet scanners only, for initial diagnosis of breast cancer and/or surgical planning for breast cancer (e.g., initial staging of axillary lymph nodes)

G0255 Current perception threshold/sensory nerve conduction test, (snct) per limb, any nerve

G0257 Unscheduled or emergency dialysis treatment for an ESRD patient in a hospital outpatient department that is not certified as an ESRD facility

G0259 Injection procedure for sacroiliac joint; arthrography

G0260 Injection procedure for sacroiliac joint; provision of anesthetic, steroid and/or other therapeutic agent, with or without arthrography

G0268 Removal of impacted cerumen (one or both ears) by physician on same date of service as audiologic function testing

G0269 Placement of occlusive device into either a venous or arterial access site, post surgical or interventional procedure (e.g., angioseal plug, vascular plug)

G0270 Medical nutrition therapy; reassessment and subsequent intervention(s) following second referral in same year for change in diagnosis, medical condition or treatment regimen (including additional hours needed for renal disease), individual, face to face with the patient, each 15 minutes

G0271 Medical nutrition therapy, reassessment and subsequent intervention(s) following second referral in same year for change in diagnosis, medical condition, or treatment regimen (including additional hours needed for renal disease), group (2 or more individuals), each 30 minutes

G0276 Blinded procedure for lumbar stenosis, percutaneous image-guided lumbar decompression (pild) or placebo-control, performed in an approved coverage with evidence development (CED) clinical trial

G0277 Hyperbaric oxygen under pressure, full body chamber, per 30 minute interval

G0278 Iliac and/or femoral artery angiography, non-selective, bilateral or ipsilateral to catheter insertion, performed at the same time as cardiac catheterization and/or coronary angiography, includes positioning or placement of the catheter in the distal aorta or ipsilateral femoral or iliac artery,

injection of dye, production of permanent images, and radiologic supervision and interpretation

G - H CODES

(list separately in addition to primary procedure)

G0279 Diagnostic digital breast tomosynthesis, unilateral or bilateral (list separately in addition to 77065 or 77066)

G0281 Electrical stimulation, (unattended), to one or more areas, for chronic stage iii and stage iv pressure ulcers, arterial ulcers, diabetic ulcers, and venous stasis ulcers not demonstrating measurable signs of healing after 30 days of conventional care, as part of a therapy plan of care

G0282 Electrical stimulation, (unattended), to one or more areas, for wound care other than described in G0281

G0283 Electrical stimulation (unattended), to one or more areas for indication(s) other than wound care, as part of a therapy plan of care

G0288 Reconstruction, computed tomographic angiography of aorta for surgical planning for vascular surgery

G0289 Arthroscopy, knee, surgical, for removal of loose body, foreign body, debridement/shaving of articular cartilage (chondroplasty) at the time of other surgical knee arthroscopy in a different compartment of the same knee

G0293 Noncovered surgical procedure(s) using conscious sedation, regional, general or spinal anesthesia in a Medicare qualifying clinical trial, per day

G0294 Noncovered procedure(s) using either no anesthesia or local anesthesia only, in a Medicare qualifying clinical trial, per day

G0295 Electromagnetic therapy, to one or more areas, for wound care other than described in G0329 or for other uses

G0296 Counseling visit to discuss need for lung cancer screening using low dose CT scan (ldct) (service is for eligibility determination and shared decision making)

G0297 Low dose CT scan (ldct) for lung cancer screening

G0299 Direct skilled nursing services of a registered nurse (RN) in the home health or hospice setting, each 15 minutes

G0300 Direct skilled nursing services of a licensed practical nurse (LPN) in the home health or hospice setting, each 15 minutes

G0302 Pre-operative pulmonary surgery services for preparation for LVRS, complete course of services, to include a minimum of 16 days of services

G0303 Pre-operative pulmonary surgery services for preparation for LVRS, 10 to 15 days of services

G0304 Pre-operative pulmonary surgery services for preparation for LVRS, 1 to 9 days of services

G0305 Post-discharge pulmonary surgery services after LVRS, minimum of 6 days of services

G0306 Complete cbc, automated (Hgb, HCT, RBC, WBC, without platelet count) and automated WBC differential count

G0307 Complete (cbc), automated (Hgb, HCT, RBC, WBC; without platelet count)

(**G0308** Creation of subcutaneous pocket with insertion of 180 day implantable interstitial glucose sensor, including system activation and patient training

Code deleted effective 12/31/2022, no HCPCS/CPT cross-reference provided.)

(**G0309** Removal of implantable interstitial glucose sensor with creation of subcutaneous pocket at different anatomic site and insertion of new 180 day implantable sensor, including system activation

Code deleted effective 12/31/2022, no HCPCS/CPT cross-reference provided.)

G0310 Immunization counseling by a physician or other qualified health care professional when the vaccine(s) is not administered on the same date of service, 5 to 15 mins time (this code is used for Medicaid billing purposes)

G0311 Immunization counseling by a physician or other qualified health care professional when the vaccine(s) is not administered on the same date of service, 16-30 mins time (this code is used for Medicaid billing purposes)

G0312 Immunization counseling by a physician or other qualify ed health care professional when the vaccine(s) is not administered on the same date of service for ages under 21, 5 to 15 mins time (this code is used for Medicaid billing purposes)

G0313 Immunization counseling by a physician or other qualified health care professional when the vaccine(s) is not administered on the same date of service for ages under 21, 16-30 mins time (this code is used for Medicaid billing purposes)

G0314 Immunization counseling by a physician or other qualified health care professional for covid-19, ages under 21, 16-30 mins time (this code is used for the Medicaid early and periodic screening, diagnostic, and treatment benefit (EPSDT)

G0315 Immunization counseling by a physician or other qualified health care professional for covid-19, ages under 21, 5-15 mins time (this code is used for the Medicaid early and periodic screening, diagnostic, and treatment benefit (EPSDT)

G0316 Prolonged hospital inpatient or observation care evaluation and management service(s) beyond the total time for the primary service (when the primary service has been selected using time on the date of the primary service); each additional 15 minutes by the physician or qualified healthcare professional, with or without direct patient contact (list separately in addition to CPT codes 99223, 99233, and 99236 for hospital inpatient or observation care evaluation and management services). (do not report G0316 on the same date of service as other prolonged services for evaluation and management 99358, 99359, 99418, 99415, 99416). (do not report G0316 for any time unit less than 15 minutes)

G0317 Prolonged nursing facility evaluation and management service(s) beyond the total time for the primary service (when the primary service has been selected using time on the date of the primary service); each additional 15 minutes by the physician or qualified healthcare professional, with or without direct patient contact (list separately in addition to CPT codes 99306, 99310 for nursing facility evaluation and management services). (do not report G0317 on the same date of service as other prolonged services for evaluation and management 99358, 99359, 99418). (do not report G0317 for any time unit less than 15 minutes)

G0318 Prolonged home or residence evaluation and management service(s) beyond the total time for the primary service (when the primary service has been selected using time on the date of the primary service); each additional 15 minutes by the physician or qualified healthcare professional, with or without direct patient contact (list separately in addition to CPT codes 99345, 99350 for home or residence evaluation and management services). (do not report G0318 on the same date of service as other prolonged services for evaluation and management 99358, 99359, 99417). (do not report G0318 for any time unit less than 15 minutes)

G0320 Home health services furnished using synchronous telemedicine rendered via a real-time two-way audio and video telecommunications system

G0321 Home health services furnished using synchronous telemedicine rendered via telephone or other real-time interactive audio-only telecommunications system

G0322 The collection of physiologic data digitally stored and/or transmitted by the patient to the home health agency (i.e., remote patient monitoring)

G0323 Care management services for behavioral health conditions, at least 20 minutes of clinical psychologist or clinical social worker time, per calendar month. (these services include the following required elements: initial assessment or follow-up monitoring, including the use of applicable validated rating scales; behavioral health care planning in relation to behavioral/psychiatric health problems, including revision for patients who are not progressing or whose status changes; facilitating and coordinating treatment such as psychotherapy, coordination with and/or referral to physicians and practitioners who are authorized by Medicare to prescribe medications and furnish e/m services, counseling and/or psychiatric consultation; and continuity of care with a designated member of the care team)

G0327 Colorectal cancer screening; blood-based biomarker

G0328 Colorectal cancer screening; fecal occult blood test, immunoassay, 1-3 simultaneous

G0329 Electromagnetic therapy, to one or more areas for chronic stage iii and stage iv pressure ulcers, arterial ulcers, diabetic ulcers and venous stasis ulcers not demonstrating measurable signs of healing after 30 days of conventional care as part of a therapy plan of care

G0330 Facility services for dental rehabilitation procedure(s) performed on a patient who requires monitored anesthesia (e.g., general, intravenous sedation (monitored anesthesia care) and use of an operating room

G0333 Pharmacy dispensing fee for inhalation drug(s); initial 30-day supply as a beneficiary

G0337 Hospice evaluation and counseling services, pre-election

G0339 Image-guided robotic linear accelerator-based stereotactic radiosurgery, complete course of therapy in one session or first session of fractionated treatment

G0340 Image-guided robotic linear accelerator-based stereotactic radiosurgery, delivery including collimator changes and custom plugging, fractionated treatment, all lesions, per session, second through fifth sessions, maximum five sessions per course of treatment

G0341 Percutaneous islet cell transplant, includes portal vein catheterization and infusion

G0342 Laparoscopy for islet cell transplant, includes portal vein catheterization and infusion

G0343 Laparotomy for islet cell transplant, includes portal vein catheterization and infusion

G0364 Bone marrow aspiration performed with bone marrow biopsy through the same incision on the same date of service

G0365 Vessel mapping of vessels for hemodialysis access (services for preoperative vessel mapping prior to creation of hemodialysis access using an autogenous hemodialysis conduit, including arterial inflow and venous outflow)

G0372 Physician service required to establish and document the need for a power mobility device

G0378 Hospital observation service, per hour

G0379 Direct admission of patient for hospital observation care

G0380 Level 1 hospital emergency department visit provided in a type b emergency department; (the ed must meet at least one of the following requirements: (1) it is licensed by the state in which it is located under applicable state law as an emergency room or emergency department; (2) it is held out to the public (by name, posted signs, advertising, or other means) as a place that provides care for emergency medical conditions on an urgent basis without requiring a previously scheduled appointment; or (3) during the calendar year immediately preceding the calendar year in which a determination under 42 CFR 489.24 is being made, based on a representative sample of patient visits that occurred during that calendar year, it provides at least one-third of all of its outpatient visits for the treatment of emergency medical conditions on an urgent basis without requiring a previously scheduled appointment)

G0381 Level 2 hospital emergency department visit provided in a type b emergency department; (the ed must meet at least one of the following requirements: (1) it is licensed by the state in which it is located under applicable state law as an emergency room or emergency department; (2) it is held out to the public (by name, posted signs, advertising, or other means) as a place that provides care for emergency medical conditions on an urgent basis without requiring a previously scheduled appointment; or (3) during the calendar year immediately preceding the calendar year in which a determination under 42 CFR 489.24 is being made, based on a representative sample of patient visits that occurred during that calendar year, it provides at least one-third of all of its outpatient visits for the treatment of emergency medical conditions on an urgent basis without requiring a previously scheduled appointment)

G0382 Level 3 hospital emergency department visit provided in a type b emergency department; (the ed must meet at least one of the following requirements: (1) it is licensed by the state in which it is located under applicable state law as an emergency room or emergency department; (2) it is held out to the public (by name, posted signs, advertising, or other means) as a place that provides care for emergency medical conditions on an urgent basis without requiring a previously scheduled appointment; or (3) during the calendar year immediately preceding the calendar year in which a determination under 42 CFR 489.24 is being made, based on a representative sample of patient visits that occurred during that calendar year, it provides at least one-third of all of its outpatient visits for the treatment of emergency medical conditions on an urgent basis without requiring a previously scheduled appointment)

G0383 Level 4 hospital emergency department visit provided in a type b emergency department; (the ed must meet at least one of the following requirements: (1) it is licensed by the state in which it is located under applicable state law as an emergency room or emergency department; (2) it is held out to the public (by name, posted signs, advertising, or other means) as a place that provides care for emergency medical conditions on an urgent basis without requiring a previously scheduled appointment; or (3) during the calendar year immediately preceding the calendar year in which a determination under 42 CFR 489.24 is being made, based on a representative sample of patient visits that occurred during that calendar year, it provides at least one-third of all of its outpatient visits for the treatment of emergency medical conditions on an urgent basis without requiring a previously scheduled appointment)

G0384 Level 5 hospital emergency department visit provided in a type b emergency department; (the ed must meet at least one of the following requirements: (1) it is licensed by the state in which it is located under applicable state law as an emergency room or emergency department; (2) it is held out to the public (by name, posted signs, advertising, or other means) as a place that provides care for emergency medical conditions on an urgent basis without requiring a previously scheduled appointment; or (3) during the calendar year immediately preceding the calendar year in which a determination under 42 CFR 489.24 is being made, based on a representative sample of patient visits that occurred during that calendar year, it provides at least one-third of all of its outpatient visits for the treatment of emergency medical conditions on an urgent basis without requiring a previously scheduled appointment)

G0389 Ultrasound b-scan and/or real time with image documentation; for abdominal aortic aneurysm (AAA) screening

G0390 Trauma response team associated with hospital critical care service

G0396 Alcohol and/or substance (other than tobacco) misuse structured assessment (e.g., audit, dast), and brief intervention 15 to 30 minutes

G0397 Alcohol and/or substance (other than tobacco) misuse structured assessment (e.g., audit, dast), and intervention, greater than 30 minutes

G0398 Home sleep study test (hst) with type ii portable monitor, unattended; minimum of 7 channels: EEG, EOG, EMG, ECG/heart rate, airflow, respiratory effort and oxygen saturation

G0399 Home sleep test (hst) with type iii portable monitor, unattended; minimum of 4 channels: 2 respiratory movement/airflow, 1 ECG/heart rate and 1 oxygen saturation

G0400 Home sleep test (hst) with type iv portable monitor, unattended; minimum of 3 channels

G0402 Initial preventive physical examination; face-to-face visit, services limited to new beneficiary during the first 12 months of Medicare enrollment

G0403 Electrocardiogram, routine ECG with 12 leads; performed as a screening for the initial preventive physical examination with interpretation and report

G0404 Electrocardiogram, routine ECG with 12 leads; tracing only, without interpretation and report, performed as a screening for the initial preventive physical examination

G0405 Electrocardiogram, routine ECG with 12 leads; interpretation and report only, performed as a screening for the initial preventive physical examination

G0406 Follow-up inpatient consultation, limited, physicians typically spend 15 minutes communicating with the patient via telehealth

G0407 Follow-up inpatient consultation, intermediate, physicians typically spend 25 minutes communicating with the patient via telehealth

G0408 Follow-up inpatient consultation, complex, physicians typically spend 35 minutes communicating with the patient via telehealth

G0409 Social work and psychological services, directly relating to and/or furthering the patient's rehabilitation goals, each 15 minutes, face-to-face; individual (services provided by a corf-qualified social worker or psychologist in a corf)

▲ **G0410** Group psychotherapy other than of a multiple-family group, in a partial hospitalization or intensive outpatient setting, approximately 45 to 50 minutes

▲ **G0411** Interactive group psychotherapy, in a partial hospitalization or intensive outpatient setting, approximately 45 to 50 minutes

G0412 Open treatment of iliac spine(s), tuberosity avulsion, or iliac wing fracture(s), unilateral or bilateral for pelvic bone fracture patterns which do not disrupt the pelvic ring includes internal fixation, when performed

G0413 Percutaneous skeletal fixation of posterior pelvic bone fracture and/or dislocation, for fracture patterns which disrupt the pelvic ring, unilateral or bilateral, (includes ilium, sacroiliac joint and/or sacrum)

G0414 Open treatment of anterior pelvic bone fracture and/or dislocation for fracture patterns which disrupt the pelvic ring, unilateral or bilateral, includes internal fixation when performed (includes pubic symphysis and/or superior/inferior rami)

G0415 Open treatment of posterior pelvic bone fracture and/or dislocation, for fracture patterns which disrupt the pelvic ring, unilateral or bilateral, includes internal fixation, when performed (includes ilium, sacroiliac joint and/or sacrum)

G0416 Surgical pathology, gross and microscopic examinations, for prostate needle biopsy, any method

G0417 Surgical pathology, gross and microscopic examination, for prostate needle biopsy, any method, 21-40 specimens

G0418 Surgical pathology, gross and microscopic examination, for prostate needle biopsy, any method, 41-60 specimens

G0419 Surgical pathology, gross and microscopic examination, for prostate needle biopsy, any method, >60 specimens

G0420 Face-to-face educational services related to the care of chronic kidney disease; individual, per session, per one hour

G0421 Face-to-face educational services related to the care of chronic kidney disease; group, per session, per one hour

G0422 Intensive cardiac rehabilitation; with or without continuous ECG monitoring with exercise, per session

G0423 Intensive cardiac rehabilitation; with or without continuous ECG monitoring; without exercise, per session

G0424 Pulmonary rehabilitation, including exercise (includes monitoring), one hour, per session, up to two sessions per day

G0425 Telehealth consultation, emergency department or initial inpatient, typically 30 minutes communicating with the patient via telehealth

G0426 Telehealth consultation, emergency department or initial inpatient, typically 50 minutes communicating with the patient via telehealth

G0427 Telehealth consultation, emergency department or initial inpatient, typically 70 minutes or more communicating with the patient via telehealth

G0428 Collagen meniscus implant procedure for filling meniscal defects (e.g., cmi, collagen scaffold, menaflex)

G - H CODES

G0429 Dermal filler injection(s) for the treatment of facial lipodystrophy syndrome (LDS) (e.g., as a result of highly active antiretroviral therapy)

G0431 Drug screen, qualitative; multiple drug classes by high complexity test method (e.g., immunoassay, enzyme assay), per patient encounter

G0432 Infectious agent antibody detection by enzyme immunoassay (EIA) technique, hiv-1 and/or hiv-2, screening

G0433 Infectious agent antibody detection by enzyme-linked immunosorbent assay (ELISA) technique, hiv-1 and/or hiv-2, screening

G0434 Drug screen, other than chromatographic; any number of drug classes, by CLIA waived test or moderate complexity test, per patient encounter

G0435 Infectious agent antibody detection by rapid antibody test, hiv-1 and/or hiv-2, screening

G0436 Smoking and tobacco cessation counseling visit for the asymptomatic patient; intermediate, greater than 3 minutes, up to 10 minutes

G0437 Smoking and tobacco cessation counseling visit for the asymptomatic patient; intensive, greater than 10 minutes

G0438 Annual wellness visit; includes a personalized prevention plan of service (PPS), initial visit

G0439 Annual wellness visit, includes a personalized prevention plan of service (PPS), subsequent visit

G0442 Annual alcohol misuse screening, 5 to 15 minutes

G0443 Brief face-to-face behavioral counseling for alcohol misuse, 15 minutes

G0444 Annual depression screening, 5 to 15 minutes

G0445 High intensity behavioral counseling to prevent sexually transmitted infection; face-to-face, individual, includes education, skills training and guidance on how to change sexual behavior; performed semi-annually, 30 minutes

G0446 Annual, face-to-face intensive behavioral therapy for cardiovascular disease, individual, 15 minutes

G0447 Face-to-face behavioral counseling for obesity, 15 minutes

G0448 Insertion or replacement of a permanent pacing cardioverter-defibrillator system with transvenous lead(s), single or dual chamber with insertion of pacing electrode, cardiac venous system, for left ventricular pacing

G0451 Development testing, with interpretation and report, per standardized instrument form

G0452 Molecular pathology procedure; physician interpretation and report

G0453 Continuous intraoperative neurophysiology monitoring, from outside the operating room (remote or nearby), per patient, (attention directed exclusively to one patient) each 15 minutes (list in addition to primary procedure)

G0454 Physician documentation of face-to-face visit for durable medical equipment determination performed by nurse practitioner, physician assistant or clinical nurse specialist

G0455 Preparation with instillation of fecal microbiota by any method, including assessment of donor specimen

G0456 Negative pressure wound therapy, (e.g., vacuum assisted drainage collection) using a mechanically-powered device, not durable medical equipment, including provision of cartridge and dressing(s), topical application(s), wound assessment, and instructions for ongoing care, per session; total wounds(s) surface area less than or equal to 50 square centimeters

G0457 Negative pressure wound therapy, (e.g., vacuum assisted drainage collection) using a mechanically-powered device, not durable medical equipment, including provision of cartridge and dressing(s), topical application(s), wound assessment, and instructions for ongoing care, per session; total wounds(s) surface area greater than 50 square centimeters

G0458 Low dose rate (LDR) prostate brachytherapy services, composite rate

G0459 Inpatient telehealth pharmacologic management, including prescription, use, and review of medication with no more than minimal medical psychotherapy

G0460 Autologous platelet rich plasma for non-diabetic chronic wounds/ulcers, including phlebotomy, centrifugation, and all other preparatory procedures, administration and dressings, per treatment

G0461 Immunohistochemistry or immunocytochemistry, per specimen; first single or multiplex antibody stain

G0462 Immunohistochemistry or immunocytochemistry, per specimen; each additional single or multiplex antibody stain (list separately in addition to code for primary procedure)

G0463 Hospital outpatient clinic visit for assessment and management of a patient

G0464 Colorectal cancer screening; stool-based DNA and fecal occult hemoglobin (e.g., KRAS, ndrG4 and bmp3)

G0465 Autologous platelet rich plasma (PRP) for diabetic chronic wounds/ulcers, using an FDA-cleared device (includes administration, dressings, phlebotomy, centrifugation, and all other preparatory procedures, per treatment)

G0466 Federally qualified health center (fqhc) visit, new patient; a medically-necessary, face-to-face encounter (one-on-one) between a new patient and a fqhc practitioner during which time one or more fqhc services are rendered and includes a typical bundle of Medicare-covered services that would be furnished per diem to a patient receiving a fqhc visit

G0467 Federally qualified health center (fqhc) visit, established patient; a medically-necessary, face-to-face encounter (one-on-one) between an established patient and a fqhc practitioner during which time one or more fqhc services are rendered and includes a typical bundle of Medicare-covered services that would be furnished per diem to a patient receiving a fqhc visit

G0468 Federally qualified health center (fqhc) visit, ippe or awv; a fqhc visit that includes an initial preventive physical examination (ippe) or annual wellness visit (awv) and includes a typical bundle of Medicare-covered services that would be furnished per diem to a patient receiving an ippe or awv

G0469 Federally qualified health center (fqhc) visit, mental health, new patient; a medically-necessary, face-to-face mental health encounter (one-on-one) between a new patient and a fqhc practitioner during which time one or more fqhc services are rendered and includes a typical bundle of Medicare-covered services that would be furnished per diem to a patient receiving a mental health visit

G0470 Federally qualified health center (fqhc) visit, mental health, established patient; a medically-necessary, face-to-face mental health encounter (one-on-one) between an established patient and a fqhc practitioner during which time one or more fqhc services are rendered and includes a typical bundle of Medicare-covered services that would be furnished per diem to a patient receiving a mental health visit

G0471 Collection of venous blood by venipuncture or urine sample by catheterization from an individual in a skilled nursing facility (SNF) or by a laboratory on behalf of a home health agency (HHA)

G0472 Hepatitis c antibody screening, for individual at high risk and other covered indication(s)

G0473 Face-to-face behavioral counseling for obesity, group (2-10), 30 minutes

G0475 HIV antigen/antibody, combination assay, screening

G0476 Infectious agent detection by nucleic acid (DNA or RNA); human papillomavirus (HPV), high-risk types (e.g., 16, 18, 31, 33, 35, 39, 45, 51, 52, 56, 58, 59, 68) for cervical cancer screening, must be performed in addition to pap test

G0477 Drug test(s), presumptive, any number of drug classes; any number of devices or procedures, (e.g., immunoassay) capable of being read by direct optical observation only (e.g., dipsticks, cups, cards, cartridges), includes sample validation when performed, per date of service

G0478 Drug test(s), presumptive, any number of drug classes; any number of devices or procedures, (e.g., immunoassay) read by instrument-assisted direct optical observation (e.g., dipsticks, cups, cards, cartridges), includes sample validation when performed, per date of service

G0479 Drug test(s), presumptive, any number of drug classes; any number of devices or procedures by instrumented chemistry analyzers utilizing immunoassay, enzyme assay, tof, maldi, ldtd, desi, dart, ghpc, gc mass spectrometry), includes sample validation when performed, per date of service

G0480 Drug test(s), definitive, utilizing (1) drug identification methods able to identify individual drugs and distinguish between structural isomers (but not necessarily stereoisomers), including, but not limited to gc/ms (any type, single or tandem) and lc/ms (any type, single or tandem and excluding immunoassays (e.g., IA, EIA, ELISA, emit, FPIA) and enzymatic methods (e.g., alcohol dehydrogenase)), (2) stable isotope or other universally recognized internal standards in all samples (e.g., to control for matrix effects, interferences and variations in signal strength), and (3) method or drug-specific calibration and matrix-matched quality control material (e.g., to control for instrument variations and mass spectral drift); qualitative or quantitative, all sources, includes specimen validity testing, per day; 1-7 drug class(es), including metabolite(s) if performed

G0481 Drug test(s), definitive, utilizing (1) drug identification methods able to identify individual drugs and distinguish between structural isomers (but not necessarily stereoisomers), including, but not limited to gc/ms (any type, single or tandem) and lc/ms (any type, single or tandem and excluding immunoassays (e.g., IA, EIA, ELISA, emit, FPIA) and enzymatic methods (e.g., alcohol dehydrogenase)), (2) stable isotope or other universally recognized internal standards in all samples (e.g., to control for matrix effects, interferences and variations in signal strength), and (3) method or drug-specific calibration and matrix-matched quality control material (e.g., to control for instrument variations and mass spectral drift); qualitative or quantitative, all sources, includes specimen validity testing, per day; 8-14 drug class(es), including metabolite(s) if performed

G0482 Drug test(s), definitive, utilizing (1) drug identification methods able to identify individual drugs and distinguish between structural isomers (but not necessarily stereoisomers), including, but not limited to gc/ms (any type, single or tandem) and lc/ms (any type, single or tandem and excluding immunoassays (e.g., IA, EIA, ELISA, emit, FPIA) and enzymatic methods (e.g., alcohol dehydrogenase)), (2) stable isotope or other universally recognized internal standards in all samples (e.g., to control for matrix effects, interferences and variations in signal strength), and (3) method or drug-specific calibration and matrix-matched quality control material (e.g., to control for instrument variations and mass spectral drift); qualitative or quantitative, all sources, includes specimen validity testing, per day; 15-21 drug class(es), including metabolite(s) if performed

G0483 Drug test(s), definitive, utilizing (1) drug identification methods able to identify individual drugs and distinguish between structural isomers (but not necessarily stereoisomers), including, but not limited to gc/ms (any type, single or tandem) and lc/ms (any type, single or tandem and excluding immunoassays (e.g., IA, EIA, ELISA, emit, FPIA) and enzymatic methods (e.g., alcohol dehydrogenase)), (2) stable isotope or other universally recognized internal standards in all samples (e.g., to control for matrix effects, interferences and variations in signal strength), and (3) method or drug-specific calibration and matrix-matched quality control material (e.g., to control for instrument variations and mass spectral drift); qualitative or quantitative, all sources, includes specimen validity testing, per day; 22 or more drug class(es), including metabolite(s) if performed

G0490 Face-to-face home health nursing visit by a rural health clinic (rhc) or federally qualified health center (fqhc) in an area with a shortage of home health agencies; (services limited to RN or LPN only)

G0491 Dialysis procedure at a Medicare certified ESRD facility for acute kidney injury without ESRD

G0492 Dialysis procedure with single evaluation by a physician or other qualified health care professional for acute kidney injury without ESRD

G0493 Skilled services of a registered nurse (RN) for the observation and assessment of the patient's condition, each 15 minutes (the change in the patient's condition requires skilled nursing personnel to identify and evaluate the patient's need for possible modification of treatment in the home health or hospice setting)

G0494 Skilled services of a licensed practical nurse (LPN) for the observation and assessment of the patient's condition, each 15 minutes (the change in the patient's condition requires skilled nursing personnel to identify and evaluate the patient's need for possible modification of treatment in the home health or hospice setting)

G0495 Skilled services of a registered nurse (RN), in the training and/or education of a patient or family member, in the home health or hospice setting, each 15 minutes

G0496 Skilled services of a licensed practical nurse (LPN), in the training and/or education of a patient or family member, in the home health or hospice setting, each 15 minutes

G0498 Chemotherapy administration, intravenous infusion technique; initiation of infusion in the office/clinic setting using office/clinic pump/supplies, with continuation of the infusion in the community setting (e.g., home, domiciliary, rest home or assisted living) using a portable pump provided by the office/clinic, includes follow up office/clinic visit at the conclusion of the infusion

G0499 Hepatitis b screening in non-pregnant, high risk individual includes hepatitis b surface antigen (HBsAg), antibodies to HBsAg (anti-HBs) and antibodies to hepatitis b core antigen (anti-HBc), and is followed by a neutralizing confirmatory test, when performed, only for an initially reactive HBsAg result

G0500 Moderate sedation services provided by the same physician or other qualified health care professional performing a gastrointestinal endoscopic service that sedation supports, requiring the presence of an independent trained observer to assist in the monitoring of the patient's level of consciousness and physiological status; initial 15 minutes of intra-service time; patient age 5 years or older (additional time may be reported with 99153, as appropriate)

G0501 Resource-intensive services for patients for whom the use of specialized mobility-assistive technology (such as adjustable height chairs or tables, patient lift, and adjustable padded leg supports) is medically necessary and used during the provision of an office/outpatient, evaluation and management visit (list separately in addition to primary service)

G0502 Initial psychiatric collaborative care management, first 70 minutes in the first calendar month of behavioral health care manager activities, in consultation with a psychiatric consultant, and directed by the treating physician or other qualified health care professional, with the following required elements: outreach to and engagement in treatment of a patient directed by the treating physician or other qualified health care professional; initial assessment of the patient, including administration of validated rating scales, with the development of an individualized treatment plan; review by the psychiatric consultant with modifications of the plan if recommended; entering patient in a registry and tracking patient follow-up and progress using the registry, with appropriate documentation, and participation in weekly caseload consultation with the psychiatric consultant; and provision of brief interventions using evidence-based techniques such as behavioral activation, motivational interviewing, and other focused treatment strategies

G0503 Subsequent psychiatric collaborative care management, first 60 minutes in a subsequent month of behavioral health care manager activities, in consultation with a psychiatric consultant, and directed by the treating physician or other qualified health care professional, with the following required elements: tracking patient follow-up and progress using the registry, with appropriate documentation; participation in weekly caseload consultation with the psychiatric consultant; ongoing collaboration with and coordination of the patient's mental health care with the treating physician or other qualified health care professional and any other treating mental health providers; additional review of progress and recommendations for changes in treatment, as indicated, including medications, based on recommendations provided by the psychiatric consultant; provision of brief interventions using evidence-based techniques such as behavioral activation, motivational interviewing, and other focused treatment strategies; monitoring of patient outcomes using validated rating scales; and relapse prevention planning with patients as they achieve remission of symptoms and/or other treatment

G0504 Initial or subsequent psychiatric collaborative care management, each additional 30 minutes in a calendar month of behavioral health care manager activities, in consultation with a psychiatric consultant, and directed by the treating physician or other qualified health care professional (list separately in addition to code for primary procedure); (use G0504 in conjunction with G0502,

G0503)

G0505 Cognition and functional assessment using standardized instruments with development of recorded care plan for the patient with cognitive impairment, history obtained from patient and/or caregiver, in office or other outpatient setting or home or domiciliary or rest home

G0506 Comprehensive assessment of and care planning for patients requiring chronic care management services (list separately in addition to primary monthly care management service)

G0507 Care management services for behavioral health conditions, at least 20 minutes of clinical staff time, directed by a physician or other qualified health care professional, per calendar month, with the following required elements: initial assessment or follow-up monitoring, including the use of applicable validated rating scales; behavioral health care planning in relation to behavioral/psychiatric health problems, including revision for patients who are not progressing or whose status changes; facilitating and coordinating treatment such as psychotherapy, pharmacotherapy, counseling and/or psychiatric consultation; and continuity of care with a designated member of the care team

G0508 Telehealth consultation, critical care, initial , physicians typically spend 60 minutes communicating with the patient and providers via telehealth

G0509 Telehealth consultation, critical care, subsequent, physicians typically spend 50 minutes communicating with the patient and providers via telehealth

G0511 Rural health clinic or federally qualified health center (rhc or fqhc) only, general care management, 20 minutes or more of clinical staff time for chronic care management services or behavioral health integration services directed by an rhc or fqhc practitioner (physician, np, pa, or CNM), per calendar month

G0512 Rural health clinic or federally qualified health center (rhc/fqhc) only, psychiatric collaborative care model (psychiatric cocm), 60 minutes or more of clinical staff time for psychiatric cocm services directed by an rhc or fqhc practitioner (physician, np, pa, or CNM) and including services furnished by a behavioral health care manager and consultation with a psychiatric consultant, per calendar month

G0513 Prolonged preventive service(s) (beyond the typical service time of the primary procedure), in the office or other outpatient setting requiring direct patient contact beyond the usual service; first 30 minutes (list separately in addition to code for preventive service)

G0514 Prolonged preventive service(s) (beyond the typical service time of the primary procedure), in the office or other outpatient setting requiring direct patient contact beyond the usual service; each additional 30 minutes (list separately in addition to code G0513 for additional 30 minutes of preventive service)

G0515 Development of cognitive skills to improve attention, memory, problem solving (includes compensatory training), direct (one-on-one) patient contact, each 15 minutes

G0516 Insertion of non-biodegradable drug delivery implants, 4 or more (services for subdermal rod implant)

G0517 Removal of non-biodegradable drug delivery implants, 4 or more (services for subdermal implants)

G0518 Removal with reinsertion, non-biodegradable drug delivery implants, 4 or more (services for subdermal implants)

G0659 Drug test(s), definitive, utilizing drug identification methods able to identify individual drugs and distinguish between structural isomers (but not necessarily stereoisomers), including but not limited to gc/ms (any type, single or tandem) and lc/ms (any type, single or tandem), excluding immunoassays (e.g., IA, EIA, ELISA, emit, FPIA) and enzymatic methods (e.g., alcohol dehydrogenase), performed without method or drug-specific calibration, without matrix-matched quality control material, or without use of stable isotope or other universally recognized internal standard(s) for each drug, drug metabolite or drug class per specimen; qualitative or quantitative, all sources, includes specimen validity testing, per day, any number of drug classes

G0908 Most recent hemoglobin (Hgb) level > 12.0 g/dl

G0909 Hemoglobin level measurement not documented; reason not given

G0910 Most recent hemoglobin level <= 12.0 g/dl

G0913 Improvement in visual function achieved within 90 days following cataract surgery

G0914 Patient care survey was not completed by patient

G0915 Improvement in visual function not achieved within 90 days following cataract surgery

G0916 Satisfaction with care achieved within 90 days following cataract surgery

G0917 Patient care survey was not completed by patient

G0918 Satisfaction with care not achieved within 90 days following cataract surgery

G0919 Influenza immunization ordered or recommended (to be given at alternate location or alternate provider); vaccine not available at time of visit

G0920 Type, anatomic location, and activity all documented

G0921 Documentation of patient reason(s) for not being able to assess (e.g., patient refuses endoscopic and/or radiologic assessment)

G0922 No documentation of disease type, anatomic location, and activity, reason not given

G1000 Clinical decision support mechanism applied pathways, as defined by the Medicare appropriate use criteria program

G1001 Clinical decision support mechanism evicore, as defined by the Medicare appropriate use criteria program

G1002 Clinical decision support mechanism medcurrent, as defined by the Medicare appropriate use criteria program

G1003 Clinical decision support mechanism medicalis, as defined by the Medicare appropriate use criteria program

G1004 Clinical decision support mechanism national decision support company, as defined by the Medicare appropriate use criteria program

G1005 Clinical decision support mechanism national imaging associates, as defined by the Medicare appropriate use criteria program

G1006 Clinical decision support mechanism test appropriate, as defined by the Medicare appropriate use criteria program

G1007 Clinical decision support mechanism aim specialty health, as defined by the Medicare appropriate use criteria program

G1008 Clinical decision support mechanism cranberry peak, as defined by the Medicare appropriate use criteria program

G1009 Clinical decision support mechanism sage health management solutions, as defined by the Medicare appropriate use criteria program

G1010 Clinical decision support mechanism stanson, as defined by the Medicare appropriate use criteria program

G1011 Clinical decision support mechanism, qualified tool not otherwise specified, as defined by the Medicare appropriate use criteria program

G1012 Clinical decision support mechanism agilemd, as defined by the Medicare appropriate use criteria program

G1013 Clinical decision support mechanism evidencecare imagingcare, as defined by the Medicare appropriate use criteria program

G1014 Clinical decision support mechanism inveniqa semantic answers in medicine, as defined by the Medicare appropriate use criteria program

G1015 Clinical decision support mechanism reliant medical group, as defined by the Medicare appropriate use criteria program

G1016 Clinical decision support mechanism speed of care, as defined by the Medicare appropriate use criteria program

G1017 Clinical decision support mechanism healthhelp, as defined by the Medicare appropriate use criteria program

G1018 Clinical decision support mechanism infinx, as defined by the Medicare appropriate use criteria program

G1019 Clinical decision support mechanism logicnets, as defined by the Medicare appropriate use criteria program

G1020 Clinical decision support mechanism curbside clinical augmented workflow, as defined by the Medicare appropriate use criteria program

G1021 Clinical decision support mechanism ehealthline clinical decision support mechanism, as defined by the Medicare appropriate use criteria program

G1022 Clinical decision support mechanism intermountain clinical decision support mechanism, as defined by the Medicare appropriate use criteria program

G1023 Clinical decision support mechanism persivia clinical decision support, as defined by the Medicare appropriate use criteria program

G1024 Clinical decision support mechanism radrite, as defined by the Medicare appropriate use criteria program

G1025 Patient-months where there are more than one Medicare capitated payment (MCP) provider listed for the month

G1026 The number of adult patient-months in the denominator who were on maintenance hemodialysis using a catheter continuously for three months or longer under the care of the same practitioner or group partner as of the last hemodialysis session of the reporting month

G1027 The number of adult patient-months in the denominator who were on maintenance hemodialysis under the care of the same practitioner or group partner as of the last hemodialysis session of the reporting month using a catheter continuously for less than three months

G1028 Take-home supply of nasal naloxone; 2-pack of 8mg per 0.1 ml nasal spray (provision of the services by a Medicare-enrolled opioid treatment program); list separately in addition to code for primary procedure

G2000 Blinded administration of convulsive therapy procedure, either electroconvulsive therapy (ECT, current covered gold standard) or magnetic seizure therapy (MST, non-covered experimental therapy), performed in an approved ide-based clinical trial, per treatment session

G2001 Brief (20 minutes) in-home visit for a new patient post-discharge. for use only in a Medicare-approved cmmi model. (services must be furnished within a beneficiary's home, domiciliary, rest home, assisted living and/or nursing facility within 90 days following discharge from an inpatient facility and no more than 9 times.)

G2002 Limited (30 minutes) in-home visit for a new patient post-discharge. for use only in a Medicare-approved cmmi model. (services must be furnished within a beneficiary's home, domiciliary, rest home, assisted living and/or nursing facility within 90 days following discharge from an inpatient facility and no more than 9 times.)

G2003 Moderate (45 minutes) in-home visit for a new patient post-discharge. for use only in a Medicare-approved cmmi model. (services must be furnished within a beneficiary's home, domiciliary, rest home, assisted living and/or nursing facility within 90 days following discharge from an inpatient facility and no more than 9 times.)

G2004 Comprehensive (60 minutes) in-home visit for a new patient post-discharge. for use only in a Medicare-approved cmmi model. (services must be furnished within a beneficiary's home,

G - H CODES

domiciliary, rest home, assisted living and/or nursing facility within 90 days following discharge from an inpatient facility and no more than 9 times.)

G2005 Extensive (75 minutes) in-home visit for a new patient post-discharge. for use only in a Medicare-approved cmmi model. (services must be furnished within a beneficiary's home, domiciliary, rest home, assisted living and/or nursing facility within 90 days following discharge from an inpatient facility and no more than 9 times.)

G2006 Brief (20 minutes) in-home visit for an existing patient post-discharge. for use only in a Medicare-approved cmmi model. (services must be furnished within a beneficiary's home, domiciliary, rest home, assisted living and/or nursing facility within 90 days following discharge from an inpatient facility and no more than 9 times.)

G2007 Limited (30 minutes) in-home visit for an existing patient post-discharge. for use only in a Medicare-approved cmmi model. (services must be furnished within a beneficiary's home, domiciliary, rest home, assisted living and/or nursing facility within 90 days following discharge from an inpatient facility and no more than 9 times.)

G2008 Moderate (45 minutes) in-home visit for an existing patient post-discharge. for use only in a Medicare-approved cmmi model. (services must be furnished within a beneficiary's home, domiciliary, rest home, assisted living and/or nursing facility within 90 days following discharge from an inpatient facility and no more than 9 times.)

G2009 Comprehensive (60 minutes) in-home visit for an existing patient post-discharge. for use only in a Medicare-approved cmmi model. (services must be furnished within a beneficiary's home, domiciliary, rest home, assisted living and/or nursing facility within 90 days following discharge from an inpatient facility and no more than 9 times.)

G2010 Remote evaluation of recorded video and/or images submitted by an established patient (e.g., store and forward), including interpretation with follow-up with the patient within 24 business hours, not originating from a related e/m service provided within the previous 7 days nor leading to an e/m service or procedure within the next 24 hours or soonest available appointment

G2011 Alcohol and/or substance (other than tobacco) misuse structured assessment (e.g., audit, dast), and brief intervention, 5-14 minutes

G2012 Brief communication technology-based service, e.g., virtual check-in, by a physician or other qualified health care professional who can report evaluation and management services, provided to an established patient, not originating from a related e/m service provided within the previous 7 days nor leading to an e/m service or procedure within the next 24 hours or soonest available appointment; 5-10 minutes of medical discussion

G2013 Extensive (75 minutes) in-home visit for an existing patient post-discharge. for use only in a Medicare-approved cmmi model. (services must be furnished within a beneficiary's home, domiciliary, rest home, assisted living and/or nursing facility within 90 days following discharge from an inpatient facility and no more than 9 times.)

G2014 Limited (30 minutes) care plan oversight. for use only in a Medicare-approved cmmi model. (services must be furnished within a beneficiary's home, domiciliary, rest home, assisted living and/or nursing facility within 90 days following discharge from an inpatient facility and no more than 9 times.)

G2015 Comprehensive (60 mins) home care plan oversight. for use only in a Medicare-approved cmmi model. (services must be furnished within a beneficiary's home, domiciliary, rest home, assisted living and/or nursing facility within 90 days following discharge from an inpatient facility.)

G2020 Services for high intensity clinical services associated with the initial engagement and outreach of beneficiaries assigned to the sip component of the PCF model (do not bill with chronic care management codes)

G2021 Health care practitioners rendering treatment in place (tip)

G2022 A model participant (ambulance supplier/provider), the beneficiary refuses services covered under the model (transport to an alternate destination/treatment in place)

G2023 Specimen collection for severe acute respiratory syndrome coronavirus 2 (sars-cov-2) (coronavirus disease [covid-19]), any specimen source

G2024 Specimen collection for severe acute respiratory syndrome coronavirus 2 (sars-cov-2) (coronavirus disease [covid-19]) from an individual in a SNF or by a laboratory on behalf of a HHA, any specimen source

G2025 Payment for a telehealth distant site service furnished by a rural health clinic (rhc) or federally qualified health center (fqhc) only

G2058 Chronic care management services, each additional 20 minutes of clinical staff time directed by a physician or other qualified health care professional, per calendar month (list separately in addition to code for primary procedure). (do not report G2058 for care management services of less than 20 minutes additional to the first 20 minutes of chronic care management services during a calendar month). (use G2058 in conjunction with 99490). (do not report 99490, G2058 in the same calendar month as 99487, 99489, 99491)).

G2061 Qualified nonphysician healthcare professional online assessment and management service, for an established patient, for up to seven days, cumulative time during the 7 days; 5-10 minutes

G2062 Qualified nonphysician healthcare professional online assessment and management service, for an established patient, for up to seven days, cumulative time during the 7 days; 11-20 minutes

G2063 Qualified nonphysician healthcare professional online assessment and management service, for an established patient, for up to seven days, cumulative time during the 7 days; 21 or more minutes

G2064 Comprehensive care management services for a single high-risk disease, e.g., principal care management, at least 30 minutes of physician or other qualified health care professional time per calendar month with the following elements: one complex chronic condition lasting at least 3 months, which is the focus of the care plan, the condition is of sufficient severity to place patient at risk of hospitalization or have been the cause of a recent hospitalization, the condition requires development or revision of disease-specific care plan, the condition requires frequent adjustments in the medication regimen, and/or the management of the condition is unusually complex due to comorbidities

G2065 Comprehensive care management for a single high-risk disease services, e.g. principal care management, at least 30 minutes of clinical staff time directed by a physician or other qualified health care professional, per calendar month with the following elements: one complex chronic condition lasting at least 3 months, which is the focus of the care plan, the condition is of sufficient severity to place patient at risk of hospitalization or have been cause of a recent hospitalization, the condition requires development or revision of disease-specific care plan, the condition requires frequent adjustments in the medication regimen, and/or the management of the condition is unusually complex due to comorbidities

(**G2066** Interrogation device evaluation(s), (remote) up to 30 days; implantable cardiovascular physiologic monitor system, implantable loop recorder system, or subcutaneous cardiac rhythm monitor system, remote data acquisition(s), receipt of transmissions and technician review, technical support and distribution of results

G2067 Medication assisted treatment, methadone; weekly bundle including dispensing and/or administration, substance use counseling, individual and group therapy, and toxicology testing, if performed (provision of the services by a Medicare-enrolled opioid treatment program)

G2068 Medication assisted treatment, buprenorphine (oral); weekly bundle including dispensing and/or administration, substance use counseling, individual and group therapy, and toxicology testing if performed (provision of the services by a Medicare-enrolled opioid treatment program)

G2069 Medication assisted treatment, buprenorphine (injectable); weekly bundle including dispensing and/or administration, substance use counseling, individual and group therapy, and toxicology testing if performed (provision of the services by a Medicare-enrolled opioid treatment program)

G2070 Medication assisted treatment, buprenorphine (implant insertion); weekly bundle including dispensing and/or administration, substance use counseling, individual and group therapy, and

G - H CODES

toxicology testing if performed (provision of the services by a Medicare-enrolled opioid treatment program)

G2071 Medication assisted treatment, buprenorphine (implant removal); weekly bundle including dispensing and/or administration, substance use counseling, individual and group therapy, and toxicology testing if performed (provision of the services by a Medicare-enrolled opioid treatment program)

G2072 Medication assisted treatment, buprenorphine (implant insertion and removal); weekly bundle including dispensing and/or administration, substance use counseling, individual and group therapy, and toxicology testing if performed (provision of the services by a Medicare-enrolled opioid treatment program)

G2073 Medication assisted treatment, naltrexone; weekly bundle including dispensing and/or administration, substance use counseling, individual and group therapy, and toxicology testing if performed (provision of the services by a Medicare-enrolled opioid treatment program)

G2074 Medication assisted treatment, weekly bundle not including the drug, including substance use counseling, individual and group therapy, and toxicology testing if performed (provision of the services by a Medicare-enrolled opioid treatment program)

G2075 Medication assisted treatment, medication not otherwise specified; weekly bundle including dispensing and/or administration, substance use counseling, individual and group therapy, and toxicology testing, if performed (provision of the services by a Medicare-enrolled opioid treatment program)

G2076 Intake activities, including initial medical examination that is a complete, fully documented physical evaluation and initial assessment by a program physician or a primary care physician, or an authorized healthcare professional under the supervision of a program physician qualified personnel that includes preparation of a treatment plan that includes the patient's short-term goals and the tasks the patient must perform to complete the short-term goals; the patient's requirements for education, vocational rehabilitation, and employment; and the medical, psycho- social, economic, legal, or other supportive services that a patient needs, conducted by qualified personnel (provision of the services by a Medicare-enrolled opioid treatment program); list separately in addition to code for primary procedure

G2077 Periodic assessment; assessing periodically by qualified personnel to determine the most appropriate combination of services and treatment (provision of the services by a Medicare-enrolled opioid treatment program); list separately in addition to code for primary procedure

G2078 Take-home supply of methadone; up to 7 additional day supply (provision of the services by a Medicare-enrolled opioid treatment program); list separately in addition to code for primary procedure

G2079 Take-home supply of buprenorphine (oral); up to 7 additional day supply (provision of the services by a Medicare-enrolled opioid treatment program); list separately in addition to code for primary procedure

G2080 Each additional 30 minutes of counseling in a week of medication assisted treatment, (provision of the services by a Medicare-enrolled opioid treatment program); list separately in addition to code for primary procedure

G2081 Patients aged 66 and older in institutional special needs plans (SNP) or residing in long-term care with a pos code 32, 33, 34, 54 or 56 for more than 90 consecutive days during the measurement period

G2082 Office or other outpatient visit for the evaluation and management of an established patient that requires the supervision of a physician or other qualified health care professional and provision of up to 56 mg of esketamine nasal self-administration, includes 2 hours post-administration observation

G2083 Office or other outpatient visit for the evaluation and management of an established patient that requires the supervision of a physician or other qualified health care professional and provision of greater than 56 mg esketamine nasal self-administration, includes 2 hours post-administration observation

G2086 Office-based treatment for opioid use disorder, including development of the treatment plan, care coordination, individual therapy and group therapy and counseling; at least 70 minutes in the first calendar month

G2087 Office-based treatment for opioid use disorder, including care coordination, individual therapy and group therapy and counseling; at least 60 minutes in a subsequent calendar month

G2088 Office-based treatment for opioid use disorder, including care coordination, individual therapy and group therapy and counseling; each additional 30 minutes beyond the first 120 minutes (list separately in addition to code for primary procedure)

G2089 Most recent hemoglobin a1c (hba1c) level 7.0 to 9.0%

G2090 Patients 66 years of age and older with at least one claim/encounter for frailty during the measurement period and a dispensed medication for dementia during the measurement period or the year prior to the measurement period

G2091 Patients 66 years of age and older with at least one claim/encounter for frailty during the measurement period and either one acute inpatient encounter with a diagnosis of advanced illness or two outpatient, observation, ed or nonacute inpatient encounters on different dates of service with an advanced illness diagnosis during the measurement period or the year prior to the measurement period

G2092 Angiotensin converting enzyme (ace) inhibitor or angiotensin receptor blocker (arb), or angiotensin receptor-neprilysin inhibitor (arni) therapy prescribed or currently being taken

G2093 Documentation of medical reason(s) for not prescribing ace inhibitor or arb or arni therapy (e.g., hypotensive patients who are at immediate risk of cardiogenic shock, hospitalized patients who have experienced marked azotemia, allergy, intolerance, other medical reasons)

G2094 Documentation of patient reason(s) for not prescribing ace inhibitor or arb or arni therapy (e.g., patient declined, other patient reasons)

(**G2095** Documentation of system reason(s) for not prescribing ace inhibitor or arb or arni therapy (e.g., other system reasons)

Code deleted effective 12/31/2022, no HCPCS/CPT cross-reference provided.)

G2096 Angiotensin converting enzyme (ace) inhibitor or angiotensin receptor blocker (arb), or angiotensin receptor-neprilysin inhibitor (arni) therapy was not prescribed, reason not given

G2097 Episodes where the patient had a competing diagnosis on or within three days after the episode date (e.g., intestinal infection, pertussis, bacterial infection, Lyme disease, otitis media, acute sinusitis, chronic sinusitis, infection of the adenoids, prostatitis, cellulitis, mastoiditis, or bone infections, acute lymphadenitis, impetigo, skin staph infections, pneumonia/gonococcal infections, venereal disease (syphilis, chlamydia, inflammatory diseases [female reproductive organs]), infections of the kidney, cystitis or UTI)

G2098 Patients 66 years of age and older with at least one claim/encounter for frailty during the measurement period and a dispensed medication for dementia during the measurement period or the year prior to the measurement period

G2099 Patients 66 years of age and older with at least one claim/encounter for frailty during the measurement period and either one acute inpatient encounter with a diagnosis of advanced illness or two outpatient, observation, ed or nonacute inpatient encounters on different dates of service with an advanced illness diagnosis during the measurement period or the year prior to the measurement period

G2100 Patients 66 years of age and older with at least one claim/encounter for frailty during the measurement period and a dispensed medication for dementia during the measurement period or the year prior to the measurement period

G2101 Patients 66 years of age and older with at least one claim/encounter for frailty during the measurement period and either one acute inpatient encounter with a diagnosis of advanced illness or two outpatient, observation, ed or nonacute inpatient encounters on different dates of service with an advanced illness diagnosis during the measurement period or the year prior to the measurement period

G2102 Dilated retinal eye exam with interpretation by an ophthalmologist or optometrist documented and reviewed

G2103 Seven standard field stereoscopic photos with interpretation by an ophthalmologist or optometrist documented and reviewed

G2104 Eye imaging validated to match diagnosis from seven standard field stereoscopic photos results documented and reviewed

G2105 Patient aged 66 or older in institutional special needs plans (SNP) or residing in long-term care with pos code 32, 33, 34, 54 or 56 for more than 90 consecutive days during the measurement period

G2106 Patients 66 years of age and older with at least one claim/encounter for frailty during the measurement period and a dispensed medication for dementia during the measurement period or the year prior to the measurement period

G2107 Patients 66 years of age and older with at least one claim/encounter for frailty during the measurement period and either one acute inpatient encounter with a diagnosis of advanced illness or two outpatient, observation, ed or nonacute inpatient encounters on different dates of service with an advanced illness diagnosis during the measurement period or the year prior to the measurement period

(**G2108** Patient aged 66 or older in institutional special needs plans (SNP) or residing in long-term care with pos code 32, 33, 34, 54 or 56 for more than 90 consecutive days during the measurement period

(**G2109** Patients 66 years of age and older with at least one claim/encounter for frailty during the measurement period and a dispensed medication for dementia during the measurement period or the year prior to the measurement period

(**G2110** Patients 66 years of age and older with at least one claim/encounter for frailty during the measurement period and either one acute inpatient encounter with a diagnosis of advanced illness or two outpatient, observation, ed or nonacute inpatient encounters on different dates of service with an advanced illness diagnosis during the measurement period or the year prior to the measurement period

G2112 Patient receiving <=5 mg daily prednisone (or equivalent), or ra activity is worsening, or glucocorticoid use is for less than 6 months

G2113 Patient receiving >5 mg daily prednisone (or equivalent) for longer than 6 months, and improvement or no change in disease activity

G2114 Patients 66-80 years of age with at least one claim/encounter for frailty during the measurement period and a dispensed medication for dementia during the measurement period or the year prior to the measurement period

G2115 Patients 66 - 80 years of age with at least one claim/encounter for frailty during the measurement period and a dispensed medication for dementia during the measurement period or the year prior to the measurement period

G2116 Patients 66 - 80 years of age with at least one claim/encounter for frailty during the measurement period and either one acute inpatient encounter with a diagnosis of advanced illness or two outpatient, observation, ed or nonacute inpatient encounters on different dates of service with an advanced illness diagnosis during the measurement period or the year prior to the measurement period

G2117 Patients 66-80 years of age with at least one claim/encounter for frailty during the measurement period and either one acute inpatient encounter with a diagnosis of advanced illness or two outpatient, observation, ed or nonacute inpatient encounters on different dates of service with an advanced illness diagnosis during the measurement period or the year prior to the measurement period

G2118 Patients 81 years of age and older with at least one claim/encounter for frailty during the measurement period

G2119 Within the past 2 years, calcium and/or vitamin d optimization has been ordered or performed

G2120 Within the past 2 years, calcium and/or vitamin d optimization has not been ordered or performed

G2121 Depression, anxiety, apathy, and psychosis assessed

G2122 Depression, anxiety, apathy, and psychosis not assessed

G2123 Patients 66-80 years of age and had at least one claim/encounter for frailty during the measurement period and either one acute inpatient encounter with a diagnosis of advanced illness or two outpatient, observation, ed or nonacute inpatient encounters on different dates of service with an advanced illness diagnosis during the measurement period or the year prior to the measurement period

G2124 Patients 66-80 years of age and had at least one claim/encounter for frailty during the measurement period and a dispensed dementia medication

G2125 Patients 81 years of age and older with at least one claim/encounter for frailty during the six months prior to the measurement period through December 31 of the measurement period

G2126 Patients 66 - 80 years of age with at least one claim/encounter for frailty during the measurement period and either one acute inpatient encounter with a diagnosis of advanced illness or two outpatient, observation, ed or nonacute inpatient encounters on different dates of service with an advanced illness diagnosis during the measurement period or the year prior to the measurement period

G2127 Patients 66-80 years of age with at least one claim/encounter for frailty during the measurement period and a dispensed medication for dementia during the measurement period or the year prior to the measurement period

G2128 Documentation of medical reason(s) for not on a daily aspirin or other antiplatelet (e.g., history of gastrointestinal bleed, intra-cranial bleed, blood disorders, idiopathic thrombocytopenic purpura (ITP), gastric bypass or documentation of active anticoagulant use during the measurement period)

G2129 Procedure-related bp's not taken during an outpatient visit. examples include same day surgery, ambulatory service center, g.i. lab, dialysis, infusion center, chemotherapy

G2130 Patients aged 66 or older in institutional special needs plans (SNP) or residing in long-term care with pos code 32, 33, 34, 54 or 56 for more than 90 days during the measurement period

G2131 Patients 81 years and older with a diagnosis of frailty

G2132 Patients 66-80 years of age with at least one claim/encounter for frailty during the measurement period and a dispensed medication for dementia during the measurement period or the year prior to the measurement period

G2133 Patients 66-80 years of age with at least one claim/encounter for frailty during the measurement period and either one acute inpatient encounter with a diagnosis of advanced illness or two outpatient, observation, ed or nonacute inpatient encounters on different dates of service with an advanced illness diagnosis during the measurement period or the year prior to the measurement period

G2134 Patients 66 years of age or older with at least one claim/encounter for frailty during the measurement period and a dispensed medication for dementia during the measurement period or the year prior to the measurement period

G2135 Patients 66 years of age or older with at least one claim/encounter for frailty during the measurement period and either one acute inpatient encounter with a diagnosis of advanced illness or two outpatient, observation, ed or nonacute inpatient encounters on different dates of service with an advanced illness diagnosis during the measurement period or the year prior to the measurement period

G - H CODES

G2136 Back pain measured by the visual analog scale (vas) or numeric pain scale at three months (6 - 20 weeks) postoperatively was less than or equal to 3.0 or back pain measured by the visual analog scale (vas) or numeric pain scale within three months preoperatively and at three months (6 - 20 weeks) postoperatively demonstrated an improvement of 5.0 points or greater

▲ **G2137** Back pain measured by the visual analog scale (vas) or numeric pain scale at three months (6 - 20 weeks) postoperatively was greater than 3.0 and back pain measured by the visual analog scale (vas) or numeric pain scale within three months preoperatively and at three months (6 - 20 weeks) postoperatively demonstrated improvement of less than 5.0 points

G2138 Back pain as measured by the visual analog scale (vas) or numeric pain scale at one year (9 to 15 months) postoperatively was less than or equal to 3.0 or back pain measured by the visual analog scale (vas) or numeric pain scale within three months preoperatively and at one year (9 to 15 months) postoperatively demonstrated an improvement of 5.0 points or greater

▲ **G2139** Back pain measured by the visual analog scale (vas) or numeric pain scale at one year (9 to 15 months) postoperatively was greater than 3.0 and back pain measured by the visual analog scale (vas) or numeric pain scale within three months preoperatively and at one year (9 to 15 months) postoperatively demonstrated improvement of less than 5.0 points

G2140 Leg pain measured by the visual analog scale (vas) or numeric pain scale at three months (6 - 20 weeks) postoperatively was less than or equal to 3.0 or leg pain measured by the visual analog scale (vas) or numeric pain scale within three months preoperatively and at three months (6 - 20 weeks) postoperatively demonstrated an improvement of 5.0 points or greater

▲ **G2141** Leg pain measured by the visual analog scale (vas) or numeric pain scale at three months (6 - 20 weeks) postoperatively was greater than 3.0 and leg pain measured by the visual analog scale (vas) or numeric pain scale within three months preoperatively and at three months (6 - 20 weeks) postoperatively demonstrated improvement of less than 5.0 points

G2142 Functional status measured by the Oswestry disability index (ODI version 2.1a) at one year (9 to 15 months) postoperatively was less than or equal to 22 or functional status measured by the ODI version 2.1a within three months preoperatively and at one year (9 to 15 months) postoperatively demonstrated an improvement of 30 points or greater

G2143 Functional status measured by the Oswestry disability index (ODI version 2.1a) at one year (9 to 15 months) postoperatively was greater than 22 and functional status measured by the ODI version 2.1a within three months preoperatively and at one year (9 to 15 months) postoperatively demonstrated an improvement of less than 30 points

G2144 Functional status measured by the Oswestry disability index (ODI version 2.1a) at three months (6-20 weeks) postoperatively was less than or equal to 22 or functional status measured by the ODI version 2.1a within three months preoperatively and at three months (6-20 weeks) postoperatively demonstrated an improvement of 30 points or greater

G2145 Functional status measured by the Oswestry disability index (ODI version 2.1a) at three months (6 - 20 weeks) postoperatively was greater than 22 and functional status measured by the ODI version 2.1a within three months preoperatively and at three months (6 - 20 weeks) postoperatively demonstrated an improvement of less than 30 points

G2146 Leg pain as measured by the visual analog scale (vas) or numeric pain scale at one year (9 to 15 months) postoperatively was less than or equal to 3.0 or leg pain measured by the visual analog scale (vas) or numeric pain scale within three months preoperatively and at one year (9 to 15 months) postoperatively demonstrated an improvement of 5.0 points or greater

▲ **G2147** Leg pain measured by the visual analog scale (vas) or numeric pain scale at one year (9 to 15 months) postoperatively was greater than 3.0 and leg pain measured by the visual analog scale (vas) or numeric pain scale within three months preoperatively and at one year (9 to 15 months) postoperatively demonstrated improvement of less than 5.0 points

G2148 Multimodal pain management was used

G2149 Documentation of medical reason(s) for not using multimodal pain management (e.g., allergy to multiple classes of analgesics, intubated patient, hepatic failure, patient reports no pain during

PACU stay, other medical reason(s))

G2150 Multimodal pain management was not used

G2151 Documentation stating patient has a diagnosis of a degenerative neurological condition such as ALS, ms, or Parkinson's diagnosed at any time before or during the episode of care

G2152 Residual score for the neck impairment successfully calculated and the score was equal to zero (0) or greater than zero (> 0)

G2153 In hospice or using hospice services during the measurement period

G2154 Patient received at least one td vaccine or one Tdap vaccine between nine years prior to the start of the measurement period and the end of the measurement period

G2155 Patient had history of at least one of the following contraindications any time during or before the measurement period: anaphylaxis due to Tdap vaccine, anaphylaxis due to td vaccine or its components; encephalopathy due to Tdap or td vaccination (post tetanus vaccination encephalitis, post diphtheria vaccination encephalitis or post pertussis vaccination encephalitis.)

G2156 Patient did not receive at least one td vaccine or one Tdap vaccine between nine years prior to the start of the measurement period and the end of the measurement period; or have history of at least one of the following contraindications any time during or before the measurement period: anaphylaxis due to Tdap vaccine, anaphylaxis due to td vaccine or its components; encephalopathy due to Tdap or td vaccination (post tetanus vaccination encephalitis, post diphtheria vaccination encephalitis or post pertussis vaccination encephalitis.)

G2157 Patients received both the 13-valent pneumococcal conjugate vaccine and the 23-valent pneumococcal polysaccharide vaccine at least 12 months apart, with the first occurrence after the age of 60 before or during the measurement period

G2158 Patient had prior pneumococcal vaccine adverse reaction any time during or before the measurement period

G2159 Patient did not receive both the 13-valent pneumococcal conjugate vaccine and the 23-valent pneumococcal polysaccharide vaccine at least 12 months apart, with the first occurrence after the age of 60 before or during measurement period; or have prior pneumococcal vaccine adverse reaction any time during or before the measurement period

G2160 Patient received at least one dose of the herpes zoster live vaccine or two doses of the herpes zoster recombinant vaccine (at least 28 days apart) anytime on or after the patient's 50th birthday before or during the measurement period

G2161 Patient had prior adverse reaction caused by zoster vaccine or its components any time during or before the measurement period

G2162 Patient did not receive at least one dose of the herpes zoster live vaccine or two doses of the herpes zoster recombinant vaccine (at least 28 days apart) anytime on or after the patient's 50th birthday before or during the measurement period; or have prior adverse reaction caused by zoster vaccine or its components any time during or before the measurement period

G2163 Patient received an influenza vaccine on or between July 1 of the year prior to the measurement period and June 30 of the measurement period

G2164 Patient had a prior influenza virus vaccine adverse reaction any time before or during the measurement period

G2165 Patient did not receive an influenza vaccine on or between July 1 of the year prior to the measurement period and June 30 of the measurement period; or did not have a prior influenza virus vaccine adverse reaction any time before or during the measurement period

G2166 Patient refused to participate at admission and/or discharge; patient unable to complete the neck fs prom at admission or discharge due to cognitive deficit, visual deficit, motor deficit, language barrier, or low reading level, and a suitable proxy/recorder is not available; patient self-discharged early; medical reason

G - H CODES

G2167 Residual score for the neck impairment successfully calculated and the score was less than zero (< 0)

G2168 Services performed by a physical therapist assistant in the home health setting in the delivery of a safe and effective physical therapy maintenance program, each 15 minutes

G2169 Services performed by an occupational therapist assistant in the home health setting in the delivery of a safe and effective occupational therapy maintenance program, each 15 minutes

(**G2170** Percutaneous arteriovenous fistula creation (AVF), direct, any site, by tissue approximation using thermal resistance energy, and secondary procedures to redirect blood flow (e.g., transluminal balloon angioplasty, coil embolization) when performed, and includes all imaging and radiologic guidance, supervision and interpretation, when performed

Code deleted effective 12/31/2022, no HCPCS/CPT cross-reference provided.)

(**G2171** Percutaneous arteriovenous fistula creation (AVF), direct, any site, using magnetic-guided arterial and venous catheters and radiofrequency energy, including flow-directing procedures (e.g., vascular coil embolization with radiologic supervision and interpretation, wen performed) and fistulogram(s), angiography, enography, and/or ultrasound, with radiologic supervision and interpretation, when performed

Code deleted effective 12/31/2022, no HCPCS/CPT cross-reference provided.)

G2172 All inclusive payment for services related to highly coordinated and integrated opioid use disorder (oud) treatment services furnished for the demonstration project

G2173 Uri episodes where the patient had a comorbid condition during the 12 months prior to or on the episode date (e.g., tuberculosis, neutropenia, cystic fibrosis, chronic bronchitis, pulmonary edema, respiratory failure, rheumatoid lung disease)

▲ **G2174** Uri episodes where the patient is taking antibiotics (table 1) in the 30 days prior to the episode date

G2175 Episodes where the patient had a comorbid condition during the 12 months prior to or on the episode date (e.g., tuberculosis, neutropenia, cystic fibrosis, chronic bronchitis, pulmonary edema, respiratory failure, rheumatoid lung disease)

G2176 Outpatient, ed, or observation visits that result in an inpatient admission

G2177 Acute bronchitis/bronchiolitis episodes when the patient had a new or refill prescription of antibiotics (table 1) in the 30 days prior to the episode date

G2178 Clinician documented that patient was not an eligible candidate for lower extremity neurological exam measure, for example patient bilateral amputee; patient has condition that would not allow them to accurately respond to a neurological exam (dementia, Alzheimer's, etc.); patient has previously documented diabetic peripheral neuropathy with loss of protective sensation

G2179 Clinician documented that patient had medical reason for not performing lower extremity neurological exam

G2180 Clinician documented that patient was not an eligible candidate for evaluation of footwear as patient is bilateral lower extremity amputee

G2181 BMI not documented due to medical reason or patient refusal of height or weight measurement

G2182 Patient receiving first-time biologic and/or immune response modifier therapy

G2183 Documentation patient unable to communicate and informant not available

G2184 Patient does not have a caregiver

G2185 Documentation caregiver is trained and certified in dementia care

G2186 Patient /caregiver dyad has been referred to appropriate resources and connection to those resources is confirmed

G2187 Patients with clinical indications for imaging of the head: head trauma

G2188 Patients with clinical indications for imaging of the head: new or change in headache above 50 years of age

G2189 Patients with clinical indications for imaging of the head: abnormal neurologic exam

G2190 Patients with clinical indications for imaging of the head: headache radiating to the neck

G2191 Patients with clinical indications for imaging of the head: positional headaches

G2192 Patients with clinical indications for imaging of the head: temporal headaches in patients over 55 years of age

G2193 Patients with clinical indications for imaging of the head: new onset headache in pre-school children or younger (<6 years of age)

G2194 Patients with clinical indications for imaging of the head: new onset headache in pediatric patients with disabilities for which headache is a concern as inferred from behavior

G2195 Patients with clinical indications for imaging of the head: occipital headache in children

G2196 Patient identified as an unhealthy alcohol user when screened for unhealthy alcohol use using a systematic screening method

G2197 Patient screened for unhealthy alcohol use using a systematic screening method and not identified as an unhealthy alcohol user

(**G2198** Documentation of medical reason(s) for not screening for unhealthy alcohol use using a systematic screening method (e.g., limited life expectancy, other medical reasons)

Code deleted effective 12/31/2022, no HCPCS/CPT cross-reference provided.)

G2199 Patient not screened for unhealthy alcohol use using a systematic screening method

G2200 Patient identified as an unhealthy alcohol user received brief counseling

(**G2201** Documentation of medical reason(s) for not providing brief counseling (e.g., limited life expectancy, other medical reasons)

Code deleted effective 12/31/2022, no HCPCS/CPT cross-reference provided.)

G2202 Patient did not receive brief counseling if identified as an unhealthy alcohol user

(**G2203** Documentation of medical reason(s) for not providing brief counseling if identified as an unhealthy alcohol user (e.g., limited life expectancy, other medical reasons)

Code deleted effective 12/31/2022, no HCPCS/CPT cross-reference provided.)

G2204 Patients between 45 and 85 years of age who received a screening colonoscopy during the performance period

G2205 Patients with pregnancy during adjuvant treatment course

G2206 Patient received adjuvant treatment course including both chemotherapy and her2-targeted therapy

G2207 Reason for not administering adjuvant treatment course including both chemotherapy and her2-targeted therapy (e.g., poor performance status (ECoG 3-4; Karnofsky <=50), cardiac contraindications, insufficient renal function, insufficient hepatic function, other active or secondary cancer diagnoses, other medical contraindications, patients who died during initial treatment course or transferred during or after initial treatment course)

G2208 Patient did not receive adjuvant treatment course including both chemotherapy and her2-targeted therapy

G2209 Patient refused to participate

G2210 Residual score for the neck impairment not measured because the patient did not complete the neck fs prom at initial evaluation and/or near discharge, reason not given

G2211 Visit complexity inherent to evaluation and management associated with medical care services that serve as the continuing focal point for all needed health care services and/or with medical care services that are part of ongoing care related to a patient's single, serious condition or a complex condition. (add-on code, list separately in addition to office/outpatient evaluation and management visit, new or established)

G - H CODES

G2212 Prolonged office or other outpatient evaluation and management service(s) beyond the maximum required time of the primary procedure which has been selected using total time on the date of the primary service; each additional 15 minutes by the physician or qualified healthcare professional, with or without direct patient contact (list separately in addition to CPT codes 99205, 99215, 99483 for office or other outpatient evaluation and management services) (do not report G2212 on the same date of service as 99358, 99359, 99415, 99416). (do not report G2212 for any time unit less than 15 minutes)

G2213 Initiation of medication for the treatment of opioid use disorder in the emergency department setting, including assessment, referral to ongoing care, and arranging access to supportive services (list separately in addition to code for primary procedure)

G2214 Initial or subsequent psychiatric collaborative care management, first 30 minutes in a month of behavioral health care manager activities, in consultation with a psychiatric consultant, and directed by the treating physician or other qualified health care professional

G2215 Take-home supply of nasal naloxone; 2-pack of 4mg per 0.1 ml nasal spray (provision of the services by a Medicare-enrolled opioid treatment program); list separately in addition to code for primary procedure

G2216 Take-home supply of injectable naloxone (provision of the services by a Medicare-enrolled opioid treatment program); list separately in addition to code for primary procedure

G2250 Remote assessment of recorded video and/or images submitted by an established patient (e.g., store and forward), including interpretation with follow-up with the patient within 24 business hours, not originating from a related service provided within the previous 7 days nor leading to a service or procedure within the next 24 hours or soonest available appointment

G2251 Brief communication technology-based service, e.g., virtual check-in, by a qualified health care professional who cannot report evaluation and management services, provided to an established patient, not originating from a related service provided within the previous 7 days nor leading to a service or procedure within the next 24 hours or soonest available appointment; 5-10 minutes of clinical discussion

G2252 Brief communication technology-based service, e.g., virtual check-in, by a physician or other qualified health care professional who can report evaluation and management services, provided to an established patient, not originating from a related e/m service provided within the previous 7 days nor leading to an e/m service or procedure within the next 24 hours or soonest available appointment; 11-20 minutes of medical discussion

G3001 Administration and supply of tositumomab, 450 mg

G3002 Chronic pain management and treatment, monthly bundle including, diagnosis; assessment and monitoring; administration of a validated pain rating scale or tool; the development, implementation, revision, and/or maintenance of a person-centered care plan that includes strengths, goals, clinical needs, and desired outcomes; overall treatment management; facilitation and coordination of any necessary behavioral health treatment; medication management; pain and health literacy counseling; any necessary chronic pain related crisis care; and ongoing communication and care coordination between relevant practitioners furnishing care, e.g. physical therapy and occupational therapy, complementary and integrative approaches, and community-based care, as appropriate. required initial face-to-face visit at least 30 minutes provided by a physician or other qualified health professional; first 30 minutes personally provided by physician or other qualified health care professional, per calendar month. (when using G3002, 30 minutes must be met or exceeded.)

G3003 Each additional 15 minutes of chronic pain management and treatment by a physician or other qualified health care professional, per calendar month. (list separately in addition to code for G3002. when using G3003, 15 minutes must be met or exceeded.)

G4000 Dermatology MIPS specialty set

G4001 Diagnostic radiology MIPS specialty set

G4002 Electrophysiology cardiac specialist MIPS specialty set

G4003	Emergency medicine MIPS specialty set
G4004	Endocrinology MIPS specialty set
G4005	Family medicine MIPS specialty set
G4006	Gastro-enterology MIPS specialty set
G4007	General surgery MIPS specialty set
G4008	Geriatrics MIPS specialty set
G4009	Hospitalists MIPS specialty set
G4010	Infectious disease MIPS specialty set
G4011	Internal medicine MIPS specialty set
G4012	Interventional radiology MIPS specialty set
G4013	Mental/behavioral and psychiatry MIPS specialty set
G4014	Nephrology MIPS specialty set
G4015	Neurology MIPS specialty set
G4016	Neurosurgical MIPS specialty set
G4017	Nutrition/dietician MIPS specialty set
G4018	Obstetrics/gynecology MIPS specialty set
G4019	Oncology/hematology MIPS specialty set
G4020	Ophthalmology/optometry MIPS specialty set
G4021	Orthopedic surgery MIPS specialty set
G4022	Otolaryngology MIPS specialty set
G4023	Pathology MIPS specialty set
G4024	Pediatrics MIPS specialty set
G4025	Physical medicine MIPS specialty set
G4026	Physical therapy/occupational therapy MIPS specialty set
G4027	Plastic surgery MIPS specialty set
G4028	Podiatry MIPS specialty set
G4029	Preventive medicine MIPS specialty set
G4030	Pulmonology MIPS specialty set
G4031	Radiation oncology MIPS specialty set
G4032	Rheumatology MIPS specialty set
G4033	Skilled nursing facility MIPS specialty set
G4034	Speech language pathology MIPS specialty set
G4035	Thoracic surgery MIPS specialty set
G4036	Urgent care MIPS specialty set
G4037	Urology MIPS specialty set
G4038	Vascular surgery MIPS specialty set
G6001	Ultrasonic guidance for placement of radiation therapy fields
G6002	Stereoscopic x-ray guidance for localization of target volume for the delivery of radiation therapy
G6003	Radiation treatment delivery, single treatment area, single port or parallel opposed ports, simple blocks or no blocks: up to 5 meV
G6004	Radiation treatment delivery, single treatment area, single port or parallel opposed ports, simple

G - H CODES

blocks or no blocks: 6-10 meV

G6005 Radiation treatment delivery, single treatment area, single port or parallel opposed ports, simple blocks or no blocks: 11-19 meV

G6006 Radiation treatment delivery, single treatment area, single port or parallel opposed ports, simple blocks or no blocks: 20 meV or greater

G6007 Radiation treatment delivery, 2 separate treatment areas, 3 or more ports on a single treatment area, use of multiple blocks: up to 5 meV

G6008 Radiation treatment delivery, 2 separate treatment areas, 3 or more ports on a single treatment area, use of multiple blocks: 6-10 meV

G6009 Radiation treatment delivery, 2 separate treatment areas, 3 or more ports on a single treatment area, use of multiple blocks: 11-19 meV

G6010 Radiation treatment delivery, 2 separate treatment areas, 3 or more ports on a single treatment area, use of multiple blocks: 20 meV or greater

G6011 Radiation treatment delivery,3 or more separate treatment areas, custom blocking, tangential ports, wedges, rotational beam, compensators, electron beam; up to 5 meV

G6012 Radiation treatment delivery,3 or more separate treatment areas, custom blocking, tangential ports, wedges, rotational beam, compensators, electron beam; 6-10 meV

G6013 Radiation treatment delivery,3 or more separate treatment areas, custom blocking, tangential ports, wedges, rotational beam, compensators, electron beam; 11-19 meV

G6014 Radiation treatment delivery,3 or more separate treatment areas, custom blocking, tangential ports, wedges, rotational beam, compensators, electron beam; 20 meV or greater

G6015 Intensity modulated treatment delivery, single or multiple fields/arcs, via narrow spatially and temporally modulated beams, binary, dynamic MLC, per treatment session

G6016 Compensator-based beam modulation treatment delivery of inverse planned treatment using 3 or more high resolution (milled or cast) compensator, convergent beam modulated fields, per treatment session

G6017 Intra-fraction localization and tracking of target or patient motion during delivery of radiation therapy (eg,3d positional tracking, gating, 3d surface tracking), each fraction of treatment

G6018 Ileoscopy, through stoma; with transendoscopic stent placement (includes predilation)

G6019 Colonoscopy through stoma; with ablation of tumor(s), polyp(s), or other lesion(s) not amenable to removal by hot biopsy forceps, bipolar cautery or snare technique

G6020 Colonoscopy through stoma; with transendoscopic stent placement (includes predilation)

G6021 Unlisted procedure, intestine

G6022 Sigmoidoscopy, flexible; with ablation of tumor(s), polyp(s), or other lesions(s) not amenable to removal by hot biopsy forceps, bipolar cautery or snare technique

G6023 Sigmoidoscopy, flexible; with transendoscopic stent placement (includes predilation)

G6024 Colonoscopy, flexible; proximal to splenic flexure; with ablation of tumor(s), polyp(s), or other lesion(s) not amenable to removal by hot biopsy forceps, bipolar cautery or snare technique

G6025 Colonoscopy, flexible, proximal to splenic flexure; with transendoscopic stent placement (includes predilation)

G6027 Anoscopy, high resolution (HRA) (with magnification and chemical agent enhancement); diagnostic, including collection of specimen(s) by brushing or washing when performed

G6028 Anoscopy, high resolution (HRA) (with magnification and chemical agent enhancement); with biopsy(ies)

G6030 Amitriptyline

G6031 Benzodiazepines

G6032 Desipramine

G6034 Doxepin

G6035 Gold

G6036 Assay of imipramine

G6037 Nortriptyline

G6038 Salicylate

G6039 Acetaminophen

G6040 Alcohol (ethanol); any specimen except breath

G6041 Alkaloids, urine, quantitative

G6042 Amphetamine or methamphetamine

G6043 Barbiturates, not elsewhere specified

G6044 Cocaine or metabolite

G6045 Dihydrocodeinone

G6046 Dihydromorphinone

G6047 Dihydrotestosterone

G6048 Dimethadione

G6049 Epiandrosterone

G6050 Ethchlorvynol

G6051 Flurazepam

G6052 Meprobamate

G6053 Methadone

G6054 Methsuximide

G6055 Nicotine

G6056 Opiate(s), drug and metabolites, each procedure

G6057 Phenothiazine

G6058 Drug confirmation, each procedure

G8126 Patient with a diagnosis of major depression documented as being treated with antidepressant medication during the entire 84 day (12 week) acute treatment phase

G8127 Patient with a diagnosis of major depression not documented as being treated with antidepressant medication during the entire 84 day (12 week) acute treatment phase

G8128 Clinician documented that patient was not an eligible candidate for antidepressant medication during the entire 12 week acute treatment phase measure

G8395 Left ventricular ejection fraction (LVEF) >= 40% or documentation as normal or mildly depressed left ventricular systolic function

G8396 Left ventricular ejection fraction (LVEF) not performed or documented

G8397 Dilated macular or fundus exam performed, including documentation of the presence or absence of macular edema and level of severity of retinopathy

G8398 Dilated macular or fundus exam not performed

G8399 Patient with documented results of a central dual-energy x-ray absorptiometry (DXA) ever being performed

G8400 Patient with central dual-energy x-ray absorptiometry (DXA) results not documented, reason not given

G8401 Clinician documented that patient was not an eligible candidate for screening

G - H CODES

G8404 Lower extremity neurological exam performed and documented

G8405 Lower extremity neurological exam not performed

G8406 Clinician documented that patient was not an eligible candidate for lower extremity neurological exam measure

G8410 Footwear evaluation performed and documented

G8415 Footwear evaluation was not performed

G8416 Clinician documented that patient was not an eligible candidate for footwear evaluation measure

G8417 BMI is documented above normal parameters, and a follow-up plan is documented

G8418 BMI is documented below normal parameters, and a follow-up plan is documented

G8419 BMI documented outside normal parameters, no follow-up plan documented, no reason given

G8420 BMI is documented within normal parameters and no follow-up plan is required

G8421 BMI not documented and no reason is given

G8422 BMI not documented, documentation the patient is not eligible for BMI calculation

G8427 Eligible clinician attests to documenting in the medical record they obtained, updated, or reviewed the patient's current medications

G8428 Current list of medications not documented as obtained, updated, or reviewed by the eligible clinician, reason not given

G8430 Documentation of a medical reason(s) for not documenting, updating, or reviewing the patient's current medications list (e.g., patient is in an urgent or emergent medical situation)

G8431 Screening for depression is documented as being positive and a follow-up plan is documented

G8432 Depression screening not documented; reason not given

G8433 Screening for depression not completed documented patient or medical reason

G8442 Pain assessment not documented as being performed, documentation the patient is not eligible for a pain assessment using a standardized tool at the time of the encounter

G8450 Beta-blocker therapy prescribed

G8451 Beta-blocker therapy for LVEF <=40% not prescribed for reasons documented by the clinician (e.g., low blood pressure, fluid overload, asthma, patients recently treated with an intravenous positive inotropic agent, allergy, intolerance, other medical reasons, patient declined, other patient reasons)

G8452 Beta-blocker therapy not prescribed

G8458 Clinician documented that patient is not an eligible candidate for genotype testing; patient not receiving antiviral treatment for hepatitis c during the measurement period (e.g., genotype test done prior to the reporting period, patient declines, patient not a candidate for antiviral treatment)

G8460 Clinician documented that patient is not an eligible candidate for quantitative RNA testing at week 12; patient not receiving antiviral treatment for hepatitis c

G8461 Patient receiving antiviral treatment for hepatitis c during the measurement period

G8464 Clinician documented that prostate cancer patient is not an eligible candidate for adjuvant hormonal therapy; low or intermediate risk of recurrence or risk of recurrence not determined

G8465 High or very high risk of recurrence of prostate cancer

G8473 Angiotensin converting enzyme (ace) inhibitor or angiotensin receptor blocker (arb) therapy prescribed

▲ **G8474** Angiotensin converting enzyme (ace) inhibitor or angiotensin receptor blocker (arb) therapy not prescribed for reasons documented by the clinician (e.g., allergy, intolerance, pregnancy, renal

failure due to ace inhibitor, diseases of the aortic or mitral valve, other medical reasons) or (e.g., patient declined, other patient reasons)

G8475 Angiotensin converting enzyme (ace) inhibitor or angiotensin receptor blocker (arb) therapy not prescribed, reason not given

G8476 Most recent blood pressure has a systolic measurement of < 140 mmHg and a diastolic measurement of < 90 mmHg

G8477 Most recent blood pressure has a systolic measurement of >= 140 mmHg and/or a diastolic measurement of >= 90 mmHg

G8478 Blood pressure measurement not performed or documented; reason not given

G8482 Influenza immunization administered or previously received

G8483 Influenza immunization was not administered for reasons documented by clinician (e.g., patient allergy or other medical reasons, patient declined or other patient reasons, vaccine not available or other system reasons)

G8484 Influenza immunization was not administered, reason not given

G8485 I intend to report the diabetes mellitus (dm) measures group

G8486 I intend to report the preventive care measures group

G8487 I intend to report the chronic kidney disease (CKD) measures group

G8489 I intend to report the coronary artery disease (cad) measures group

G8490 I intend to report the rheumatoid arthritis (ra) measures group

G8491 I intend to report the HIV/aids measures group

G8492 I intend to report the perioperative care measures group

G8493 I intend to report the back pain measures group

G8494 All quality actions for the applicable measures in the diabetes mellitus (dm) measures group have been performed for this patient

G8495 All quality actions for the applicable measures in the chronic kidney disease (CKD) measures group have been performed for this patient

G8496 All quality actions for the applicable measures in the preventive care measures group have been performed for this patient

G8497 All quality actions for the applicable measures in the coronary artery bypass graft (CABG) measures group have been performed for this patient

G8498 All quality actions for the applicable measures in the coronary artery disease (cad) measures group have been performed for this patient

G8499 All quality actions for the applicable measures in the rheumatoid arthritis (ra) measures group have been performed for this patient

G8500 All quality actions for the applicable measures in the HIV/aids measures group have been performed for this patient

G8501 All quality actions for the applicable measures in the perioperative care measures group have been performed for this patient

G8502 All quality actions for the applicable measures in the back pain measures group have been performed for this patient

G8506 Patient receiving angiotensin converting enzyme (ace) inhibitor or angiotensin receptor blocker (arb) therapy

G8509 Pain assessment documented as positive using a standardized tool, follow-up plan not documented, reason not given

G8510 Screening for depression is documented as negative, a follow-up plan is not required

G8511 Screening for depression documented as positive, follow-up plan not documented, reason not given

G8530 Autogenous av fistula received

G8531 Clinician documented that patient was not an eligible candidate for autogenous av fistula

G8532 Clinician documented that patient received vascular access other than autogenous av fistula, reason not given

▲ **G8535** Elder maltreatment screen not documented; documentation that patient is not eligible for the elder maltreatment screen at the time of the encounter related to one of the following reasons: (1) patient refuses to participate in the screening and has reasonable decisional capacity for self-protection, or (2) patient is in an urgent or emergent situation where time is of the essence and to delay treatment to perform the screening would jeopardize the patient's health status

G8536 No documentation of an elder maltreatment screen, reason not given

G8539 Functional outcome assessment documented as positive using a standardized tool and a care plan based on identified deficiencies is documented within two days of the functional outcome assessment

G8540 Functional outcome assessment not documented as being performed, documentation the patient is not eligible for a functional outcome assessment using a standardized tool at the time of the encounter

G8541 Functional outcome assessment using a standardized tool not documented, reason not given

G8542 Functional outcome assessment using a standardized tool is documented; no functional deficiencies identified, care plan not required

G8543 Documentation of a positive functional outcome assessment using a standardized tool; care plan not documented within two days of assessment, reason not given

G8544 I intend to report the coronary artery bypass graft (CABG) measures group

G8545 I intend to report the hepatitis c measures group

G8547 I intend to report the ischemic vascular disease (IVD) measures group

G8548 I intend to report the heart failure (hf) measures group

G8549 All quality actions for the applicable measures in the hepatitis c measures group have been performed for this patient

G8551 All quality actions for the applicable measures in the heart failure (hf) measures group have been performed for this patient

G8552 All quality actions for the applicable measures in the ischemic vascular disease (IVD) measures group have been performed for this patient

G8559 Patient referred to a physician (preferably a physician with training in disorders of the ear) for an otologic evaluation

G8560 Patient has a history of active drainage from the ear within the previous 90 days

G8561 Patient is not eligible for the referral for otologic evaluation for patients with a history of active drainage measure

G8562 Patient does not have a history of active drainage from the ear within the previous 90 days

G8563 Patient not referred to a physician (preferably a physician with training in disorders of the ear) for an otologic evaluation, reason not given

G8564 Patient was referred to a physician (preferably a physician with training in disorders of the ear) for an otologic evaluation, reason not specified)

G8565 Verification and documentation of sudden or rapidly progressive hearing loss

G8566 Patient is not eligible for the "referral for otologic evaluation for sudden or rapidly progressive hearing loss" measure

G8567 Patient does not have verification and documentation of sudden or rapidly progressive hearing loss

G8568 Patient was not referred to a physician (preferably a physician with training in disorders of the ear) for an otologic evaluation, reason not given

G8569 Prolonged postoperative intubation (> 24 hrs) required

G8570 Prolonged postoperative intubation (> 24 hrs) not required

G8571 Development of deep sternal wound infection/mediastinitis within 30 days postoperatively

G8572 No deep sternal wound infection/mediastinitis

G8573 Stroke following isolated CABG surgery

G8574 No stroke following isolated CABG surgery

G8575 Developed postoperative renal failure or required dialysis

G8576 No postoperative renal failure/dialysis not required

G8577 Re-exploration required due to mediastinal bleeding with or without tamponade, graft occlusion, valve dysfunction or other cardiac reason

G8578 Re-exploration not required due to mediastinal bleeding with or without tamponade, graft occlusion, valve dysfunction or other cardiac reason

G8579 Antiplatelet medication at discharge

G8580 Antiplatelet medication contraindicated

G8581 No antiplatelet medication at discharge

G8582 Beta-blocker at discharge

G8583 Beta-blocker contraindicated

G8584 No beta-blocker at discharge

G8585 Anti-lipid treatment at discharge

G8586 Anti-lipid treatment contraindicated

G8587 No anti-lipid treatment at discharge

G8593 Lipid profile results documented and reviewed (must include total cholesterol, HDL-c, triglycerides and calculated LDL-c)

G8594 Lipid profile not performed; reason not given

G8595 Most recent LDL-c < 100 mg/dl

G8597 Most recent LDL-c >= 100 mg/dl

G8598 Aspirin or another antiplatelet therapy used

G8599 Aspirin or another antiplatelet therapy not used, reason not given

G8600 IV thrombolytic therapy initiated within 4.5 hours (<= 270 minutes) of time last known well

▲ **G8601** Iv thrombolytic therapy not initiated within 4.5 hours (<= 270 minutes) of time last known well for reasons documented by clinician (e.g., patient enrolled in clinical trial for stroke, patient admitted for elective carotid intervention)

G8602 IV thrombolytic therapy not initiated within 4.5 hours (<= 270 minutes) of time last known well, reason not given

G8627 Surgical procedure performed within 30 days following cataract surgery for major complications (e.g., retained nuclear fragments, endophthalmitis, dislocated or wrong power IOL, retinal detachment, or wound dehiscence)

G8628 Surgical procedure not performed within 30 days following cataract surgery for major complications (e.g., retained nuclear fragments, endophthalmitis, dislocated or wrong power IOL, retinal detachment, or wound dehiscence)

G8629 Documentation of order for prophylactic parenteral antibiotic to be given within one hour (if fluoroquinolone or vancomycin, two hours) prior to surgical incision (or start of procedure when no incision is required)

G8630 Documentation that administration of prophylactic parenteral antibiotics was initiated within one hour (if fluoroquinolone or vancomycin, two hours) prior to surgical incision (or start of procedure when no incision is required), as ordered

G8631 Clinician documented that patient was not an eligible candidate for ordering prophylactic parenteral antibiotics to be given within one hour (if fluoroquinolone or vancomycin, two hours) prior to surgical incision (or start of procedure when no incision is required)

G8632 Prophylactic parenteral antibiotics were not ordered to be given or given within one hour (if fluoroquinolone or vancomycin, two hours) prior to the surgical incision (or start of procedure when no incision is required), reason not given

G8633 Pharmacologic therapy (other than minerals/vitamins) for osteoporosis prescribed

G8634 Clinician documented patient not an eligible candidate to receive pharmacologic therapy for osteoporosis

G8635 Pharmacologic therapy for osteoporosis was not prescribed, reason not given

G8645 I intend to report the asthma measures group

G8646 All quality actions for the applicable measures in the asthma measures group have been performed for this patient

G8647 Residual score for the knee impairment successfully calculated and the score was equal to zero (0) or greater than zero (> 0)

G8648 Residual score for the knee impairment successfully calculated and the score was less than zero (< 0)

G8649 Risk-adjusted functional status change residual score for the knee impairment not measured because the patient did not complete the fs status survey near discharge, patient not appropriate

G8650 Residual score for the knee impairment not measured because the patient did not complete the lepf prom at initial evaluation and/or near discharge, reason not given

G8651 Residual score for the hip impairment successfully calculated and the score was equal to zero (0) or greater than zero (> 0)

G8652 Residual score for the hip impairment successfully calculated and the score was less than zero (< 0)

G8653 Risk-adjusted functional status change residual scores for the hip impairment not measured because the patient did not complete the fs status survey near discharge, patient not appropriate

G8654 Residual score for the hip impairment not measured because the patient did not complete the lepf prom at initial evaluation and/or near discharge, reason not given

G8655 Residual score for the lower leg, foot or ankle impairment successfully calculated and the score was equal to zero (0) or greater than zero (> 0)

G8656 Residual score for the lower leg, foot or ankle impairment successfully calculated and the score was less than zero (< 0)

G8657 Risk-adjusted functional status change residual score for the lower leg, foot or ankle impairment not measured because the patient did not complete the fs status survey near discharge, patient not appropriate

G8658 Residual score for the lower leg, foot or ankle impairment not measured because the patient did not complete the lepf prom at initial evaluation and/or near discharge, reason not given

G8659 Residual score for the low back impairment successfully calculated and the score was equal to zero (0) or greater than zero (> 0)

G8660 Residual score for the low back impairment successfully calculated and the score was less than zero (< 0)

G8661 Risk-adjusted functional status change residual score for the low back impairment not measured because the patient did not complete the fs status survey near discharge, patient not appropriate

G8662 Residual score for the low back impairment not measured because the patient did not complete the low back fs prom at initial evaluation and/or near discharge, reason not given

G8663 Residual score for the shoulder impairment successfully calculated and the score was equal to zero (0) or greater than zero (> 0)

G8664 Residual score for the shoulder impairment successfully calculated and the score was less than zero (< 0)

G8665 Risk-adjusted functional status change residual score for the shoulder impairment not measured because the patient did not complete the fs status survey near discharge, patient not appropriate

G8666 Residual score for the shoulder impairment not measured because the patient did not complete the shoulder fs prom at initial evaluation and/or near discharge, reason not given

G8667 Residual score for the elbow, wrist or hand impairment successfully calculated and the score was equal to zero (0) or greater than zero (> 0)

G8668 Residual score for the elbow, wrist or hand impairment successfully calculated and the score was less than zero (< 0)

G8669 Risk-adjusted functional status change residual score for the elbow, wrist or hand impairment not measured because the patient did not complete the fs status survey near discharge, patient not appropriate

G8670 Residual score for the elbow, wrist or hand impairment not measured because the patient did not complete the elbow/wrist/hand fs prom at initial evaluation and/or near discharge, reason not given

G8671 Risk-adjusted functional status change residual score for the neck, cranium, mandible, thoracic spine, ribs or other general orthopedic impairment successfully calculated and the score was equal to zero (0) or greater than zero (> 0)

G8672 Risk-adjusted functional status change residual score for the neck, cranium, mandible, thoracic spine, ribs or other general orthopedic impairment successfully calculated and the score was less than zero (< 0)

G8673 Risk-adjusted functional status change residual score for the neck, cranium, mandible, thoracic spine, ribs or other general orthopedic impairment not measured because the patient did not complete the fs status survey near discharge, patient not appropriate

G8674 Risk-adjusted functional status change residual score for the neck, cranium, mandible, thoracic spine, ribs or other general orthopedic impairment not measured because the patient did not complete the general orthopedic fs prom at initial evaluation and/or near discharge, reason not given

G8682 LVF testing documented as being performed prior to discharge or in the previous 12 months

G8683 LVF testing not performed prior to discharge or in the previous 12 months for a medical or patient documented reason

G8685 LVF testing not documented as being performed prior to discharge or in the previous 12 months, reason not given

G8694 Left ventricular ejection fraction (LVEF) < = 40% or documentation of moderate or severe lvsd

G8696 Antithrombotic therapy prescribed at discharge

G8697 Antithrombotic therapy not prescribed for documented reasons (e.g., patient had stroke during hospital stay, patient expired during inpatient stay, other medical reason(s)); (e.g., patient left against medical advice, other patient reason(s))

G8698 Antithrombotic therapy was not prescribed at discharge, reason not given

G8699 Rehabilitation services (occupational, physical or speech) ordered at or prior to discharge

G8700 Rehabilitation services (occupational, physical or speech) not indicated at or prior to discharge

G8701 Rehabilitation services were not ordered, reason not otherwise specified

G8702 Documentation that prophylactic antibiotics were given within 4 hours prior to surgical incision or intraoperatively

G8703 Documentation that prophylactic antibiotics were neither given within 4 hours prior to surgical incision nor intraoperatively

G8704 12-lead electrocardiogram (ECG) performed

G8705 Documentation of medical reason(s) for not performing a 12-lead electrocardiogram (ECG)

G8706 Documentation of patient reason(s) for not performing a 12-lead electrocardiogram (ECG)

G8707 12-lead electrocardiogram (ECG) not performed; reason not given

G8708 Patient not prescribed antibiotic

G8709 URI episodes when the patient had competing diagnoses on or three days after the episode date (e.g., intestinal infection, pertussis, bacterial infection, Lyme disease, otitis media, acute sinusitis, acute pharyngitis, acute tonsillitis, chronic sinusitis, infection of the pharynx/larynx/tonsils/ adenoids, prostatitis, cellulitis, mastoiditis, or bone infections, acute lymphadenitis, impetigo, skin staph infections, pneumonia/gonococcal infections, venereal disease (syphilis, chlamydia, inflammatory diseases [female reproductive organs]), infections of the kidney, cystitis or UTI, and acne)

G8710 Patient prescribed antibiotic

G8711 Prescribed antibiotic on or within 3 days after the episode date

G8712 Antibiotic not prescribed or dispensed

G8713 Spkt/v greater than or equal to 1.2 (single-pool clearance of urea [kt] / volume [v])

G8714 Hemodialysis treatment performed exactly three times per week for > 90 days

G8717 Spkt/v less than 1.2 (single-pool clearance of urea [kt] / volume [v]), reason not given

G8718 Total kt/v greater than or equal to 1.7 per week (total clearance of urea [kt] / volume [v])

G8720 Total kt/v less than 1.7 per week (total clearance of urea [kt] / volume [v])

G8721 Pt category (primary tumor), pn category (regional lymph nodes), and histologic grade were documented in pathology report

G8722 Documentation of medical reason(s) for not including the pt category, the pn category or the histologic grade in the pathology report (e.g., re-excision without residual tumor; non-carcinomas anal canal)

G8723 Specimen site is other than anatomic location of primary tumor

G8724 Pt category, pn category and histologic grade were not documented in the pathology report, reason not given

G8725 Fasting lipid profile performed (triglycerides, LDL-c, HDL-c and total cholesterol)

G8726 Clinician has documented reason for not performing fasting lipid profile (e.g., patient declined, other patient reasons)

G8728 Fasting lipid profile not performed; reason not given

G8730 Pain assessment documented as positive using a standardized tool and a follow-up plan is documented

G8731 Pain assessment using a standardized tool is documented as negative, no follow-up plan required

G8732 No documentation of pain assessment, reason not given

G8733 Elder maltreatment screen documented as positive, and a follow-up plan is documented

G8734 Elder maltreatment screen documented as negative; follow-up is not required

G8735 Elder maltreatment screen documented as positive, follow-up plan not documented, reason not given

G8736 Most current LDL-c <100mg/dl

G8737 Most current LDL-c >=100mg/dl

G8738 Left ventricular ejection fraction (LVEF) < 40% or documentation of severely or moderately depressed left ventricular systolic function

G8739 Left ventricular ejection fraction (LVEF) >= 40% or documentation as normal or mildly depressed left ventricular systolic function

G8740 Left ventricular ejection fraction (LVEF) not performed or assessed, reason not given

G8749 Absence of signs of melanoma (tenderness, jaundice, localized neurologic signs such as weakness, or any other sign suggesting systemic spread) or absence of symptoms of melanoma (cough, dyspnea, pain, paresthesia, or any other symptom suggesting the possibility of systemic spread of melanoma)

G8751 Smoking status and exposure to second hand smoke in the home not assessed, reason not given

G8752 Most recent systolic blood pressure < 140 mmHg

G8753 Most recent systolic blood pressure >= 140 mmHg

G8754 Most recent diastolic blood pressure < 90 mmHg

G8755 Most recent diastolic blood pressure >= 90 mmHg

G8756 No documentation of blood pressure measurement, reason not given

G8757 All quality actions for the applicable measures in the chronic obstructive pulmonary disease (COPD) measures group have been performed for this patient

G8758 All quality actions for the applicable measures in the inflammatory bowel disease (IBD) measures group have been performed for this patient

G8759 All quality actions for the applicable measures in the sleep apnea measures group have been performed for this patient

G8761 All quality actions for the applicable measures in the dementia measures group have been performed for this patient

G8762 All quality actions for the applicable measures in the Parkinson's disease measures group have been performed for this patient

G8763 All quality actions for the applicable measures in the hypertension (HTN) measures group have been performed for this patient

G8764 All quality actions for the applicable measures in the cardiovascular prevention measures group have bee performed for this patient

G8765 All quality actions for the applicable measures in the cataract measures group have been performed for this patient

G8767 Lipid panel results documented and reviewed (must include total cholesterol, HDL-c, triglycerides and calculated LDL-c)

G8768 Documentation of medical reason(s) for not performing lipid profile (e.g., patients with palliative goals or for whom treatment of hypertension with standard treatment goals is not clinically appropriate)

G8769 Lipid profile not performed; reason not given

G8770 Urine protein test result documented and reviewed

G8771 Documentation of diagnosis of chronic kidney disease

G8772 Documentation of medical reason(s) for not performing urine protein test (e.g., patients with palliative goals or for whom treatment of hypertension with standard treatment goals is not clinically appropriate)

G8773 Urine protein test was not performed, reason not given

G8774 Serum creatinine test result documented and reviewed

G8775 Documentation of medical reason(s) for not performing serum creatinine test (e.g., patients with palliative goals or for whom treatment of hypertension with standard treatment goals is not clinically appropriate)

G8776 Serum creatinine test not performed; reason not given

G8777 Diabetes screening test performed

G8778 Documentation of medical reason(s) for not performing diabetes screening test (e.g., patients with a diagnosis of diabetes, or with palliative goals or for whom treatment of hypertension with standard treatment goals is not clinically appropriate)

G8779 Diabetes screening test not performed; reason not given

G8780 Counseling for diet and physical activity performed

G8781 Documentation of medical reason(s) for patient not receiving counseling for diet and physical activity (e.g., patients with palliative goals or for whom treatment of hypertension with standard treatment goals is not clinically appropriate)

G8782 Counseling for diet and physical activity not performed reason not given

G8783 Normal blood pressure reading documented, follow-up not required

G8784 Patient not eligible (e.g., documentation the patient is not eligible due to active diagnosis of hypertension, patient refuses, urgent or emergent situation)

G8785 Blood pressure reading not documented, reason not given

G8797 Specimen site other than anatomic location of esophagus

G8798 Specimen site other than anatomic location of prostate

G8806 Performance of trans-abdominal or trans-vaginal ultrasound and pregnancy location documented

▲ **G8807** Trans-abdominal or trans-vaginal ultrasound not performed for reasons documented by clinician (e.g., patient has a documented intrauterine pregnancy [IUP])

G8808 Trans-abdominal or trans-vaginal ultrasound not performed; reason not given

G8809 Rh-immunoglobulin (RhoGAM) ordered

G8810 Rh-immunoglobulin (RhoGAM) not ordered for reasons documented by clinician (e.g., patient had prior documented receipt of RhoGAM within 12 weeks, patient refusal)

G8811 Documentation rh-immunoglobulin (RhoGAM) was not ordered, reason not given

G8815 Documented reason in the medical records for why the statin therapy was not prescribed (i.e., lower extremity bypass was for a patient with non-atherosclerotic disease)

G8816 Statin medication prescribed at discharge

(**G8818** Patient discharge to home no later than post-operative day #7
Code deleted effective 12/31/2023, no HCPCS/CPT cross-reference provided.)

G8818 Patient discharge to home no later than post-operative day #7

(**G8825** Patient not discharged to home by post-operative day #7
Code deleted effective 12/31/2023, no HCPCS/CPT cross-reference provided.)

G8826 Patient discharged to home no later than post-operative day #2 following EVAR

G8833 Patient not discharged to home by post-operative day #2 following EVAR

G8834 Patient discharged to home no later than post-operative day #2 following CEA

G8838 Patient not discharged to home by post-operative day #2 following CEA

G8839 Sleep apnea symptoms assessed, including presence or absence of snoring and daytime sleepiness

G8840 Documentation of reason(s) for not documenting an assessment of sleep symptoms (e.g., patient didn't have initial daytime sleepiness, patient visited between initial testing and initiation of therapy)

G8841 Sleep apnea symptoms not assessed; reason not given

G8842 Apnea hypopnea index (ahi), respiratory disturbance index (RDI) or respiratory event index (rei) documented or measured within 2 months of initial evaluation for suspected obstructive sleep apnea

G8843 Documentation of reason(s) for not measuring an apnea hypopnea index (ahi), a respiratory disturbance index (RDI), or a respiratory event index (rei) within 2 months of initial evaluation for suspected obstructive sleep apnea (e.g., medical, neurological, or psychiatric disease that prohibits successful completion of a sleep study, patients for whom a sleep study would present a bigger risk than benefit or would pose an undue burden, dementia, patients who decline ahi/RDI/rei measurement, patients who had a financial reason for not completing testing, test was ordered but not completed, patients decline because their insurance (payer) does not cover the expense))

G8844 Apnea hypopnea index (ahi), respiratory disturbance index (RDI), or respiratory event index (rei) not documented or measured within 2 months of initial evaluation for suspected obstructive sleep apnea, reason not given

G8845 Positive airway pressure therapy prescribed

G8846 Moderate or severe obstructive sleep apnea (apnea hypopnea index (ahi) or respiratory disturbance index (RDI) of 15 or greater)

G8848 Mild obstructive sleep apnea (apnea hypopnea index (ahi) or respiratory disturbance index (RDI) of less than 15)

G8849 Documentation of reason(s) for not prescribing positive airway pressure therapy (e.g., patient unable to tolerate, alternative therapies use, patient declined, financial, insurance coverage)

G8850 Positive airway pressure therapy not prescribed; reason not given

▲ **G8851** Adherence to therapy was assessed at least annually through an objective informatics system or through self-reporting (if objective reporting is not available, documented)

(**G8852** Positive airway pressure therapy was prescribed
Code deleted effective 12/31/2023, no HCPCS/CPT cross-reference provided.)

G8853 Positive airway pressure therapy not prescribed

▲ **G8854** Documentation of reason(s) for not objectively reporting adherence to evidence-based therapy (e.g., patients who have been diagnosed with a terminal or advanced disease with an expected life span of less than 6 months, patients who decline therapy, patients who do not return for follow-up at least annually, patients unable to access/afford therapy, patient's insurance will not cover therapy)

▲ **G8855** Adherence to therapy was not assessed at least annually through an objective informatics system or through self-reporting (if objective reporting is not available), reason not given

G8856 Referral to a physician for an otologic evaluation performed

G8857 Patient is not eligible for the referral for otologic evaluation measure (e.g., patients who are already under the care of a physician for acute or chronic dizziness)

G8858 Referral to a physician for an otologic evaluation not performed, reason not given

G8859 Patient receiving corticosteroids greater than or equal to 10mg/day for 60 or greater consecutive days

G8860 Patients who have received dose of corticosteroids greater than or equal to 10mg/day for 60 or greater consecutive days

G8861 Within the past 2 years, central dual-energy x-ray absorptiometry (DXA) ordered and documented, review of systems and medication history or pharmacologic therapy (other than minerals/vitamins) for osteoporosis prescribed

G8862 Patients not receiving corticosteroids greater than or equal to 10mg/day for 60 or greater consecutive days

G8863 Patients not assessed for risk of bone loss; reason not given

G - H CODES

G8864 Pneumococcal vaccine administered or previously received

G8865 Documentation of medical reason(s) for not administering or previously receiving pneumococcal vaccine (e.g., patient allergic reaction, potential adverse drug reaction)

G8866 Documentation of patient reason(s) for not administering or previously receiving pneumococcal vaccine (e.g., patient refusal)

G8867 Pneumococcal vaccine not administered or previously received; reason not given

G8868 Patients receiving a first course of anti-TNF therapy

G8869 Patient has documented immunity to hepatitis b and initiating anti-TNF therapy

G8870 Hepatitis b vaccine injection administered or previously received and is receiving a first course of anti-TNF therapy

G8871 Patient not receiving a first course of anti-TNF therapy

G8872 Excised tissue evaluated by imaging intraoperatively to confirm successful inclusion of targeted lesion

G8873 Patients with needle localization specimens which are not amenable to intraoperative imaging such as MRI needle wire localization, or targets which are tentatively identified on mammogram or ultrasound which do not contain a biopsy marker, but which can be verified on intraoperative inspection or pathology (e.g., needle biopsy site where the biopsy marker is remote from the actual biopsy site)

G8874 Excised tissue not evaluated by imaging intraoperatively to confirm successful inclusion of targeted lesion

G8875 Clinician diagnosed breast cancer preoperatively by a minimally invasive biopsy method

G8876 Documentation of reason(s) for not performing minimally invasive biopsy to diagnose breast cancer preoperatively (e.g., lesion too close to skin, implant, chest wall, etc., lesion could not be adequately visualized for needle biopsy, patient condition prevents needle biopsy [weight, breast thickness, etc.], duct excision without imaging abnormality, prophylactic mastectomy, reduction mammoplasty, excisional biopsy performed by another physician)

G8877 Clinician did not attempt to achieve the diagnosis of breast cancer preoperatively by a minimally invasive biopsy method, reason not given

G8878 Sentinel lymph node biopsy procedure performed

G8879 Clinically node negative (t1n0m0 or t2n0m0) invasive breast cancer

G8880 Documentation of reason(s) sentinel lymph node biopsy not performed (e.g., reasons could include but not limited to; non-invasive cancer, incidental discovery of breast cancer on prophylactic mastectomy, incidental discovery of breast cancer on reduction mammoplasty, pre-operative biopsy proven lymph node (ln) metastases, inflammatory carcinoma, stage 3 locally advanced cancer, recurrent invasive breast cancer, clinically node positive after neoadjuvant systemic therapy, patient refusal after informed consent, patient with significant age, comorbidities, or limited life expectancy and favorable tumor; adjuvant systemic therapy unlikely to change)

G8881 Stage of breast cancer is greater than t1n0m0 or t2n0m0

G8882 Sentinel lymph node biopsy procedure not performed; reason not given

(**G8883** Biopsy results reviewed, communicated, tracked and documented
Code deleted effective 12/31/2023, no HCPCS/CPT cross-reference provided.)

(**G8884** Clinician documented reason that patient's biopsy results were not reviewed
Code deleted effective 12/31/2023, no HCPCS/CPT cross-reference provided.)

(**G8885** Biopsy results not reviewed, communicated, tracked or documented
Code deleted effective 12/31/2023, no HCPCS/CPT cross-reference provided.)

G8886 Most recent blood pressure under control

G - H CODES

G8887 Documentation of medical reason(s) for most recent blood pressure not being under control (e.g., patients with palliative goals or for whom treatment of hypertension with standard treatment goals is not clinically appropriate)

G8888 Most recent blood pressure not under control, results documented and reviewed

G8889 No documentation of blood pressure measurement, reason not given

G8890 Most recent LDL-c under control, results documented and reviewed

G8891 Documentation of medical reason(s) for most recent LDL-c not under control (e.g., patients with palliative goals for whom treatment of hypertension with standard treatment goals is not clinically appropriate)

G8892 Documentation of medical reason(s) for not performing LDL-c test (e.g., patients with palliative goals or for whom treatment of hypertension with standard treatment goals is not clinically appropriate)

G8893 Most recent LDL-c not under control, results documented and reviewed

G8894 LDL-c not performed; reason not given

G8895 Oral aspirin or other antithrombotic therapy prescribed

G8896 Documentation of medical reason(s) for not prescribing oral aspirin or other antithrombotic therapy (e.g., patient documented to be low risk or patient with terminal illness or treatment of hypertension with standard treatment goals is not clinically appropriate, or for whom risk of aspirin or other antithrombotic therapy exceeds potential benefits such as for individuals whose blood pressure is poorly controlled)

G8897 Oral aspirin or other antithrombotic therapy was not prescribed, reason not given

G8898 I intend to report the chronic obstructive pulmonary disease (COPD) measures group

G8899 I intend to report the inflammatory bowel disease (IBD) measures group

G8900 I intend to report the sleep apnea measures group

G8902 I intend to report the dementia measures group

G8903 I intend to report the Parkinson's disease measures group

G8904 I intend to report the hypertension (HTN) measures group

G8905 I intend to report the cardiovascular prevention measures group

G8906 I intend to report the cataract measures group

G8907 Patient documented not to have experienced any of the following events: a burn prior to discharge; a fall within the facility; wrong site/side/patient/procedure/implant event; or a hospital transfer or hospital admission upon discharge from the facility

G8908 Patient documented to have received a burn prior to discharge

G8909 Patient documented not to have received a burn prior to discharge

G8910 Patient documented to have experienced a fall within ASC

G8911 Patient documented not to have experienced a fall within ambulatory surgical center

G8912 Patient documented to have experienced a wrong site, wrong side, wrong patient, wrong procedure or wrong implant event

G8913 Patient documented not to have experienced a wrong site, wrong side, wrong patient, wrong procedure or wrong implant event

G8914 Patient documented to have experienced a hospital transfer or hospital admission upon discharge from ASC

G8915 Patient documented not to have experienced a hospital transfer or hospital admission upon discharge from ASC

G8916 Patient with preoperative order for iv antibiotic surgical site infection (SSI) prophylaxis, antibiotic initiated on time

G8917 Patient with preoperative order for iv antibiotic surgical site infection (SSI) prophylaxis, antibiotic not initiated on time

G8918 Patient without preoperative order for iv antibiotic surgical site infection (SSI) prophylaxis

G8923 Left ventricular ejection fraction (LVEF) <= 40% or documentation of moderately or severely depressed left ventricular systolic function

▲ **G8924** Spirometry results documented (fev1/FVC < 70%)

G8925 Spirometry test results demonstrate fev1 >= 60% fev1/FVC >= 70%, predicted or patient does not have COPD symptoms

G8926 Spirometry test not performed or documented; reason not given

G8927 Adjuvant chemotherapy referred, prescribed or previously received for AJCC stage iii, colon cancer

G8928 Adjuvant chemotherapy not prescribed or previously received, for documented reasons (e.g., medical co-morbidities, diagnosis date more than 5 years prior to the current visit date, patient's diagnosis date is within 120 days of the end of the 12 month reporting period, patient's cancer has metastasized, medical contraindication/allergy, poor performance status, other medical reasons, patient refusal, other patient reasons, patient is currently enrolled in a clinical trial that precludes prescription of chemotherapy, other system reasons)

G8929 Adjuvant chemotherapy not prescribed or previously received; reason not given

G8930 Assessment of depression severity at the initial evaluation

G8931 Assessment of depression severity not documented; reason not given

G8932 Suicide risk assessed at the initial evaluation

G8933 Suicide risk not assessed at the initial evaluation; reason not given

G8934 Left ventricular ejection fraction (LVEF) <=40% or documentation of moderately or severely depressed left ventricular systolic function

G8935 Clinician prescribed angiotensin converting enzyme (ace) inhibitor or angiotensin receptor blocker (arb) therapy

▲ **G8936** Clinician documented that patient was not an eligible candidate for angiotensin converting enzyme (ace) inhibitor or angiotensin receptor blocker (arb) therapy (eg, allergy, intolerance, pregnancy, renal failure due to ace inhibitor, diseases of the aortic or mitral valve, other medical reasons) or (eg, patient declined, other patient reasons)

G8937 Clinician did not prescribe angiotensin converting enzyme (ace) inhibitor or angiotensin receptor blocker (arb) therapy, reason not given

G8938 BMI is documented as being outside of normal parameters, follow-up plan is not documented, documentation the patient is not eligible

G8939 Pain assessment documented as positive, follow-up plan not documented, documentation the patient is not eligible at the time of the encounter

G8940 Screening for depression documented as positive, a follow-up plan not completed, documented reason

(**G8941** Elder maltreatment screen documented as positive, follow-up plan not documented, documentation the patient is not eligible for follow-up plan at the time of the encounter
Code deleted effective 12/31/2023, no HCPCS/CPT cross-reference provided.)

▲ **G8942** Functional outcome assessment using a standardized tool is documented within the previous 30 days and a care plan, based on identified deficiencies is documented within two days of the functional outcome assessment

G - H CODES

G8943 LDL-c result not present or not within 12 months prior

G8944 AJCC melanoma cancer stage 0 through iic melanoma

G8946 Minimally invasive biopsy method attempted but not diagnostic of breast cancer (e.g., high risk lesion of breast such as atypical ductal hyperplasia, lobular neoplasia, atypical lobular hyperplasia, lobular carcinoma in situ, atypical columnar hyperplasia, flat epithelial atypia, radial scar, complex sclerosing lesion, papillary lesion, or any lesion with spindle cells)

G8947 One or more neuropsychiatric symptoms

G8948 No neuropsychiatric symptoms

G8949 Documentation of patient reason(s) for patient not receiving counseling for diet and physical activity (e.g., patient is not willing to discuss diet or exercise interventions to help control blood pressure, or the patient said he/she refused to make these changes)

G8950 Elevated or hypertensive blood pressure reading documented, and the indicated follow-up is documented

G8951 Pre-hypertensive or hypertensive blood pressure reading documented, indicated follow-up not documented, documentation the patient is not eligible

G8952 Elevated or hypertensive blood pressure reading documented, indicated follow-up not documented, reason not given

G8953 All quality actions for the applicable measures in the oncology measures group have been performed for this patient

G8955 Most recent assessment of adequacy of volume management documented

G8956 Patient receiving maintenance hemodialysis in an outpatient dialysis facility

G8957 Patient not receiving maintenance hemodialysis in an outpatient dialysis facility

G8958 Assessment of adequacy of volume management not documented reason not given

G8959 Clinician treating major depressive disorder communicates to clinician treating comorbid condition

G8960 Clinician treating major depressive disorder did not communicate to clinician treating comorbid condition, reason not given

G8961 Cardiac stress imaging test primarily performed on low-risk surgery patient for preoperative evaluation within 30 days preceding this surgery

G8962 Cardiac stress imaging test performed on patient for any reason including those who did not have low risk surgery or test that was performed more than 30 days preceding low risk surgery

(**G8963** Cardiac stress imaging performed primarily for monitoring of asymptomatic patient who had PCI within 2 years
Code deleted effective 12/31/2023, no HCPCS/CPT cross-reference provided.)

(**G8964** Cardiac stress imaging test performed primarily for any other reason than monitoring of asymptomatic patient who had PCI within 2 years (e.g., symptomatic patient, patient greater than 2 years since PCI, initial evaluation, etc)
Code deleted effective 12/31/2023, no HCPCS/CPT cross-reference provided.)

G8965 Cardiac stress imaging test primarily performed on low CHD risk patient for initial detection and risk assessment

G8966 Cardiac stress imaging test performed on symptomatic or higher than low CHD risk patient or for any reason other than initial detection and risk assessment

G8967 FDA approved oral anticoagulant is prescribed

▲ **G8968** Documentation of medical reason(s) for not prescribing an FDA-approved anticoagulant (e.g., present or planned atrial appendage occlusion or ligation or patient being currently enrolled in a clinical trial related to AF/atrial flutter treatment)

G8969 Documentation of patient reason(s) for not prescribing an oral anticoagulant that is FDA approved for the prevention of thromboembolism (e.g., patient preference for not receiving anticoagulation)

G - H CODES

G8970 No risk factors or one moderate risk factor for thromboembolism

G8971 Warfarin or another oral anticoagulant that is FDA approved not prescribed, reason not given

G8972 One or more high risk factors for thromboembolism or more than one moderate risk factor for thromboembolism

G8973 Most recent hemoglobin (Hgb) level < 10 g/dl

G8974 Hemoglobin level measurement not documented; reason not given

G8975 Documentation of medical reason(s) for patient having a hemoglobin level < 10 g/dl (e.g., patients who have non-renal etiologies of anemia [e.g., sickle cell anemia or other hemoglobinopathies, hypersplenism, primary bone marrow disease, anemia related to chemotherapy for diagnosis of malignancy, postoperative bleeding, active bloodstream or peritoneal infection], other medical reasons)

G8976 Most recent hemoglobin (Hgb) level >= 10 g/dl

G8977 I intend to report the oncology measures group

G8978 Mobility: walking & moving around functional limitation, current status, at therapy episode outset and at reporting intervals

G8979 Mobility: walking & moving around functional limitation, projected goal status, at therapy episode outset, at reporting intervals, and at discharge or to end reporting

G8980 Mobility: walking & moving around functional limitation, discharge status, at discharge from therapy or to end reporting

G8981 Changing & maintaining body position functional limitation, current status, at therapy episode outset and at reporting intervals

G8982 Changing & maintaining body position functional limitation, projected goal status, at therapy episode outset, at reporting intervals, and at discharge or to end reporting

G8983 Changing & maintaining body position functional limitation, discharge status, at discharge from therapy or to end reporting

G8984 Carrying, moving & handling objects functional limitation, current status, at therapy episode outset and at reporting intervals

G8985 Carrying, moving and handling objects, projected goal status, at therapy episode outset, at reporting intervals, and at discharge or to end reporting

G8986 Carrying, moving & handling objects functional limitation, discharge status, at discharge from therapy or to end reporting

G8987 Self care functional limitation, current status, at therapy episode outset and at reporting intervals

G8988 Self care functional limitation, projected goal status, at therapy episode outset, at reporting intervals, and at discharge or to end reporting

G8989 Self care functional limitation, discharge status, at discharge from therapy or to end reporting

G8990 Other physical or occupational therapy primary functional limitation, current status, at therapy episode outset and at reporting intervals

G8991 Other physical or occupational therapy primary functional limitation, projected goal status, at therapy episode outset, at reporting intervals, and at discharge or to end reporting

G8992 Other physical or occupational therapy primary functional limitation, discharge status, at discharge from therapy or to end reporting

G8993 Other physical or occupational therapy subsequent functional limitation, current status, at therapy episode outset and at reporting intervals

G8994 Other physical or occupational therapy subsequent functional limitation, projected goal status, at therapy episode outset, at reporting intervals, and at discharge or to end reporting

G8995 Other physical or occupational therapy subsequent functional limitation, discharge status, at discharge from therapy or to end reporting

G8996 Swallowing functional limitation, current status at therapy episode outset and at reporting intervals

G8997 Swallowing functional limitation, projected goal status, at therapy episode outset, at reporting intervals, and at discharge or to end reporting

G8998 Swallowing functional limitation, discharge status, at discharge from therapy or to end reporting

G8999 Motor speech functional limitation, current status at therapy episode outset and at reporting intervals

G9001 Coordinated care fee, initial rate

G9002 Coordinated care fee, maintenance rate

G9003 Coordinated care fee, risk adjusted high, initial

G9004 Coordinated care fee, risk adjusted low, initial

G9005 Coordinated care fee, risk adjusted maintenance

G9006 Coordinated care fee, home monitoring

G9007 Coordinated care fee, scheduled team conference

G9008 Coordinated care fee, physician coordinated care oversight services

G9009 Coordinated care fee, risk adjusted maintenance, level 3

G9010 Coordinated care fee, risk adjusted maintenance, level 4

G9011 Coordinated care fee, risk adjusted maintenance, level 5

G9012 Other specified case management service not elsewhere classified

G9013 ESRD demo basic bundle level I

G9014 ESRD demo expanded bundle including venous access and related services

G9016 Smoking cessation counseling, individual, in the absence of or in addition to any other evaluation and management service, per session (6-10 minutes) [demo project code only]

G9017 Amantadine hydrochloride, oral, per 100 mg (for use in a Medicare-approved demonstration project)

G9018 Zanamivir, inhalation powder, administered through inhaler, per 10 mg (for use in a Medicare-approved demonstration project)

G9019 Oseltamivir phosphate, oral, per 75 mg (for use in a Medicare-approved demonstration project)

G9020 Rimantadine hydrochloride, oral, per 100 mg (for use in a Medicare-approved demonstration project)

G9033 Amantadine hydrochloride, oral brand, per 100 mg (for use in a Medicare-approved demonstration project)

G9034 Zanamivir, inhalation powder, administered through inhaler, brand, per 10 mg (for use in a Medicare-approved demonstration project)

G9035 Oseltamivir phosphate, oral, brand, per 75 mg (for use in a Medicare-approved demonstration project)

G9036 Rimantadine hydrochloride, oral, brand, per 100 mg (for use in a Medicare-approved demonstration project)

G9050 Oncology; primary focus of visit; work-up, evaluation, or staging at the time of cancer diagnosis or recurrence (for use in a Medicare-approved demonstration project)

G9051 Oncology; primary focus of visit; treatment decision-making after disease is staged or restaged, discussion of treatment options, supervising/coordinating active cancer directed therapy or managing consequences of cancer directed therapy (for use in a Medicare-approved demonstration project)

G9052 Oncology; primary focus of visit; surveillance for disease recurrence for patient who has completed definitive cancer-directed therapy and currently lacks evidence of recurrent disease; cancer directed therapy might be considered in the future (for use in a Medicare-approved demonstration project)

G9053 Oncology; primary focus of visit; expectant management of patient with evidence of cancer for whom no cancer directed therapy is being administered or arranged at present; cancer directed therapy might be considered in the future (for use in a Medicare-approved demonstration project)

G9054 Oncology; primary focus of visit; supervising, coordinating or managing care of patient with terminal cancer or for whom other medical illness prevents further cancer treatment; includes symptom management, end-of-life care planning, management of palliative therapies (for use in a Medicare-approved demonstration project)

G9055 Oncology; primary focus of visit; other, unspecified service not otherwise listed (for use in a Medicare-approved demonstration project)

G9056 Oncology; practice guidelines; management adheres to guidelines (for use in a Medicare-approved demonstration project)

G9057 Oncology; practice guidelines; management differs from guidelines as a result of patient enrollment in an institutional review board approved clinical trial (for use in a Medicare-approved demonstration project)

G9058 Oncology; practice guidelines; management differs from guidelines because the treating physician disagrees with guideline recommendations (for use in a Medicare-approved demonstration project)

G9059 Oncology; practice guidelines; management differs from guidelines because the patient, after being offered treatment consistent with guidelines, has opted for alternative treatment or management, including no treatment (for use in a Medicare-approved demonstration project)

G9060 Oncology; practice guidelines; management differs from guidelines for reason(s) associated with patient comorbid illness or performance status not factored into guidelines (for use in a Medicare-approved demonstration project)

G9061 Oncology; practice guidelines; patient's condition not addressed by available guidelines (for use in a Medicare-approved demonstration project)

G9062 Oncology; practice guidelines; management differs from guidelines for other reason(s) not listed (for use in a Medicare-approved demonstration project)

G9063 Oncology; disease status; limited to non-small cell lung cancer; extent of disease initially established as stage I (prior to neo-adjuvant therapy, if any) with no evidence of disease progression, recurrence, or metastases (for use in a Medicare-approved demonstration project)

G9064 Oncology; disease status; limited to non-small cell lung cancer; extent of disease initially established as stage ii (prior to neo-adjuvant therapy, if any) with no evidence of disease progression, recurrence, or metastases (for use in a Medicare-approved demonstration project)

G9065 Oncology; disease status; limited to non-small cell lung cancer; extent of disease initially established as stage iii a (prior to neo-adjuvant therapy, if any) with no evidence of disease progression, recurrence, or metastases (for use in a Medicare-approved demonstration project)

G9066 Oncology; disease status; limited to non-small cell lung cancer; stage iii b- iv at diagnosis, metastatic, locally recurrent, or progressive (for use in a Medicare-approved demonstration project)

G9067 Oncology; disease status; limited to non-small cell lung cancer; extent of disease unknown, staging in progress, or not listed (for use in a Medicare-approved demonstration project)

G9068 Oncology; disease status; limited to small cell and combined small cell/non-small cell; extent of disease initially established as limited with no evidence of disease progression, recurrence, or metastases (for use in a Medicare-approved demonstration project)

G9069 Oncology; disease status; small cell lung cancer, limited to small cell and combined small cell/non-small cell; extensive stage at diagnosis, metastatic, locally recurrent, or progressive (for use in a Medicare-approved demonstration project)

G9070 Oncology; disease status; small cell lung cancer, limited to small cell and combined small cell/non-small; extent of disease unknown, staging in progress, or not listed (for use in a Medicare-approved demonstration project)

G9071 Oncology; disease status; invasive female breast cancer (does not include ductal carcinoma in situ); adenocarcinoma as predominant cell type; stage I or stage iia-iib; or t3, n1, m0; and er and/or pr positive; with no evidence of disease progression, recurrence, or metastases (for use in a Medicare-approved demonstration project)

G9072 Oncology; disease status; invasive female breast cancer (does not include ductal carcinoma in situ); adenocarcinoma as predominant cell type; stage I, or stage iia-iib; or t3, n1, m0; and er and pr negative; with no evidence of disease progression, recurrence, or metastases (for use in a Medicare-approved demonstration project)

G9073 Oncology; disease status; invasive female breast cancer (does not include ductal carcinoma in situ); adenocarcinoma as predominant cell type; stage iiia-iiib; and not t3, n1, m0; and er and/or pr positive; with no evidence of disease progression, recurrence, or metastases (for use in a Medicare-approved demonstration project)

G9074 Oncology; disease status; invasive female breast cancer (does not include ductal carcinoma in situ); adenocarcinoma as predominant cell type; stage iiia-iiib; and not t3, n1, m0; and er and pr negative; with no evidence of disease progression, recurrence, or metastases (for use in a Medicare-approved demonstration project)

G9075 Oncology; disease status; invasive female breast cancer (does not include ductal carcinoma in situ); adenocarcinoma as predominant cell type; m1 at diagnosis, metastatic, locally recurrent, or progressive (for use in a Medicare-approved demonstration project)

G9077 Oncology; disease status; prostate cancer, limited to adenocarcinoma as predominant cell type; t1-t2c and Gleason 2-7 and PSA < or equal to 20 at diagnosis with no evidence of disease progression, recurrence, or metastases (for use in a Medicare-approved demonstration project)

G9078 Oncology; disease status; prostate cancer, limited to adenocarcinoma as predominant cell type; t2 or t3a Gleason 8-10 or PSA > 20 at diagnosis with no evidence of disease progression, recurrence, or metastases (for use in a Medicare-approved demonstration project)

G9079 Oncology; disease status; prostate cancer, limited to adenocarcinoma as predominant cell type; t3b-t4, any n; any t, n1 at diagnosis with no evidence of disease progression, recurrence, or metastases (for use in a Medicare-approved demonstration project)

G9080 Oncology; disease status; prostate cancer, limited to adenocarcinoma; after initial treatment with rising PSA or failure of PSA decline (for use in a Medicare-approved demonstration project)

G9083 Oncology; disease status; prostate cancer, limited to adenocarcinoma; extent of disease unknown, staging in progress, or not listed (for use in a Medicare-approved demonstration project)

G9084 Oncology; disease status; colon cancer, limited to invasive cancer, adenocarcinoma as predominant cell type; extent of disease initially established as t1-3, n0, m0 with no evidence of disease progression, recurrence, or metastases (for use in a Medicare-approved demonstration project)

G9085 Oncology; disease status; colon cancer, limited to invasive cancer, adenocarcinoma as predominant cell type; extent of disease initially established as t4, n0, m0 with no evidence of disease progression, recurrence, or metastases (for use in a Medicare-approved demonstration project)

G9086 Oncology; disease status; colon cancer, limited to invasive cancer, adenocarcinoma as predominant cell type; extent of disease initially established as t1-4, n1-2, m0 with no evidence of disease progression, recurrence, or metastases (for use in a Medicare-approved demonstration project)

G9087 Oncology; disease status; colon cancer, limited to invasive cancer, adenocarcinoma as predominant cell type; m1 at diagnosis, metastatic, locally recurrent, or progressive with current clinical, radiologic, or biochemical evidence of disease (for use in a Medicare-approved demonstration project)

G9088 Oncology; disease status; colon cancer, limited to invasive cancer, adenocarcinoma as predominant cell type; m1 at diagnosis, metastatic, locally recurrent, or progressive without current clinical, radiologic, or biochemical evidence of disease (for use in a Medicare-approved demonstration project)

G9089 Oncology; disease status; colon cancer, limited to invasive cancer, adenocarcinoma as predominant cell type; extent of disease unknown, staging in progress, or not listed (for use in a Medicare-approved demonstration project)

G9090 Oncology; disease status; rectal cancer, limited to invasive cancer, adenocarcinoma as predominant cell type; extent of disease initially established as t1-2, n0, m0 (prior to neo-adjuvant therapy, if any) with no evidence of disease progression, recurrence, or metastases (for use in a Medicare-approved demonstration project)

G9091 Oncology; disease status; rectal cancer, limited to invasive cancer, adenocarcinoma as predominant cell type; extent of disease initially established as t3, n0, m0 (prior to neo-adjuvant therapy, if any) with no evidence of disease progression, recurrence, or metastases (for use in a Medicare-approved demonstration project)

G9092 Oncology; disease status; rectal cancer, limited to invasive cancer, adenocarcinoma as predominant cell type; extent of disease initially established as t1-3, n1-2, m0 (prior to neo-adjuvant therapy, if any) with no evidence of disease progression, recurrence or metastases (for use in a Medicare-approved demonstration project)

G9093 Oncology; disease status; rectal cancer, limited to invasive cancer, adenocarcinoma as predominant cell type; extent of disease initially established as t4, any n, m0 (prior to neo-adjuvant therapy, if any) with no evidence of disease progression, recurrence, or metastases (for use in a Medicare-approved demonstration project)

G9094 Oncology; disease status; rectal cancer, limited to invasive cancer, adenocarcinoma as predominant cell type; m1 at diagnosis, metastatic, locally recurrent, or progressive (for use in a Medicare-approved demonstration project)

G9095 Oncology; disease status; rectal cancer, limited to invasive cancer, adenocarcinoma as predominant cell type; extent of disease unknown, staging in progress, or not listed (for use in a Medicare-approved demonstration project)

G9096 Oncology; disease status; esophageal cancer, limited to adenocarcinoma or squamous cell carcinoma as predominant cell type; extent of disease initially established as t1-t3, n0-n1 or nx (prior to neo-adjuvant therapy, if any) with no evidence of disease progression, recurrence, or metastases (for use in a Medicare-approved demonstration project)

G9097 Oncology; disease status; esophageal cancer, limited to adenocarcinoma or squamous cell carcinoma as predominant cell type; extent of disease initially established as t4, any n, m0 (prior to neo-adjuvant therapy, if any) with no evidence of disease progression, recurrence, or metastases (for use in a Medicare-approved demonstration project)

G9098 Oncology; disease status; esophageal cancer, limited to adenocarcinoma or squamous cell carcinoma as predominant cell type; m1 at diagnosis, metastatic, locally recurrent, or progressive (for use in a Medicare-approved demonstration project)

G9099 Oncology; disease status; esophageal cancer, limited to adenocarcinoma or squamous cell carcinoma as predominant cell type; extent of disease unknown, staging in progress, or not listed (for use in a Medicare-approved demonstration project)

G9100 Oncology; disease status; gastric cancer, limited to adenocarcinoma as predominant cell type; post r0 resection (with or without neoadjuvant therapy) with no evidence of disease recurrence, progression, or metastases (for use in a Medicare-approved demonstration project)

G9101 Oncology; disease status; gastric cancer, limited to adenocarcinoma as predominant cell type; post r1 or r2 resection (with or without neoadjuvant therapy) with no evidence of disease progression, or metastases (for use in a Medicare-approved demonstration project)

G9102 Oncology; disease status; gastric cancer, limited to adenocarcinoma as predominant cell type; clinical or pathologic m0, unresectable with no evidence of disease progression, or metastases (for use in a Medicare-approved demonstration project)

G9103 Oncology; disease status; gastric cancer, limited to adenocarcinoma as predominant cell type;

clinical or pathologic m1 at diagnosis, metastatic, locally recurrent, or progressive (for use in a Medicare-approved demonstration project)

G9104 Oncology; disease status; gastric cancer, limited to adenocarcinoma as predominant cell type; extent of disease unknown, staging in progress, or not listed (for use in a Medicare-approved demonstration project)

G9105 Oncology; disease status; pancreatic cancer, limited to adenocarcinoma as predominant cell type; post r0 resection without evidence of disease progression, recurrence, or metastases (for use in a Medicare-approved demonstration project)

G9106 Oncology; disease status; pancreatic cancer, limited to adenocarcinoma; post r1 or r2 resection with no evidence of disease progression, or metastases (for use in a Medicare-approved demonstration project)

G9107 Oncology; disease status; pancreatic cancer, limited to adenocarcinoma; unresectable at diagnosis, m1 at diagnosis, metastatic, locally recurrent, or progressive (for use in a Medicare-approved demonstration project)

G9108 Oncology; disease status; pancreatic cancer, limited to adenocarcinoma; extent of disease unknown, staging in progress, or not listed (for use in a Medicare-approved demonstration project)

G9109 Oncology; disease status; head and neck cancer, limited to cancers of oral cavity, pharynx and larynx with squamous cell as predominant cell type; extent of disease initially established as t1-t2 and n0, m0 (prior to neo-adjuvant therapy, if any) with no evidence of disease progression, recurrence, or metastases (for use in a Medicare-approved demonstration project)

G9110 Oncology; disease status; head and neck cancer, limited to cancers of oral cavity, pharynx and larynx with squamous cell as predominant cell type; extent of disease initially established as t3-4 and/or n1-3, m0 (prior to neo-adjuvant therapy, if any) with no evidence of disease progression, recurrence, or metastases (for use in a Medicare-approved demonstration project)

G9111 Oncology; disease status; head and neck cancer, limited to cancers of oral cavity, pharynx and larynx with squamous cell as predominant cell type; m1 at diagnosis, metastatic, locally recurrent, or progressive (for use in a Medicare-approved demonstration project)

G9112 Oncology; disease status; head and neck cancer, limited to cancers of oral cavity, pharynx and larynx with squamous cell as predominant cell type; extent of disease unknown, staging in progress, or not listed (for use in a Medicare-approved demonstration project)

G9113 Oncology; disease status; ovarian cancer, limited to epithelial cancer; pathologic stage IA-b (grade 1) without evidence of disease progression, recurrence, or metastases (for use in a Medicare-approved demonstration project)

G9114 Oncology; disease status; ovarian cancer, limited to epithelial cancer; pathologic stage IA-b (grade 2-3); or stage ic (all grades); or stage ii; without evidence of disease progression, recurrence, or metastases (for use in a Medicare-approved demonstration project)

G9115 Oncology; disease status; ovarian cancer, limited to epithelial cancer; pathologic stage iii-iv; without evidence of progression, recurrence, or metastases (for use in a Medicare-approved demonstration project)

G9116 Oncology; disease status; ovarian cancer, limited to epithelial cancer; evidence of disease progression, or recurrence, and/or platinum resistance (for use in a Medicare-approved demonstration project)

G9117 Oncology; disease status; ovarian cancer, limited to epithelial cancer; extent of disease unknown, staging in progress, or not listed (for use in a Medicare-approved demonstration project)

G9123 Oncology; disease status; chronic myelogenous leukemia, limited to Philadelphia chromosome positive and/or bcr-abl positive; chronic phase not in hematologic, cytogenetic, or molecular remission (for use in a Medicare-approved demonstration project)

G9124 Oncology; disease status; chronic myelogenous leukemia, limited to Philadelphia chromosome positive and/or bcr-abl positive; accelerated phase not in hematologic cytogenetic, or molecular remission (for use in a Medicare-approved demonstration project)

G9125 Oncology; disease status; chronic myelogenous leukemia, limited to Philadelphia chromosome positive and/or bcr-abl positive; blast phase not in hematologic, cytogenetic, or molecular remission (for use in a Medicare-approved demonstration project)

G9126 Oncology; disease status; chronic myelogenous leukemia, limited to Philadelphia chromosome positive and/or bcr-abl positive; in hematologic, cytogenetic, or molecular remission (for use in a Medicare-approved demonstration project)

G9128 Oncology; disease status; limited to multiple myeloma, systemic disease; smoldering, stage I (for use in a Medicare-approved demonstration project)

G9129 Oncology; disease status; limited to multiple myeloma, systemic disease; stage ii or higher (for use in a Medicare-approved demonstration project)

G9130 Oncology; disease status; limited to multiple myeloma, systemic disease; extent of disease unknown, staging in progress, or not listed (for use in a Medicare-approved demonstration project)

G9131 Oncology; disease status; invasive female breast cancer (does not include ductal carcinoma in situ); adenocarcinoma as predominant cell type; extent of disease unknown, staging in progress, or not listed (for use in a Medicare-approved demonstration project)

G9132 Oncology; disease status; prostate cancer, limited to adenocarcinoma; hormone-refractory/androgen-independent (e.g., rising PSA on anti-androgen therapy or post-orchiectomy); clinical metastases (for use in a Medicare-approved demonstration project)

G9133 Oncology; disease status; prostate cancer, limited to adenocarcinoma; hormone-responsive; clinical metastases or m1 at diagnosis (for use in a Medicare-approved demonstration project)

G9134 Oncology; disease status; non-Hodgkin's lymphoma, any cellular classification; stage I, ii at diagnosis, not relapsed, not refractory (for use in a Medicare-approved demonstration project)

G9135 Oncology; disease status; non-Hodgkin's lymphoma, any cellular classification; stage iii, iv, not relapsed, not refractory (for use in a Medicare-approved demonstration project)

G9136 Oncology; disease status; non-Hodgkin's lymphoma, transformed from original cellular diagnosis to a second cellular classification (for use in a Medicare-approved demonstration project)

G9137 Oncology; disease status; non-Hodgkin's lymphoma, any cellular classification; relapsed/refractory (for use in a Medicare-approved demonstration project)

G9138 Oncology; disease status; non-Hodgkin's lymphoma, any cellular classification; diagnostic evaluation, stage not determined, evaluation of possible relapse or non-response to therapy, or not listed (for use in a Medicare-approved demonstration project)

G9139 Oncology; disease status; chronic myelogenous leukemia, limited to Philadelphia chromosome positive and/or bcr-abl positive; extent of disease unknown, staging in progress, not listed (for use in a Medicare-approved demonstration project)

G9140 Frontier extended stay clinic demonstration; for a patient stay in a clinic approved for the CMS demonstration project; the following measures should be present: the stay must be equal to or greater than 4 hours; weather or other conditions must prevent transfer or the case falls into a category of monitoring and observation cases that are permitted by the rules of the demonstration; there is a maximum frontier extended stay clinic (fesc) visit of 48 hours, except in the case when weather or other conditions prevent transfer; payment is made on each period up to 4 hours, after the first 4 hours

G9143 Warfarin responsiveness testing by genetic technique using any method, any number of specimen(s)

G9147 Outpatient intravenous insulin treatment (oivit) either pulsatile or continuous, by any means, guided by the results of measurements for: respiratory quotient; and/or, urine urea nitrogen (uun); and/or, arterial, venous or capillary glucose; and/or potassium concentration

G9148 National committee for quality assurance - level 1 medical home

G9149 National committee for quality assurance - level 2 medical home

G9150 National committee for quality assurance - level 3 medical home

G9151 Mapcp demonstration - state provided services

G9152 Mapcp demonstration - community health teams

G9153 Mapcp demonstration - physician incentive pool

G9156 Evaluation for wheelchair requiring face to face visit with physician

G9157 Transesophageal doppler measurement of cardiac output (including probe placement, image acquisition, and interpretation per course of treatment) for monitoring purposes

G9158 Motor speech functional limitation, discharge status, at discharge from therapy or to end reporting

G9159 Spoken language comprehension functional limitation, current status at therapy episode outset and at reporting intervals

G9160 Spoken language comprehension functional limitation, projected goal status at therapy episode outset, at reporting intervals, and at discharge or to end reporting

G9161 Spoken language comprehension functional limitation, discharge status, at discharge from therapy or to end reporting

G9162 Spoken language expression functional limitation, current status at therapy episode outset and at reporting intervals

G9163 Spoken language expression functional limitation, projected goal status at therapy episode outset, at reporting intervals, and at discharge or to end reporting

G9164 Spoken language expression functional limitation, discharge status at discharge from therapy or to end reporting

G9165 Attention functional limitation, current status at therapy episode outset and at reporting intervals

G9166 Attention functional limitation, projected goal status at therapy episode outset, at reporting intervals, and at discharge or to end reporting

G9167 Attention functional limitation, discharge status at discharge from therapy or to end reporting

G9168 Memory functional limitation, current status at therapy episode outset and at reporting intervals

G9169 Memory functional limitation, projected goal status at therapy episode outset, at reporting intervals, and at discharge or to end reporting

G9170 Memory functional limitation, discharge status at discharge from therapy or to end reporting

G9171 Voice functional limitation, current status at therapy episode outset and at reporting intervals

G9172 Voice functional limitation, projected goal status at therapy episode outset, at reporting intervals, and at discharge or to end reporting

G9173 Voice functional limitation, discharge status at discharge from therapy or to end reporting

G9174 Other speech language pathology functional limitation, current status at therapy episode outset and at reporting intervals

G9175 Other speech language pathology functional limitation, projected goal status at therapy episode outset, at reporting intervals, and at discharge or to end reporting

G9176 Other speech language pathology functional limitation, discharge status at discharge from therapy or to end reporting

G9186 Motor speech functional limitation, projected goal status at therapy episode outset, at reporting intervals, and at discharge or to end reporting

G9187 Bundled payments for care improvement initiative home visit for patient assessment performed by a qualified health care professional for individuals not considered homebound including, but not limited to, assessment of safety, falls, clinical status, fluid status, medication reconciliation/ management, patient compliance with orders/plan of care, performance of activities of daily living, appropriateness of care setting; (for use only in the Medicare-approved bundled payments for care improvement initiative); may not be billed for a 30-day period covered by a transitional care management code

G9188 Beta-blocker therapy not prescribed; reason not given

G9189 Beta-blocker therapy prescribed or currently being taken

G9190 Documentation of medical reason(s) for not prescribing beta-blocker therapy (e.g., allergy, intolerance, other medical reasons)

G9191 Documentation of patient reason(s) for not prescribing beta-blocker therapy (e.g., patient declined, other patient reasons)

(**G9192** Documentation of system reason(s) for not prescribing beta-blocker therapy (eg, other reasons attributable to the health care system)
Code deleted effective 12/31/2023, no HCPCS/CPT cross-reference provided.)

G9193 Clinician documented that patient with a diagnosis of major depression was not an eligible candidate for antidepressant medication treatment or patient did not have a diagnosis of major depression

G9194 Patient with a diagnosis of major depression documented as being treated with antidepressant medication during the entire 180 day (6 month) continuation treatment phase

G9195 Patient with a diagnosis of major depression not documented as being treated with antidepressant medication during the entire 180 day (6 months) continuation treatment phase

(**G9196** Documentation of medical reason(s) for not ordering a first or second generation cephalosporin for antimicrobial prophylaxis (e.g., patients enrolled in clinical trials, patients with documented infection prior to surgical procedure of interest, patients who were receiving antibiotics more than 24 hours prior to surgery [except colon surgery patients taking oral prophylactic antibiotics], patients who were receiving antibiotics within 24 hours prior to arrival [except colon surgery patients taking oral prophylactic antibiotics], other medical reason(s))
Code deleted effective 12/31/2022, no HCPCS/CPT cross-reference provided.)

(**G9197** Documentation of order for first or second generation cephalosporin for antimicrobial prophylaxis
Code deleted effective 12/31/2022, no HCPCS/CPT cross-reference provided.)

(**G9198** Order for first or second generation cephalosporin for antimicrobial prophylaxis was not documented, reason not given
Code deleted effective 12/31/2022, no HCPCS/CPT cross-reference provided.)

G9199 Venous thromboembolism (VTE) prophylaxis did not administer the day of or the day after hospital admission for documented reasons (e.g., patient is ambulatory, patient expired during inpatient stay, patient already on warfarin or another anticoagulant, other medical reason(s) or e.g., patient left against medical advice, other patient reason(s))

G9200 Venous thromboembolism (VTE) prophylaxis was not administered the day of or the day after hospital admission, reason not given

G9201 Venous thromboembolism (VTE) prophylaxis administered the day of or the day after hospital admission

G9202 Patients with a positive hepatitis c antibody test

G9203 RNA testing for hepatitis c documented as performed within 12 months prior to initiation of antiviral treatment for hepatitis c

G9204 RNA testing for hepatitis c was not documented as performed within 12 months prior to initiation of antiviral treatment for hepatitis c, reason not given

G9205 Patient starting antiviral treatment for hepatitis c during the measurement period

G9206 Patient starting antiviral treatment for hepatitis c during the measurement period

G9207 Hepatitis c genotype testing documented as performed within 12 months prior to initiation of antiviral treatment for hepatitis c

G9208 Hepatitis c genotype testing was not documented as performed within 12 months prior to initiation of antiviral treatment for hepatitis c, reason not given

G9209 Hepatitis c quantitative RNA testing documented as performed between 4-12 weeks after the initiation of antiviral treatment

G9210 Hepatitis c quantitative RNA testing not performed between 4-12 weeks after the initiation of antiviral treatment for documented reason(s) (e.g., patients whose treatment was discontinued during the testing period prior to testing, other medical reasons, patient declined, other patient reasons)

G9211 Hepatitis c quantitative RNA testing was not documented as performed between 4-12 weeks after the initiation of antiviral treatment, reason not given

G9212 Dsm-ivtm criteria for major depressive disorder documented at the initial evaluation

G9213 DSM-iv-tr criteria for major depressive disorder not documented at the initial evaluation, reason not otherwise specified

G9214 Cd4+ cell count or cd4+ cell percentage results documented

G9215 Cd4+ cell count, or percentage not documented as performed, reason not given

G9216 PCP prophylaxis was not prescribed at time of diagnosis of HIV, reason not given

G9217 PCP prophylaxis was not prescribed within 3 months of low cd4+ cell count below 200 cells/mm3, reason not given

G9218 PCP prophylaxis was not prescribed within 3 months of low cd4+ cell count below 500 cells/mm3 or a cd4 percentage below 15%, reason not given

G9219 Pneumocystis jiroveci pneumonia prophylaxis not prescribed within 3 months of low cd4+ cell count below 200 cells/mm3 for medical reason (i.e., patient's cd4+ cell count above threshold within 3 months after cd4+ cell count below threshold, indicating that the patient's cd4+ levels are within an acceptable range and the patient does not require PCP prophylaxis)

G9220 Pneumocystis jiroveci pneumonia prophylaxis not prescribed within 3 months of low cd4+ cell count below 500 cells/mm3 or a cd4 percentage below 15% for medical reason (i.e., patient's cd4+ cell count above threshold within 3 months after cd4+ cell count below threshold, indicating that the patient's cd4+ levels are within an acceptable range and the patient does not require PCP prophylaxis)

G9221 Pneumocystis jiroveci pneumonia prophylaxis prescribed

G9222 Pneumocystis jiroveci pneumonia prophylaxis prescribed within 3 months of low cd4+ cell count below 200 cells/mm3

G9223 Pneumocystis jiroveci pneumonia prophylaxis prescribed within 3 months of low cd4+ cell count below 500 cells/mm3 or a cd4 percentage below 15%

G9224 Documentation of medical reason for not performing foot exam (e.g., patient with bilateral foot/leg amputation)

G9225 Foot exam was not performed, reason not given

G9226 Foot examination performed (includes examination through visual inspection, sensory exam with 10-g monofilament plus testing any one of the following: vibration using 128-hz tuning fork, pinprick sensation, ankle reflexes, or vibration perception threshold, and pulse exam; report when all of the 3 components are completed)

G9227 Functional outcome assessment documented, care plan not documented, documentation the patient is not eligible for a care plan at the time of the encounter

G9228 Chlamydia, gonorrhea and syphilis screening results documented (report when results are present for all of the 3 screenings)

(**G9229** Chlamydia, gonorrhea, and syphilis screening results not documented (patient refusal is the only allowed exception)

Code deleted effective 12/31/2023, no HCPCS/CPT cross-reference provided.)

G - H CODES

G9230 Chlamydia, gonorrhea, and syphilis not screened; reason not given

G9231 Documentation of end stage renal disease (ESRD), dialysis, renal transplant before or during the measurement period or pregnancy during the measurement period

G9232 Clinician treating major depressive disorder did not communicate to clinician treating comorbid condition for specified patient reason (e.g., patient is unable to communicate the diagnosis of a comorbid condition; the patient is unwilling to communicate the diagnosis of a comorbid condition; or the patient is unaware of the comorbid condition, or any other specified patient reason)

G9233 All quality actions for the applicable measures in the total knee replacement measures group have been performed for this patient

G9234 I intend to report the total knee replacement measures group

G9235 All quality actions for the applicable measures in the general surgery measures group have been performed for this patient

G9236 All quality actions for the applicable measures in the optimizing patient exposure to ionizing radiation measures group have been performed for this patient

G9237 I intend to report the general surgery measures group

G9238 I intend to report the optimizing patient exposure to ionizing radiation measures group

G9239 Documentation of reasons for patient initiating maintenance hemodialysis with a catheter as the mode of vascular access (e.g., patient has a maturing arteriovenous fistula (AVF)/arteriovenous graft (avg), time-limited trial of hemodialysis, other medical reasons, patient declined AVF/avg, other patient reasons, patient followed by reporting nephrologist for fewer than 90 days, other system reasons)

G9240 Patient whose mode of vascular access is a catheter at the time maintenance hemodialysis is initiated

G9241 Patient whose mode of vascular access is not a catheter at the time maintenance hemodialysis is initiated

G9242 Documentation of viral load equal to or greater than 200 copies/ml or viral load not performed

G9243 Documentation of viral load less than 200 copies/ml

G9244 Antiretroviral therapy not prescribed

G9245 Antiretroviral therapy prescribed

G9246 Patient did not have at least one medical visit in each 6 month period of the 24 month measurement period, with a minimum of 60 days between medical visits

G9247 Patient had at least one medical visit in each 6 month period of the 24 month measurement period, with a minimum of 60 days between medical visits

G9248 Patient did not have a medical visit in the last 6 months

G9249 Patient had a medical visit in the last 6 months

(G9250 Documentation of patient pain brought to a comfortable level within 48 hours from initial assessment
Code deleted effective 12/31/2022, no HCPCS/CPT cross-reference provided.)

(G9251 Documentation of patient with pain not brought to a comfortable level within 48 hours from initial assessment
Code deleted effective 12/31/2022, no HCPCS/CPT cross-reference provided.)

G9252 Adenoma(s) or other neoplasm detected during screening colonoscopy

G9253 Adenoma(s) or other neoplasm not detected during screening colonoscopy

G9254 Documentation of patient discharged to home later than post-operative day 2 following case

G9255 Documentation of patient discharged to home no later than post operative day 2 following case

G - H CODES

G9256 Documentation of patient death following case

G9257 Documentation of patient stroke following case

G9258 Documentation of patient stroke following CEA

G9259 Documentation of patient survival and absence of stroke following case

G9260 Documentation of patient death following CEA

G9261 Documentation of patient survival and absence of stroke following CEA

G9262 Documentation of patient death in the hospital following endovascular AAA repair

G9263 Documentation of patient discharged alive following endovascular AAA repair

G9264 Documentation of patient receiving maintenance hemodialysis for greater than or equal to 90 days with a catheter for documented reasons (e.g., other medical reasons, patient declined arteriovenous fistula (AVF)/arteriovenous graft (avg), other patient reasons)

G9265 Patient receiving maintenance hemodialysis for greater than or equal to 90 days with a catheter as the mode of vascular access

G9266 Patient receiving maintenance hemodialysis for greater than or equal to 90 days without a catheter as the mode of vascular access

G9267 Documentation of patient with one or more complications or mortality within 30 days

G9268 Documentation of patient with one or more complications within 90 days

G9269 Documentation of patient without one or more complications and without mortality within 30 days

G9270 Documentation of patient without one or more complications within 90 days

G9271 LDL value < 100

G9272 LDL value >= 100

G9273 Blood pressure has a systolic value of < 140 and a diastolic value of < 90

G9274 Blood pressure has a systolic value of =140 and a diastolic value of = 90 or systolic value < 140 and diastolic value = 90 or systolic value = 140 and diastolic value < 90

G9275 Documentation that patient is a current non-tobacco user

G9276 Documentation that patient is a current tobacco user

G9277 Documentation that the patient is on daily aspirin or anti-platelet or has documentation of a valid contraindication or exception to aspirin/anti-platelet; contraindications/exceptions include anti-coagulant use, allergy to aspirin or anti-platelets, history of gastrointestinal bleed and bleeding disorder; additionally, the following exceptions documented by the physician as a reason for not taking daily aspirin or anti-platelet are acceptable (use of non-steroidal anti-inflammatory agents, documented risk for drug interaction, uncontrolled hypertension defined as >180 systolic or >110 diastolic or gastroesophageal reflux)

G9278 Documentation that the patient is not on daily aspirin or anti-platelet regimen

G9279 Pneumococcal screening performed and documentation of vaccination received prior to discharge

G9280 Pneumococcal vaccination not administered prior to discharge; reason not specified

G9281 Screening performed and documentation that vaccination not indicated/patient refusal

G9282 Documentation of medical reason(s) for not reporting the histological type or NSCLC-nos classification with an explanation (e.g., biopsy taken for other purposes in a patient with a history of non-small cell lung cancer or other documented medical reasons)

G9283 Non small cell lung cancer biopsy and cytology specimen report documents classification into specific histologic type or classified as NSCLC-nos with an explanation

G9284 Non small cell lung cancer biopsy and cytology specimen report does not document classification into specific histologic type or classified as NSCLC-nos with an explanation

G9285 Specimen site other than anatomic location of lung or is not classified as non small cell lung cancer

G9286 Antibiotic regimen prescribed within 10 days after onset of symptoms

G9287 Antibiotic regimen not prescribed within 10 days after onset of symptoms

G9288 Documentation of medical reason(s) for not reporting the histological type or NSCLC-nos classification with an explanation (e.g., a solitary fibrous tumor in a person with a history of non-small cell carcinoma or other documented medical reasons)

G9289 Non small cell lung cancer biopsy and cytology specimen report documents classification into specific histologic type or classified as NSCLC-nos with an explanation

G9290 Non small cell lung cancer biopsy and cytology specimen report does not document classification into specific histologic type or classified as NSCLC-nos with an explanation

G9291 Specimen site other than anatomic location of lung, is not classified as non small cell lung cancer or classified as NSCLC-nos

G9292 Documentation of medical reason(s) for not reporting pt category and a statement on thickness and ulceration and for pt1, mitotic rate (e.g., negative skin biopsies in a patient with a history of melanoma or other documented medical reasons)

G9293 Pathology report does not include the pt category and a statement on thickness and ulceration and for pt1, mitotic rate

G9294 Pathology report includes the pt category and a statement on thickness and ulceration and for pt1, mitotic rate

G9295 Specimen site other than anatomic cutaneous location

G9296 Patients with documented shared decision-making including discussion of conservative (non-surgical) therapy (e.g., NSAIDs, analgesics, weight loss, exercise, injections) prior to the procedure

G9297 Shared decision-making including discussion of conservative (non-surgical) therapy (e.g., NSAIDs, analgesics, weight loss, exercise, injections) prior to the procedure, not documented, reason not given

G9298 Patients who are evaluated for venous thromboembolic and cardiovascular risk factors within 30 days prior to the procedure (e.g., history of DVT, pe, mi, arrhythmia and stroke)

G9299 Patients who are not evaluated for venous thromboembolic and cardiovascular risk factors within 30 days prior to the procedure (e.g., history of DVT, pe, mi, arrhythmia and stroke, reason not given)

G9300 Documentation of medical reason(s) for not completely infusing the prophylactic antibiotic prior to the inflation of the proximal tourniquet (e.g., a tourniquet was not used)

G9301 Patients who had the prophylactic antibiotic completely infused prior to the inflation of the proximal tourniquet

G9302 Prophylactic antibiotic not completely infused prior to the inflation of the proximal tourniquet; reason not given

G9303 Operative report does not identify the prosthetic implant specifications including the prosthetic implant manufacturer, the brand name of the prosthetic implant and the size of each prosthetic implant, reason not given

G9304 Operative report identifies the prosthetic implant specifications including the prosthetic implant manufacturer, the brand name of the prosthetic implant and the size of each prosthetic implant

G9305 Intervention for presence of leak of endoluminal contents through an anastomosis not required

G9306 Intervention for presence of leak of endoluminal contents through an anastomosis required

G9307 No return to the operating room for a surgical procedure, for complications of the principal operative procedure, within 30 days of the principal operative procedure

G9308 Unplanned return to the operating room for a surgical procedure, for complications of the principal operative procedure, within 30 days of the principal operative procedure

G9309 No unplanned hospital readmission within 30 days of principal procedure

G9310 Unplanned hospital readmission within 30 days of principal procedure

G9311 No surgical site infection

G9312 Surgical site infection

G9313 Amoxicillin, with or without clavulanate, not prescribed as first line antibiotic at the time of diagnosis for documented reason

G9314 Amoxicillin, with or without clavulanate, not prescribed as first line antibiotic at the time of diagnosis, reason not given

G9315 Amoxicillin, with or without clavulanate, prescribed as a first line antibiotic at the time of diagnosis

G9316 Documentation of patient-specific risk assessment with a risk calculator based on multi-institutional clinical data, the specific risk calculator used, and communication of risk assessment from risk calculator with the patient or family

G9317 Documentation of patient-specific risk assessment with a risk calculator based on multi-institutional clinical data, the specific risk calculator used, and communication of risk assessment from risk calculator with the patient or family not completed

G9318 Imaging study named according to standardized nomenclature

G9319 Imaging study not named according to standardized nomenclature; reason not given

G9320 Documentation of medical reason(s) for not naming CT studies according to a standardized nomenclature provided (e.g., CT studies performed for radiation treatment planning or image-guided radiation treatment delivery)

G9321 Count of previous CT (any type of CT) and cardiac nuclear medicine (myocardial perfusion) studies documented in the 12-month period prior to the current study

G9322 Count of previous CT and cardiac nuclear medicine (myocardial perfusion) studies not documented in the 12-month period prior to the current study, reason not given

G9323 Documentation of medical reason(s) for not counting previous CT and cardiac nuclear medicine (myocardial perfusion) studies (e.g., CT studies performed for radiation treatment planning or image-guided radiation treatment delivery)

G9324 All necessary data elements not included; reason not given

G9325 CT studies not reported to a radiation dose index registry due to medical reasons (e.g., CT studies performed for radiation treatment planning or image-guided radiation treatment delivery)

G9326 CT studies performed not reported to a radiation dose index registry that is capable of collecting at a minimum all necessary data elements, reason not given

G9327 CT studies performed reported to a radiation dose index registry that is capable of collecting at a minimum all necessary data elements

G9328 DICOM format image data availability not documented in final report due to medical reasons (e.g., CT studies performed for radiation treatment planning or image-guided radiation treatment delivery)

G9329 DICOM format image data available to non-affiliated external healthcare facilities or entities on a secure, media free, reciprocally searchable basis with patient authorization for at least a 12-month period after the study not documented in final report, reason not given

G9340 Final report documented that DICOM format image data available to non-affiliated external healthcare facilities or entities on a secure, media free, reciprocally searchable basis with patient authorization for at least a 12-month period after the study

G9341 Search conducted for prior patient CT studies completed at non-affiliated external healthcare facilities or entities within the past 12-months and are available through a secure, authorized, media-free, shared archive prior to an imaging study being performed

G9342 Search not conducted prior to an imaging study being performed for prior patient CT studies completed at non-affiliated external healthcare facilities or entities within the past 12-months and are available through a secure, authorized, media-free, shared archive, reason not given

G9343 Due to medical reasons, search not conducted for DICOM format images for prior patient CT imaging studies completed at non-affiliated external healthcare facilities or entities within the past 12 months that are available through a secure, authorized, media-free, shared archive (e.g., CT studies performed for radiation treatment planning or image-guided radiation treatment delivery)

G9344 Due to system reasons search not conducted for DICOM format images for prior patient CT imaging studies completed at non-affiliated external healthcare facilities or entities within the past 12 months that are available through a secure, authorized, media-free, shared archive (e.g., non-affiliated external healthcare facilities or entities does not have archival abilities through a shared archival system)

G9345 Follow-up recommendations documented according to recommended guidelines for incidentally detected pulmonary nodules (e.g., follow-up CT imaging studies needed or that no follow-up is needed) based at a minimum on nodule size and patient risk factors

G9346 Follow-up recommendations not documented according to recommended guidelines for incidentally detected pulmonary nodules due to medical reasons (e.g., patients with known malignant disease, patients with unexplained fever, CT studies performed for radiation treatment planning or image-guided radiation treatment delivery)

G9347 Follow-up recommendations not documented according to recommended guidelines for incidentally detected pulmonary nodules, reason not given

G9348 CT scan of the paranasal sinuses ordered at the time of diagnosis for documented reasons

G9349 CT scan of the paranasal sinuses ordered at the time of diagnosis or received within 28 days after date of diagnosis

G9350 CT scan of the paranasal sinuses not ordered at the time of diagnosis or received within 28 days after date of diagnosis

G9351 More than one CT scan of the paranasal sinuses ordered or received within 90 days after diagnosis

G9352 More than one CT scan of the paranasal sinuses ordered or received within 90 days after the date of diagnosis, reason not given

G9353 More than one CT scan of the paranasal sinuses ordered or received within 90 days after the date of diagnosis for documented reasons (e.g., patients with complications, second CT obtained prior to surgery, other medical reasons)

G9354 One CT scan or no CT scan of the paranasal sinuses ordered within 90 days after the date of diagnosis

G9355 Elective delivery (without medical indication) by cesarean birth or induction of labor not performed (< 39 weeks of gestation)

G9356 Elective delivery (without medical indication) by cesarean birth or induction of labor performed (< 39 weeks of gestation)

G9357 Post-partum screenings, evaluations and education performed

G9358 Post-partum screenings, evaluations and education not performed

(G9359 Documentation of negative or managed positive tb screen with further evidence that tb is not active prior to treatment with a biologic immune response modifier

Code deleted effective 12/31/2022, no HCPCS/CPT cross-reference provided.)

(G9360 No documentation of negative or managed positive tb screen

Code deleted effective 12/31/2022, no HCPCS/CPT cross-reference provided.)

G9361 Medical indication for delivery by cesarean birth or induction of labor (<39 weeks of gestation) [documentation of reason(s) for elective delivery (e.g., hemorrhage and placental complications, hypertension, preeclampsia and eclampsia, rupture of membranes (premature or prolonged), maternal conditions complicating pregnancy/delivery, fetal conditions complicating pregnancy/delivery, late pregnancy, prior uterine surgery, or participation in clinical trial)]

G9362 Duration of monitored anesthesia care (mac) or peripheral nerve block (pnb) without the use of general anesthesia during an applicable procedure 60 minutes or longer, as documented in the anesthesia record

G9363 Duration of monitored anesthesia care (mac) or peripheral nerve block (pnb) without the use of general anesthesia during an applicable procedure or general or neuraxial anesthesia less than 60 minutes, as documented in the anesthesia record

G9364 Sinusitis caused by, or presumed to be caused by, bacterial infection

G9365 One high-risk medication ordered

G9366 One high-risk medication not ordered

G9367 At least two orders for high-risk medications from the same drug class

G9368 At least two orders for high-risk medications from the same drug class not ordered

G9369 Individual filled at least two prescriptions for any antipsychotic medication and had a PDC of 0.8 or greater

G9370 Individual who did not fill at least two prescriptions for any antipsychotic medication or did not have a PDC of 0.8 or greater

G9376 Patient continued to have the retina attached at the 6 months follow up visit (+/- 1 month) following only one surgery

G9377 Patient did not have the retina attached after 6 months following only one surgery

G9378 Patient continued to have the retina attached at the 6 months follow up visit (+/- 1 month)

G9379 Patient did not achieve flat retinas six months post surgery

▲ **G9380** Patient offered assistance with end of life issues or existing end of life plan was reviewed or updated during the measurement period

G9381 Documentation of medical reason(s) for not offering assistance with end of life issues (e.g., patient in hospice care, patient in terminal phase) during the measurement period

▲ **G9382** Patient not offered assistance with end of life issues or existing end of life plan was not reviewed or updated during the measurement period

G9383 Patient received screening for HCV infection within the 12 month reporting period

G9384 Documentation of medical reason(s) for not receiving annual screening for HCV infection (e.g., decompensated cirrhosis indicating advanced disease [i.e., ascites, esophageal variceal bleeding, hepatic encephalopathy], hepatocellular carcinoma, waitlist for organ transplant, limited life expectancy, other medical reasons)

G9385 Documentation of patient reason(s) for not receiving annual screening for HCV infection (e.g., patient declined, other patient reasons)

G9386 Screening for HCV infection not received within the 12 month reporting period, reason not given

G9389 Unplanned rupture of the posterior capsule requiring vitrectomy during cataract surgery

G9390 No unplanned rupture of the posterior capsule requiring vitrectomy during cataract surgery

G9391 Patient achieves refraction +-1 d for the eye that underwent cataract surgery, measured at the one month follow up visit

G9392 Patient does not achieve refraction +-1 d for the eye that underwent cataract surgery, measured at the one month follow up visit

G9393 Patient with an initial phq-9 score greater than nine who achieves remission at twelve months as demonstrated by a twelve month (+/- 30 days) phq-9 score of less than five

G - H CODES

G9394 Patient who had a diagnosis of bipolar disorder or personality disorder, death, permanent nursing home resident or receiving hospice or palliative care any time during the measurement or assessment period

G9395 Patient with an initial phq-9 score greater than nine who did not achieve remission at twelve months as demonstrated by a twelve month (+/- 30 days) phq-9 score greater than or equal to five

G9396 Patient with an initial phq-9 score greater than nine who was not assessed for remission at twelve months (+/- 30 days)

G9399 Documentation in the patient record of a discussion between the physician/clinician and the patient that includes all of the following: treatment choices appropriate to genotype, risks and benefits, evidence of effectiveness, and patient preferences toward the outcome of the treatment

G9400 Documentation of medical or patient reason(s) for not discussing treatment options; medical reasons: patient is not a candidate for treatment due to advanced physical or mental health comorbidity (including active substance use); currently receiving antiviral treatment; successful antiviral treatment (with sustained virologic response) prior to reporting period; other documented medical reasons; patient reasons: patient unable or unwilling to participate in the discussion or other patient reasons

G9401 No documentation in the patient record of a discussion between the physician or other qualified healthcare professional and the patient that includes all of the following: treatment choices appropriate to genotype, risks and benefits, evidence of effectiveness, and patient preferences toward treatment

G9402 Patient received follow-up within 30 days after discharge

G9403 Clinician documented reason patient was not able to complete 30 day follow-up from acute inpatient setting discharge (e.g., patient death prior to follow-up visit, patient non-compliant for visit follow-up)

G9404 Patient did not receive follow-up within 30 days after discharge

G9405 Patient received follow-up within 7 days after discharge

G9406 Clinician documented reason patient was not able to complete 7 day follow-up from acute inpatient setting discharge (i.e., patient death prior to follow-up visit, patient non-compliance for visit follow-up)

G9407 Patient did not receive follow-up within 7 days after discharge

G9408 Patients with cardiac tamponade and/or pericardiocentesis occurring within 30 days

G9409 Patients without cardiac tamponade and/or pericardiocentesis occurring within 30 days

G9410 Patient admitted within 180 days, status post cied implantation, replacement, or revision with an infection requiring device removal or surgical revision

G9411 Patient not admitted within 180 days, status post cied implantation, replacement, or revision with an infection requiring device removal or surgical revision

G9412 Patient admitted within 180 days, status post cied implantation, replacement, or revision with an infection requiring device removal or surgical revision

G9413 Patient not admitted within 180 days, status post cied implantation, replacement, or revision with an infection requiring device removal or surgical revision

G9414 Patient had one dose of meningococcal vaccine (serogroups a, c, w, y) on or between the patient's 11th and 13th birthdays

G9415 Patient did not have one dose of meningococcal vaccine (serogroups a, c, w, y) on or between the patient's 11th and 13th birthdays

G9416 Patient had one tetanus, diphtheria toxoids and acellular pertussis vaccine (Tdap) on or between the patient's 10th and 13th birthdays

G9417 Patient did not have one tetanus, diphtheria toxoids and acellular pertussis vaccine (Tdap) on or between the patient's 10th and 13th birthdays

G9418 Primary non-small cell lung cancer lung biopsy and cytology specimen report documents classification into specific histologic type following iaslc guidance or classified as NSCLC-nos with an explanation

G9419 Documentation of medical reason(s) for not including the histological type or NSCLC-nos classification with an explanation (e.g., specimen insufficient or non-diagnostic, specimen does not contain cancer, or other documented medical reasons)

G9420 Specimen site other than anatomic location of lung or is not classified as primary non-small cell lung cancer

G9421 Primary non-small cell lung cancer lung biopsy and cytology specimen report does not document classification into specific histologic type or histologic type does not follow iaslc guidance or is classified as NSCLC-nos but without an explanation

G9422 Primary lung carcinoma resection report documents pt category, pn category and for non-small cell lung cancer, histologic type (e.g., squamous cell carcinoma, adenocarcinoma and not NSCLC-nos)

G9423 Documentation of medical reason for not including pt category, pn category and histologic type [for patient with appropriate exclusion criteria (e.g., metastatic disease, benign tumors, malignant tumors other than carcinomas, inadequate surgical specimens)]

G9424 Specimen site other than anatomic location of lung, or classified as NSCLC-nos

G9425 Primary lung carcinoma resection report does not document pt category, pn category and for non-small cell lung cancer, histologic type (e.g., squamous cell carcinoma, adenocarcinoma)

G9426 Improvement in median time from ed arrival to initial ed oral or parenteral pain medication administration performed for ed admitted patients

G9427 Improvement in median time from ed arrival to initial ed oral or parenteral pain medication administration not performed for ed admitted patients

G9428 Pathology report includes the pt category, thickness, ulceration and mitotic rate, peripheral and deep margin status and presence or absence of microsatellitosis for invasive tumors

G9429 Documentation of medical reason(s) for not including pt category, thickness, ulceration and mitotic rate, peripheral and deep margin status and presence or absence of microsatellitosis for invasive tumors (e.g., negative skin biopsies, insufficient tissue, or other documented medical reasons)

G9430 Specimen site other than anatomic cutaneous location

G9431 Pathology report does not include the pt category, thickness, ulceration and mitotic rate, peripheral and deep margin status and presence or absence of microsatellitosis for invasive tumors

G9432 Asthma well-controlled based on the act, c-act, acq, or ataq score and results documented

G9433 Death, permanent nursing home resident or receiving hospice or palliative care any time during the measurement period

G9434 Asthma not well-controlled based on the act, c-act, acq, or ataq score, or specified asthma control tool not used, reason not given

G9435 Aspirin prescribed at discharge

G9436 Aspirin not prescribed for documented reasons (e.g., allergy, medical intolerance, history of bleed)

G9437 Aspirin not prescribed at discharge

G9438 P2y inhibitor prescribed at discharge

G9439 P2y inhibitor not prescribed for documented reasons (e.g., allergy, medical intolerance, history of bleed)

G9440 P2y inhibitor not prescribed at discharge

G - H CODES

G9441 Statin prescribed at discharge

G9442 Statin not prescribed for documented reasons (e.g., allergy, medical intolerance)

G9443 Statin not prescribed at discharge

G9448 Patients who were born in the years 1945 to 1965

G9449 History of receiving blood transfusions prior to 1992

G9450 History of injection drug use

(G9451 Patient received one-time screening for HCV infection
Code deleted effective 12/31/2023, no HCPCS/CPT cross-reference provided.)

▲ G9452 Documentation of medical reason(s) for not receiving HCV antibody test due to limited life expectancy

Code deleted effective 12/31/2023, no HCPCS/CPT cross-reference provided.)

(G9453 Documentation of patient reason(s) for not receiving one-time screening for HCV infection (e.g., patient declined, other patient reasons)
Code deleted effective 12/31/2023, no HCPCS/CPT cross-reference provided.)

(G9454 One-time screening for HCV infection not received within 12-month reporting period and no documentation of prior screening for HCV infection, reason not given

G9455 Patient underwent abdominal imaging with ultrasound, contrast enhanced CT or contrast MRI for HCC

G9456 Documentation of medical or patient reason(s) for not ordering or performing screening for HCC. medical reason: comorbid medical conditions with expected survival < 5 years, hepatic decompensation and not a candidate for liver transplantation, or other medical reasons; patient reasons: patient declined or other patient reasons (e.g., cost of tests, time related to accessing testing equipment)

G9457 Patient did not undergo abdominal imaging and did not have a documented reason for not undergoing abdominal imaging in the submission period

G9458 Patient documented as tobacco user and received tobacco cessation intervention (must include at least one of the following: advice given to quit smoking or tobacco use, counseling on the benefits of quitting smoking or tobacco use, assistance with or referral to external smoking or tobacco cessation support programs, or current enrollment in smoking or tobacco use cessation program) if identified as a tobacco user

G9459 Currently a tobacco non-user

G9460 Tobacco assessment or tobacco cessation intervention not performed; reason not given

G9463 I intend to report the sinusitis measures group

G9464 All quality actions for the applicable measures in the sinusitis measures group have been performed for this patient

G9465 I intend to report the acute otitis externa (aoe) measures group

G9466 All quality actions for the applicable measures in the aoe measures group have been performed for this patient

G9467 Patient who have received or are receiving corticosteroids greater than or equal to 10 mg/day of prednisone equivalents for 60 or greater consecutive days or a single prescription equating to 600 mg prednisone or greater for all fills within the last twelve months

G9468 Patient not receiving corticosteroids greater than or equal to 10 mg/day of prednisone equivalents for 60 or greater consecutive days or a single prescription equating to 600 mg prednisone or greater for all fills

G9469 Patients who have received or are receiving corticosteroids greater than or equal to 10 mg/day of prednisone equivalents for 90 or greater consecutive days or a single prescription equating to 900 mg prednisone or greater for all fills

G9470 Patients not receiving corticosteroids greater than or equal to 10 mg/day of prednisone equivalents for 60 or greater consecutive days or a single prescription equating to 600 mg prednisone or greater for all fills

G9471 Within the past 2 years, central dual-energy x-ray absorptiometry (DXA) not ordered or documented

G9472 Within the past 2 years, central dual-energy x-ray absorptiometry (DXA) not ordered and documented, no review of systems and no medication history or pharmacologic therapy (other than minerals/vitamins) for osteoporosis prescribed

G9473 Services performed by chaplain in the hospice setting, each 15 minutes

G9474 Services performed by dietary counselor in the hospice setting, each 15 minutes

G9475 Services performed by other counselor in the hospice setting, each 15 minutes

G9476 Services performed by volunteer in the hospice setting, each 15 minutes

G9477 Services performed by care coordinator in the hospice setting, each 15 minutes

G9478 Services performed by other qualified therapist in the hospice setting, each 15 minutes

G9479 Services performed by qualified pharmacist in the hospice setting, each 15 minutes

G9480 Admission to Medicare care choice model program (mccm)

G9481 Remote in-home visit for the evaluation and management of a new patient for use only in a Medicare-approved CMS innovation center demonstration project, which requires these 3 key components: a problem focused history; a problem focused examination; and straightforward medical decision making, furnished in real time using interactive audio and video technology. counseling and coordination of care with other physicians, other qualified health care professionals or agencies are provided consistent with the nature of the problem(s) and the needs of the patient or the family or both. usually, the presenting problem(s) are self limited or minor. typically, 10 minutes are spent with the patient or family or both via real time, audio and video intercommunications technology

G9482 Remote in-home visit for the evaluation and management of a new patient for use only in a Medicare-approved CMS innovation center demonstration project, which requires these 3 key components: an expanded problem focused history; an expanded problem focused examination; straightforward medical decision making, furnished in real time using interactive audio and video technology. counseling and coordination of care with other physicians, other qualified health care professionals or agencies are provided consistent with the nature of the problem(s) and the needs of the patient or the family or both. usually, the presenting problem(s) are of low to moderate severity. typically, 20 minutes are spent with the patient or family or both via real time, audio and video intercommunications technology

G9483 Remote in-home visit for the evaluation and management of a new patient for use only in a Medicare-approved CMS innovation center demonstration project, which requires these 3 key components: a detailed history; a detailed examination; medical decision making of low complexity, furnished in real time using interactive audio and video technology. counseling and coordination of care with other physicians, other qualified health care professionals or agencies are provided consistent with the nature of the problem(s) and the needs of the patient or the family or both. usually, the presenting problem(s) are of moderate severity. typically, 30 minutes are spent with the patient or family or both via real time, audio and video intercommunications technology

G9484 Remote in-home visit for the evaluation and management of a new patient for use only in a Medicare-approved CMS innovation center demonstration project, which requires these 3 key components: a comprehensive history; a comprehensive examination; medical decision making of moderate complexity, furnished in real time using interactive audio and video technology. counseling and coordination of care with other physicians, other qualified health care professionals or agencies are provided consistent with the nature of the problem(s) and the needs of the patient or the family or both. usually, the presenting problem(s) are of moderate to high severity. typically, 45 minutes are spent with the patient or family or both via real time, audio and video intercommunications technology

G9485 Remote in-home visit for the evaluation and management of a new patient for use only in a Medicare-approved CMS innovation center demonstration project, which requires these 3 key components: a comprehensive history; a comprehensive examination; medical decision making of high complexity, furnished in real time using interactive audio and video technology. counseling and coordination of care with other physicians, other qualified health care professionals or agencies are provided consistent with the nature of the problem(s) and the needs of the patient or the family or both. usually, the presenting problem(s) are of moderate to high severity. typically, 60 minutes are spent with the patient or family or both via real time, audio and video intercommunications technology

G9486 Remote in-home visit for the evaluation and management of an established patient for use only in a Medicare-approved CMS innovation center demonstration project, which requires at least 2 of the following 3 key components: a problem focused history; a problem focused examination; straightforward medical decision making, furnished in real time using interactive audio and video technology. Counseling and coordination of care with other physicians, other qualified health care professionals or agencies are provided consistent with the nature of the problem(s) and the needs of the patient or the family or both. usually, the presenting problem(s) are self limited or minor. typically, 10 minutes are spent with the patient or family or both via real time, audio and video intercommunications technology

G9487 Remote in-home visit for the evaluation and management of an established patient for use only in a Medicare-approved CMS innovation center demonstration project, which requires at least 2 of the following 3 key components: an expanded problem focused history; an expanded problem focused examination; medical decision making of low complexity, furnished in real time using interactive audio and video technology. Counseling and coordination of care with other physicians, other qualified health care professionals or agencies are provided consistent with the nature of the problem(s) and the needs of the patient or the family or both. usually, the presenting problem(s) are of low to moderate severity. typically, 15 minutes are spent with the patient or family or both via real time, audio and video intercommunications technology

G9488 Remote in-home visit for the evaluation and management of an established patient for use only in a Medicare-approved CMS innovation center demonstration project, which requires at least 2 of the following 3 key components: a detailed history; a detailed examination; medical decision making of moderate complexity, furnished in real time using interactive audio and video technology. Counseling and coordination of care with other physicians, other qualified health care professionals or agencies are provided consistent with the nature of the problem(s) and the needs of the patient or the family or both. usually, the presenting problem(s) are of moderate to high severity. typically, 25 minutes are spent with the patient or family or both via real time, audio and video intercommunications technology

G9489 Remote in-home visit for the evaluation and management of an established patient for use only in a Medicare-approved coms innovation center demonstration project, which requires at least 2 of the following 3 key components: a comprehensive history; a comprehensive examination; medical decision making of high complexity, furnished in real time using interactive audio and video technology. Counseling and coordination of care with other physicians, other qualified health care professionals or agencies are provided consistent with the nature of the problem(s) and the needs of the patient or the family or both. usually, the presenting problem(s) are of moderate to high severity. typically, 40 minutes are spent with the patient or family or both via real time, audio and video intercommunications technology

G9490 CMS innovation center models, home visit for patient assessment performed by clinical staff for an individual not considered homebound, including, but not necessarily limited to patient assessment of clinical status, safety/fall prevention, functional status/ambulation, medication reconciliation/ management, compliance with orders/plan of care, performance of activities of daily living, and ensuring beneficiary connections to community and other services. (for use only in Medicare-approved CMS innovation center models); may not be billed for a 30 day period covered by a transitional care management code

G9496 Documentation of reason for not detecting adenoma(s) or other neoplasm. (e.g., neoplasm detected is only diagnosed as traditional serrated adenoma, sessile serrated polyp, or sessile serrated adenoma

G9497 Received instruction from the anesthesiologist or proxy prior to the day of surgery to abstain from

G - H CODES

smoking on the day of surgery

G9498 Antibiotic regimen prescribed

G9499 Patient did not start or is not receiving antiviral treatment for hepatitis c during the measurement period

G9500 Radiation exposure indices documented in final report for procedure using fluoroscopy

G9501 Radiation exposure indices not documented in final report for procedure using fluoroscopy, reason not given

G9502 Documentation of medical reason for not performing foot exam (i.e., patients who have had either a bilateral amputation above or below the knee, or both a left and right amputation above or below the knee before or during the measurement period)

G9503 Patient taking tamsulosin hydrochloride

G9504 Documented reason for not assessing hepatitis b virus (HBV) status (e.g., patient not initiating anti-TNF therapy, patient declined) prior to initiating anti-TNF therapy

G9505 Antibiotic regimen prescribed within 10 days after onset of symptoms for documented medical reason

(**G9506** Biologic immune response modifier prescribed

Code deleted effective 12/31/2022, no HCPCS/CPT cross-reference provided.)

G9507 Documentation that the patient is on a statin medication or has documentation of a valid contraindication or exception to statin medications; contraindications/exceptions that can be defined by diagnosis codes include pregnancy during the measurement period, active liver disease, rhabdomyolysis, end stage renal disease on dialysis and heart failure; provider documented contraindications/exceptions include breastfeeding during the measurement period, woman of child-bearing age not actively taking birth control, allergy to statin, drug interaction (HIV protease inhibitors, nefazodone, cyclosporine, gemfibrozil, and danazol) and intolerance (with supporting documentation of trying a statin at least once within the last 5 years or diagnosis codes for myositis or toxic myopathy related to drugs)

G9508 Documentation that the patient is not on a statin medication

G9509 Adult patients 18 years of age or older with major depression or dysthymia who reached remission at twelve months as demonstrated by a twelve month (+/-60 days) phq-9 or phq-9m score of less than 5

G9510 Adult patients 18 years of age or older with major depression or dysthymia who did not reach remission at twelve months as demonstrated by a twelve month (+/-60 days) phq-9 or phq-9m score of less than 5. either phq- 9 or phq-9m score was not assessed or is greater than or equal to 5

G9511 Index event date phq-9 or phq-9m score greater than 9 documented during the twelve month denominator identification period

G9512 Individual had a PDC of 0.8 or greater

G9513 Individual did not have a PDC of 0.8 or greater

G9514 Patient required a return to the operating room within 90 days of surgery

G9515 Patient did not require a return to the operating room within 90 days of surgery

G9516 Patient achieved an improvement in visual acuity, from their preoperative level, within 90 days of surgery

G9517 Patient did not achieve an improvement in visual acuity, from their preoperative level, within 90 days of surgery, reason not given

G9518 Documentation of active injection drug use

G9519 Patient achieves final refraction (spherical equivalent) +/- 1.0 diopters of their planned refraction within 90 days of surgery

G9520 Patient does not achieve final refraction (spherical equivalent) +/- 1.0 diopters of their planned

G - H CODES

refraction within 90 days of surgery

G9521 Total number of emergency department visits and inpatient hospitalizations less than two in the past 12 months

G9522 Total number of emergency department visits and inpatient hospitalizations equal to or greater than two in the past 12 months or patient not screened, reason not given

G9523 Patient discontinued from hemodialysis or peritoneal dialysis

G9524 Patient was referred to hospice care

G9525 Documentation of patient reason(s) for not referring to hospice care (e.g., patient declined, other patient reasons)

G9526 Patient was not referred to hospice care, reason not given

G9529 Patient with minor blunt head trauma had an appropriate indication(s) for a head CT

G9530 Patient presented with a minor blunt head trauma and had a head CT ordered for trauma by an emergency care provider

G9531 Patient has documentation of ventricular shunt, brain tumor, multisystem trauma, or is currently taking an antiplatelet medication including: abciximab, anagrelide, cangrelor, cilostazol, clopidogrel, dipyridamole, eptifibatide, prasugrel, ticlopidine, ticagrelor, tirofiban, or vorapaxar

G9532 Patient had a head CT for trauma ordered by someone other than an emergency care provider or was ordered for a reason other than trauma

G9533 Patient with minor blunt head trauma did not have an appropriate indication(s) for a head CT

G9534 Advanced brain imaging (CTA, CT, MRA or MRI) was not ordered

G9535 Patients with a normal neurological examination

G9536 Documentation of medical reason(s) for ordering an advanced brain imaging study (i.e., patient has an abnormal neurological examination; patient has the coexistence of seizures, or both; recent onset of severe headache; change in the type of headache; signs of increased intracranial pressure (e.g., papilledema, absent venous pulsations on funduscopic examination, altered mental status, focal neurologic deficits, signs of meningeal irritation); HIV-positive patients with a new type of headache; immunocompromised patient with unexplained headache symptoms; patient on coagulopathy/anti-coagulation or anti-platelet therapy; very young patients with unexplained headache symptoms)

G9537 Imaging needed as part of a clinical trial; or other clinician ordered the study

G9538 Advanced brain imaging (CTA, CT, MRA or MRI) was ordered

G9539 Intent for potential removal at time of placement

G9540 Patient alive 3 months post procedure

G9541 Filter removed within 3 months of placement

G9542 Documented re-assessment for the appropriateness of filter removal within 3 months of placement

G9543 Documentation of at least two attempts to reach the patient to arrange a clinical re-assessment for the appropriateness of filter removal within 3 months of placement

G9544 Patients that do not have the filter removed, documented re-assessment for the appropriateness of filter removal, or documentation of at least two attempts to reach the patient to arrange a clinical re-assessment for the appropriateness of filter removal within 3 months of placement

G9547 Cystic renal lesion that is simple appearing (Bosniak I or ii) , or adrenal lesion less than or equal to 1.0 cm or adrenal lesion greater than 1.0 cm but less than or equal to 4.0 cm classified as likely benign by unenhanced CT or washout protocol CT, or MRI with in- and opposed-phase sequences or other equivalent institutional imaging protocols

G9548 Final reports for imaging studies stating no follow-up imaging is recommended

G9549 Documentation of medical reason(s) that follow-up imaging is indicated (e.g., patient has lymphadenopathy, signs of metastasis or an active diagnosis or history of cancer, and other medical reason(s))

G9550 Final reports for imaging studies with follow-up imaging recommended, or final reports that do not include a specific recommendation of no follow-up

G9551 Final reports for imaging studies without an incidentally found lesion noted

G9552 Incidental thyroid nodule < 1.0 cm noted in report

G9553 Prior thyroid disease diagnosis

G9554 Final reports for CT, CTA, MRI or MRA of the chest or neck with follow-up imaging recommended

G9555 Documentation of medical reason(s) for recommending follow up imaging (e.g., patient has multiple endocrine neoplasia, patient has cervical lymphadenopathy, other medical reason(s))

G9556 Final reports for CT, CTA, MRI or MRA of the chest or neck with follow-up imaging not recommended

G9557 Final reports for CT, CTA, MRI or MRA studies of the chest or neck without an incidentally found thyroid nodule < 1.0 cm noted or no nodule found

G9558 Patient treated with a beta-lactam antibiotic as definitive therapy

G9559 Documentation of medical reason(s) for not prescribing a beta-lactam antibiotic (e.g., allergy, intolerance to beta-lactam antibiotics)

G9560 Patient not treated with a beta-lactam antibiotic as definitive therapy; reason not given

G9561 Patients prescribed opiates for longer than six weeks

G9562 Patients who had a follow-up evaluation conducted at least every three months during opioid therapy

G9563 Patients who did not have a follow-up evaluation conducted at least every three months during opioid therapy

G9572 Index date phq-score greater than 9 documented during the twelve month denominator identification period

G9573 Adult patients 18 years of age or older with major depression or dysthymia who did not reach remission at six months as demonstrated by a six month (+/-60 days) phq-9 or phq-9m score of less than five

G9574 Adult patients 18 years of age or older with major depression or dysthymia who did not reach remission at six months as demonstrated by a six month (+/-60 days) phq-9 or phq-9m score of less than five; either phq-9 or phq-9m score was not assessed or is greater than or equal to five

G9577 Patients prescribed opiates for longer than six weeks

G9578 Documentation of signed opioid treatment agreement at least once during opioid therapy

G9579 No documentation of signed an opioid treatment agreement at least once during opioid therapy

G9580 Door to puncture time of 90 minutes or less

G9581 Door to puncture time of greater than 2 hours for reasons documented by clinician (e.g., patients who are transferred from one institution to another with a known diagnosis of CVA for endovascular stroke treatment; hospitalized patients with newly diagnosed CVA considered for endovascular stroke treatment)

G9582 Door to puncture time of greater than 90 minutes, no reason given

G9583 Patients prescribed opiates for longer than six weeks

G9584 Patient evaluated for risk of misuse of opiates by using a brief validated instrument (e.g., opioid risk tool, soapp-r) or patient interviewed at least once during opioid therapy

G9585 Patient not evaluated for risk of misuse of opiates by using a brief validated instrument (e.g.,

G - H CODES

opioid risk tool, soapp-r) or patient not interviewed at least once during opioid therapy

G9593 Pediatric patient with minor blunt head trauma classified as low risk according to the pecarn prediction rules

G9594 Patient presented with a minor blunt head trauma and had a head CT ordered for trauma by an emergency care provider

G9595 Patient has documentation of ventricular shunt, brain tumor, or coagulopathy

(**G9596** Pediatric patient had a head CT for trauma ordered by someone other than an emergency care provider or was ordered for a reason other than trauma
Code deleted effective 12/31/2023, no HCPCS/CPT cross-reference provided.)

G9597 Pediatric patient with minor blunt head trauma not classified as low risk according to the pecarn prediction rules

G9598 Aortic aneurysm 5.5 - 5.9 cm maximum diameter on centerline formatted CT or minor diameter on axial formatted CT

G9599 Aortic aneurysm 6.0 cm or greater maximum diameter on centerline formatted CT or minor diameter on axial formatted CT

G9600 Symptomatic AAAS that required urgent/emergent (non-elective) repair

G9601 Patient discharge to home no later than post-operative day #7

G9602 Patient not discharged to home by post-operative day #7

G9603 Patient survey score improved from baseline following treatment

G9604 Patient survey results not available

G9605 Patient survey score did not improve from baseline following treatment

G9606 Intraoperative cystoscopy performed to evaluate for lower tract injury

G9607 Documented medical reasons for not performing intraoperative cystoscopy (e.g., urethral pathology precluding cystoscopy, any patient who has a congenital or acquired absence of the urethra) or in the case of patient death

G9608 Intraoperative cystoscopy not performed to evaluate for lower tract injury

G9609 Documentation of an order for anti-platelet agents

G9610 Documentation of medical reason(s) in the patient's record for not ordering anti-platelet agents

G9611 Order for anti-platelet agents was not documented in the patient's record, reason not given

(**G9612** Photodocumentation of two or more cecal landmarks to establish a complete examination
Code deleted effective 12/31/2023, no HCPCS/CPT cross-reference provided.)

(**G9613** Documentation of post-surgical anatomy (e.g., right hemicolectomy, ileocecal resection, etc.)
Code deleted effective 12/31/2023, no HCPCS/CPT cross-reference provided.)

(**G9614** Photodocumentation of less than two cecal landmarks (i.e., no cecal landmarks or only one cecal landmark) to establish a complete examination
Code deleted effective 12/31/2023, no HCPCS/CPT cross-reference provided.)

G9615 Preoperative assessment documented

G9616 Documentation of reason(s) for not documenting a preoperative assessment (e.g., patient with a gynecologic or other pelvic malignancy noted at the time of surgery)

G9617 Preoperative assessment not documented; reason not given

(**G9618** Documentation of screening for uterine malignancy or those that had an ultrasound and/or endometrial sampling of any kind
Code deleted effective 12/31/2022, no HCPCS/CPT cross-reference provided.)

G9619 Documentation of reason(s) for not screening for uterine malignancy (e.g., prior hysterectomy)

(**G9620** Patient not screened for uterine malignancy, or those that have not had an ultrasound and/or

endometrial sampling of any kind, reason not given
Code deleted effective 12/31/2022, no HCPCS/CPT cross-reference provided.)

G9621 Patient identified as an unhealthy alcohol user when screened for unhealthy alcohol use using a systematic screening method and received brief counseling

G9622 Patient not identified as an unhealthy alcohol user when screened for unhealthy alcohol use using a systematic screening method

(**G9623** Documentation of medical reason(s) for not screening for unhealthy alcohol use (e.g., limited life expectancy, other medical reasons)
Code deleted effective 12/31/2022, no HCPCS/CPT cross-reference provided.)

G9624 Patient not screened for unhealthy alcohol use using a systematic screening method or patient did not receive brief counseling if identified as an unhealthy alcohol user

G9625 Patient sustained bladder injury at the time of surgery or discovered subsequently up to 30 days post-surgery

G9626 Documented medical reason for not reporting bladder injury (e.g., gynecologic or other pelvic malignancy documented, concurrent surgery involving bladder pathology, injury that occurs during a urinary incontinence procedure, patient death from non-medical causes not related to surgery, patient died during procedure without evidence of bladder injury)

G9627 Patient did not sustain bladder injury at the time of surgery nor discovered subsequently up to 30 days post-surgery

G9628 Patient sustained bowel injury at the time of surgery or discovered subsequently up to 30 days post-surgery

G9629 Documented medical reasons for not reporting bowel injury (e.g., gynecologic or other pelvic malignancy documented, planned (e.g., not due to an unexpected bowel injury) resection and/or re-anastomosis of bowel, or patient death from non-medical causes not related to surgery, patient died during procedure without evidence of bowel injury)

G9630 Patient did not sustain a bowel injury at the time of surgery nor discovered subsequently up to 30 days post-surgery

(**G9631** Patient sustained ureter injury at the time of surgery or discovered subsequently up to 30 days post-surgery
Code deleted effective 12/31/2022, no HCPCS/CPT cross-reference provided.)

(**G9632** Documented medical reasons for not reporting ureter injury (e.g., gynecologic or other pelvic malignancy documented, concurrent surgery involving bladder pathology, injury that occurs during a urinary incontinence procedure, patient death from non-medical causes not related to surgery, patient died during procedure without evidence of ureter injury)
Code deleted effective 12/31/2022, no HCPCS/CPT cross-reference provided.)

(**G9633** Patient did not sustain ureter injury at the time of surgery nor discovered subsequently up to 30 days post-surgery
Code deleted effective 12/31/2022, no HCPCS/CPT cross-reference provided.)

G9634 Health-related quality of life assessed with tool during at least two visits and quality of life score remained the same or improved

G9635 Health-related quality of life not assessed with tool for documented reason(s) (e.g., patient has a cognitive or neuropsychiatric impairment that impairs his/her ability to complete the HRQoL survey, patient has the inability to read and/or write in order to complete the HRQoL questionnaire)

G9636 Health-related quality of life not assessed with tool during at least two visits or quality of life score declined

G - H CODES

G9637 Final reports with documentation of one or more dose reduction techniques (e.g., automated exposure control, adjustment of the ma and/or kv according to patient size, use of iterative reconstruction technique)

G9638 Final reports without documentation of one or more dose reduction techniques (e.g., automated exposure control, adjustment of the ma and/or kv according to patient size, use of iterative reconstruction technique)

G9639 Major amputation or open surgical bypass not required within 48 hours of the index endovascular lower extremity revascularization procedure

G9640 Documentation of planned hybrid or staged procedure

G9641 Major amputation or open surgical bypass required within 48 hours of the index endovascular lower extremity revascularization procedure

G9642 Current smoker (e.g., cigarette, cigar, pipe, e-cigarette or marijuana)

G9643 Elective surgery

G9644 Patients who abstained from smoking prior to anesthesia on the day of surgery or procedure

G9645 Patients who did not abstain from smoking prior to anesthesia on the day of surgery or procedure

G9646 Patients with 90 day MRS score of 0 to 2

G9647 Patients in whom MRS score could not be obtained at 90 day follow-up

G9648 Patients with 90 day MRS score greater than 2

G9649 Psoriasis assessment tool documented meeting any one of the specified benchmarks (e.g., (PGA; 5-point or 6-point scale), body surface area (BSA), psoriasis area and severity index (PASI) and/or dermatology life quality index) (DLQI))

G9650 Documentation that the patient declined therapy change or has documented contraindications (e.g., experienced adverse effects or lack of efficacy with all other therapy options) in order to achieve better disease control as measured by PGA, BSA, PASI, or DLQI

G9651 Psoriasis assessment tool documented not meeting any one of the specified benchmarks (e.g., (PGA; 5-point or 6-point scale), body surface area (BSA), psoriasis area and severity index (PASI) and/or dermatology life quality index) (DLQI)) or psoriasis assessment tool not documented

G9652 Patient has been treated with a systemic or biologic medication for psoriasis for at least six months

G9653 Patient has not been treated with a systemic or biologic medication for psoriasis for at least six months

G9654 Monitored anesthesia care (mac)

G9655 A transfer of care protocol or handoff tool/checklist that includes the required key handoff elements is used

G9656 Patient transferred directly from anesthetizing location to PACU or other non-ICU location

G9657 Transfer of care during an anesthetic or to the intensive care unit

G9658 A transfer of care protocol or handoff tool/checklist that includes the required key handoff elements is not used

G9659 Patients greater than or equal to 86 years of age who underwent a screening colonoscopy and did not have a history of colorectal cancer or other valid medical reason for the colonoscopy, including: iron deficiency anemia, lower gastrointestinal bleeding, Crohn's disease (i.e., regional enteritis), familial adenomatous polyposis, lynch syndrome (i.e., hereditary non-polyposis colorectal cancer), inflammatory bowel disease, ulcerative colitis, abnormal finding of gastrointestinal tract, or changes in bowel habits

G9660 Documentation of medical reason(s) for a colonoscopy performed on a patient greater than or equal to 86 years of age (e.g., iron deficiency anemia, lower gastrointestinal bleeding, Crohn's disease (i.e., regional enteritis), familial history of adenomatous polyposis, lynch syndrome (i.e., hereditary non-polyposis colorectal cancer), inflammatory bowel disease, ulcerative colitis, abnormal finding of gastrointestinal tract, or changes in bowel habits)

G9661 Patients greater than or equal to 86 years of age who received a colonoscopy for an assessment of signs/symptoms of GI tract illness, and/or because the patient meets high risk criteria, and/or to follow-up on previously diagnosed advanced lesions

G9662 Previously diagnosed or have a diagnosis of clinical ASCVD, including ASCVD procedure

G9663 Any LDL-c laboratory result >= 190 mg/dl

G9664 Patients who are currently statin therapy users or received an order (prescription) for statin therapy

G9665 Patients who are not currently statin therapy users or did not receive an order (prescription) for statin therapy

G9666 Patient's highest fasting or direct LDL-c laboratory test result in the measurement period or two years prior to the beginning of the measurement period is 70-189 mg/dl

G9667 Documentation of medical reason(s) for not currently being a statin therapy user or receive an order (prescription) for statin therapy (e.g., patient with adverse effect, allergy or intolerance to statin medication therapy, patients who have an active diagnosis of pregnancy or who are breastfeeding, patients who are receiving palliative care, patients with active liver disease or hepatic disease or insufficiency, patients with end stage renal disease (ESRD), and patients with diabetes who have a fasting or direct LDL-c laboratory test result < 70 mg/dl and are not taking statin therapy)

G9669 I intend to report the multiple chronic conditions measures group

G9670 All quality actions for the applicable measures in the multiple chronic conditions measures group have been performed for this patient

G9671 I intend to report the diabetic retinopathy measures group

G9672 All quality actions for the applicable measures in the diabetic retinopathy measures group have been performed for this patient

G9673 I intend to report the cardiovascular prevention measures group

G9674 Patients with clinical ASCVD diagnosis

G9675 Patients who have ever had a fasting or direct laboratory result of LDL-c = 190 mg/dl

G9676 Patients aged 40 to 75 years at the beginning of the measurement period with type 1 or type 2 diabetes and with an LDL-c result of 70-189 mg/dl recorded as the highest fasting or direct laboratory test result in the measurement year or during the two years prior to the beginning of the measurement period

G9677 All quality actions for the applicable measures in the cardiovascular prevention measures group have been performed for this patient

G9678 Oncology care model (ocm) monthly enhanced oncology services (meos) payment for ocm enhanced services. g9678 payments may only be made to ocm practitioners for ocm beneficiaries for the furnishment of enhanced services as defined in the ocm participation agreement

G9679 This code is for onsite acute care treatment of a nursing facility resident with pneumonia; may only be billed once per day per beneficiary

G9680 This code is for onsite acute care treatment of a nursing facility resident with CHF; may only be billed once per day per beneficiary

G9681 This code is for onsite acute care treatment of a resident with COPD or asthma; may only be billed once per day per beneficiary

G9682 This code is for the onsite acute care treatment a nursing facility resident with a skin infection; may only be billed once per day per beneficiary

G9683 Facility service(s) for the onsite acute care treatment of a nursing facility resident with fluid or electrolyte disorder. (may only be billed once per day per beneficiary). this service is for a demonstration project

G9684 This code is for the onsite acute care treatment of a nursing facility resident for a UTI; may only be

G - H CODES

billed once per day per beneficiary

G9685 Physician service or other qualified health care professional for the evaluation and management of a beneficiary's acute change in condition in a nursing facility. this service is for a demonstration project

G9686 Onsite nursing facility conference, which is separate and distinct from an evaluation and management visit, including qualified practitioner and at least one member of the nursing facility interdisciplinary care team

G9687 Hospice services provided to patient any time during the measurement period

G9688 Patients using hospice services any time during the measurement period

G9689 Patient admitted for performance of elective carotid intervention

G9690 Patient receiving hospice services any time during the measurement period

G9691 Patient had hospice services any time during the measurement period

G9692 Hospice services received by patient any time during the measurement period

G9693 Patient use of hospice services any time during the measurement period

G9694 Hospice services utilized by patient any time during the measurement period

G9695 Long-acting inhaled bronchodilator prescribed

▲ **G9696** Documentation of medical reason(s) for not prescribing a long-acting inhaled bronchodilator (e.g., patient intolerance or history of side effects)

(**G9697** Documentation of patient reason(s) for not prescribing a long-acting inhaled bronchodilator Code deleted effective 12/31/2023, no HCPCS/CPT cross-reference provided.)

▲ **G9698** Documentation of system reason(s) for not prescribing a long-acting inhaled bronchodilator (e.g., cost of treatment or lack of insurance)

G9699 Long-acting inhaled bronchodilator not prescribed, reason not otherwise specified

G9700 Patients who use hospice services any time during the measurement period

G9701 Children who are taking antibiotics in the 30 days prior to the date of the encounter during which the diagnosis was established

G9702 Patients who use hospice services any time during the measurement period

▲ **G9703** Episodes where the patient is taking antibiotics (table 1) in the 30 days prior to the episode date

G9704 AJCC breast cancer stage i: t1 mic or t1a documented

G9705 AJCC breast cancer stage i: t1b (tumor > 0.5 cm but <= 1 cm in greatest dimension) documented

G9706 Low (or very low) risk of recurrence, prostate cancer

G9707 Patient received hospice services any time during the measurement period

G9708 Women who had a bilateral mastectomy or who have a history of a bilateral mastectomy or for whom there is evidence of a right and a left unilateral mastectomy

G9709 Hospice services used by patient any time during the measurement period

G9710 Patient was provided hospice services any time during the measurement period

G9711 Patients with a diagnosis or past history of total colectomy or colorectal cancer

G9712 Documentation of medical reason(s) for prescribing or dispensing antibiotic (e.g., intestinal infection, pertussis, bacterial infection, Lyme disease, otitis media, acute sinusitis, acute pharyngitis, acute tonsillitis, chronic sinusitis, infection of the pharynx/larynx/tonsils/adenoids, prostatitis, cellulitis/ mastoiditis/bone infections, acute lymphadenitis, impetigo, skin staph infections, pneumonia, gonococcal infections/venereal disease (syphilis, chlamydia, inflammatory diseases [female reproductive organs]), infections of the kidney, cystitis/UTI, acne, HIV disease/asymptomatic HIV, cystic fibrosis, disorders of the immune system, malignancy neoplasms, chronic bronchitis, emphysema, bronchiectasis, extrinsic allergic alveolitis, chronic airway obstruction, chronic obstructive asthma, pneumoconiosis and other lung disease due to external agents, other diseases of the respiratory system, and tuberculosis

G9713 Patients who use hospice services any time during the measurement period

G9714 Patient is using hospice services any time during the measurement period

(**G9715** Patients who use hospice services any time during the measurement period
Code deleted effective 12/31/2023, no HCPCS/CPT cross-reference provided.)

G9716 BMI is documented as being outside of normal parameters, follow-up plan is not completed for documented medical reason

▲ **G9717** Documentation stating the patient has had a diagnosis of bipolar disorder

(**G9718** Hospice services for patient provided any time during the measurement period
Code deleted effective 12/31/2022, no HCPCS/CPT cross-reference provided.)

G9719 Patient is not ambulatory, bed ridden, immobile, confined to chair, wheelchair bound, dependent on helper pushing wheelchair, independent in wheelchair or minimal help in wheelchair

G9720 Hospice services for patient occurred any time during the measurement period

G9721 Patient not ambulatory, bed ridden, immobile, confined to chair, wheelchair bound, dependent on helper pushing wheelchair, independent in wheelchair or minimal help in wheelchair

G9722 Documented history of renal failure or baseline serum creatinine >= 4.0 mg/dl; renal transplant recipients are not considered to have preoperative renal failure, unless, since transplantation the cr has been or is 4.0 or higher

G9723 Hospice services for patient received any time during the measurement period

G9724 Patients who had documentation of use of anticoagulant medications overlapping the measurement year

(**G9725** Patients who use hospice services any time during the measurement period
Code deleted effective 12/31/2023, no HCPCS/CPT cross-reference provided.)

G9726 Patient refused to participate

G9727 Patient unable to complete the lepf prom at initial evaluation and/or discharge due to blindness, illiteracy, severe mental incapacity or language incompatibility and an adequate proxy is not available

G9728 Patient refused to participate

G9729 Patient unable to complete the lepf prom at initial evaluation and/or discharge due to blindness, illiteracy, severe mental incapacity or language incompatibility and an adequate proxy is not available

G9730 Patient refused to participate

G9731 Patient unable to complete the lepf prom at initial evaluation and/or discharge due to blindness, illiteracy, severe mental incapacity or language incompatibility and an adequate proxy is not available

G9732 Patient refused to participate

G9733 Patient unable to complete the low back fs prom at initial evaluation and/or discharge due to blindness, illiteracy, severe mental incapacity or language incompatibility and an adequate proxy is not available

G9734 Patient refused to participate

G9735 Patient unable to complete the shoulder fs prom at initial evaluation and/or discharge due to blindness, illiteracy, severe mental incapacity or language incompatibility and an adequate proxy is not available

G9736 Patient refused to participate

G9737 Patient unable to complete the elbow/wrist/hand fs prom at initial evaluation and/or discharge due to blindness, illiteracy, severe mental incapacity or language incompatibility and an adequate proxy is not available

G9738 Patient refused to participate

G9739 Patient unable to complete the general orthopedic fs prom at initial evaluation and/or discharge due to blindness, illiteracy, severe mental incapacity or language incompatibility and an adequate proxy is not available

G9740 Hospice services given to patient any time during the measurement period

G9741 Patients who use hospice services any time during the measurement period

G9742 Psychiatric symptoms assessed

G9743 Psychiatric symptoms not assessed; reason not otherwise specified

G9744 Patient not eligible due to active diagnosis of hypertension

G9745 Documented reason for not screening or recommending a follow-up for high blood pressure

G9746 Patient has mitral stenosis or prosthetic heart valves, or patient has transient or reversible cause of af (e.g., pneumonia, hyperthyroidism, pregnancy, cardiac surgery)

G9747 Patient is undergoing palliative dialysis with a catheter

G9748 Patient approved by a qualified transplant program and scheduled to receive a living donor kidney transplant

G9749 Patient is undergoing palliative dialysis with a catheter

G9750 Patient approved by a qualified transplant program and scheduled to receive a living donor kidney transplant

G9751 Patient died at any time during the 24-month measurement period

G9752 Emergency surgery

G9753 Documentation of medical reason for not conducting a search for DICOM format images for prior patient CT imaging studies completed at non-affiliated external healthcare facilities or entities within the past 12 months that are available through a secure, authorized, media-free, shared archive (e.g., trauma, acute myocardial infarction, stroke, aortic aneurysm where time is of the essence)

G9754 A finding of an incidental pulmonary nodule

G9755 Documentation of medical reason(s) for not including a recommended interval and modality for follow-up or for no follow-up, and source of recommendations (e.g., patients with unexplained fever, immunocompromised patients who are at risk for infection)

G9756 Surgical procedures that included the use of silicone oil

G9757 Surgical procedures that included the use of silicone oil

G9758 Patient in hospice at any time during the measurement period

G9759 History of preoperative posterior capsule rupture

G9760 Patients who use hospice services any time during the measurement period

G9761 Patients who use hospice services any time during the measurement period

G9762 Patient had at least two HPV vaccines (with at least 146 days between the two) or three HPV vaccines on or between the patient's 9th and 13th birthdays

G9763 Patient did not have at least two HPV vaccines (with at least 146 days between the two) or three HPV vaccines on or between the patient's 9th and 13th birthdays

G9764 Patient has been treated with a systemic medication for psoriasis vulgaris

G9765 Documentation that the patient declined change in medication or alternative therapies were unavailable, has documented contraindications, or has not been treated with a systemic medication for at least six consecutive months (e.g., experienced adverse effects or lack of efficacy with all other therapy options) in order to achieve better disease control as measured by PGA, BSA, PASI, or DLQI

G9766 Patients who are transferred from one institution to another with a known diagnosis of CVA for endovascular stroke treatment

G9767 Hospitalized patients with newly diagnosed CVA considered for endovascular stroke treatment

G9768 Patients who utilize hospice services any time during the measurement period

G9769 Patient had a bone mineral density test in the past two years or received osteoporosis medication or therapy in the past 12 months

G9770 Peripheral nerve block (pnb)

▲ **G9771** At least 1 body temperature measurement equal to or greater than 35.5 degrees Celsius (or 95.9 degrees Fahrenheit) achieved within the 30 minutes immediately before or 15 minutes immediately after anesthesia end time

▲ **G9772** Documentation of medical reason(s) for not achieving at least 1 body temperature measurement equal to or greater than 35.5 degrees Celsius (or 95.9 degrees Fahrenheit) within the 30 minutes immediately before or 15 minutes immediately after anesthesia end time (e.g., emergency cases, intentional hypothermia, etc.)

▲ **G9773** At least 1 body temperature measurement equal to or greater than 35.5 degrees Celsius (or 95.9 degrees Fahrenheit) not achieved within the 30 minutes immediately before or 15 minutes immediately after anesthesia end time, reason not given

(**G9774** Patients who have had a hysterectomy

Code deleted effective 12/31/2022, no HCPCS/CPT cross-reference provided.)

G9775 Patient received at least 2 prophylactic pharmacologic anti-emetic agents of different classes preoperatively and/or intraoperatively

G9776 Documentation of medical reason for not receiving at least 2 prophylactic pharmacologic anti-emetic agents of different classes preoperatively and/or intraoperatively (e.g., intolerance or other medical reason)

G9777 Patient did not receive at least 2 prophylactic pharmacologic anti-emetic agents of different classes preoperatively and/or intraoperatively

(**G9778** Patients who have a diagnosis of pregnancy at any time during the measurement period

Code deleted effective 12/31/2022, no HCPCS/CPT cross-reference provided.)

▲ **G9779** Patients who are breastfeeding at any time during the performance period

▲ **G9780** Patients who have a diagnosis of rhabdomyolysis at any time during the performance period

G9781 Documentation of medical reason(s) for not currently being a statin therapy user or receiving an order (prescription) for statin therapy (e.g., patients with statin-associated muscle symptoms or an allergy to statin medication therapy, patients who are receiving palliative or hospice care, patients with active liver disease or hepatic disease or insufficiency, patients with end stage renal disease [ESRD], or other medical reasons)

G9782 History of or active diagnosis of familial hypercholesterolemia

G9783 Documentation of patients with diabetes who have a most recent fasting or direct LDL- c laboratory test result < 70 mg/dl and are not taking statin therapy

G9784 Pathologists/dermatopathologists providing a second opinion on a biopsy

G9785 Pathology report diagnosing cutaneous basal cell carcinoma, squamous cell carcinoma, or melanoma (to include in situ disease) sent from the pathologist/ dermatopathologist to the biopsying clinician for review within 7 days from the time when the tissue specimen was received by the pathologist

G - H CODES

G9786 Pathology report diagnosing cutaneous basal cell carcinoma, squamous cell carcinoma, or melanoma (to include in situ disease) was not sent from the pathologist/ dermatopathologist to the biopsying clinician for review within 7 days from the time when the tissue specimen was received by the pathologist

G9787 Patient alive as of the last day of the measurement year

G9788 Most recent bp is less than or equal to 140/90 mm hg

G9789 Blood pressure recorded during inpatient stays, emergency room visits, or urgent care visits

G9790 Most recent bp is greater than 140/90 mm hg, or blood pressure not documented

G9791 Most recent tobacco status is tobacco free

G9792 Most recent tobacco status is not tobacco free

G9793 Patient is currently on a daily aspirin or other antiplatelet

G9794 Documentation of medical reason(s) for not on a daily aspirin or other antiplatelet (e.g., history of gastrointestinal bleed, intra-cranial bleed, idiopathic thrombocytopenic purpura (ITP), gastric bypass or documentation of active anticoagulant use during the measurement period)

G9795 Patient is not currently on a daily aspirin or other antiplatelet

G9796 Patient is currently on a statin therapy

G9797 Patient is not on a statin therapy

G9798 Discharge(s) for AMI between July 1 of the year prior measurement period to June 30 of the measurement period

G9799 Patients with a medication dispensing event indicator of a history of asthma any time during the patient's history through the end of the measure period

G9800 Patients who are identified as having an intolerance or allergy to beta-blocker therapy

G9801 Hospitalizations in which the patient was transferred directly to a non-acute care facility for any diagnosis

G9802 Patients who use hospice services any time during the measurement period

G9803 Patient prescribed at least a 135 day treatment within the 180-day measurement interval with beta-blockers post-discharge for AMI

G9804 Patient was not prescribed at least a 135 day treatment within the 180-day measurement interval with beta-blockers post-discharge for AMI

G9805 Patients who use hospice services any time during the measurement period

G9806 Patients who received cervical cytology or an HPV test

G9807 Patients who did not receive cervical cytology or an HPV test

(**G9808** Any patients who had no asthma controller medications dispensed during the measurement year
Code deleted effective 12/31/2022, no HCPCS/CPT cross-reference provided.)

(**G9809** Patients who use hospice services any time during the measurement period
Code deleted effective 12/31/2022, no HCPCS/CPT cross-reference provided.)

(**G9810** Patient achieved a PDC of at least 75% for their asthma controller medication
Code deleted effective 12/31/2022, no HCPCS/CPT cross-reference provided.)

(**G9811** Patient did not achieve a PDC of at least 75% for their asthma controller medication
Code deleted effective 12/31/2022, no HCPCS/CPT cross-reference provided.)

G9812 Patient died including all deaths occurring during the hospitalization in which the operation was performed, even if after 30 days, and those deaths occurring after discharge from the hospital, but within 30 days of the procedure

G9813 Patient did not die within 30 days of the procedure or during the index hospitalization

G9814 Death occurring during the index acute care hospitalization

G9815 Death did not occur during the index acute care hospitalization

G9816 Death occurring after discharge from the hospital but within 30 days post procedure

G9817 Death did not occur after discharge from the hospital within 30 days post procedure

G9818 Documentation of sexual activity

G9819 Patients who use hospice services any time during the measurement period

G9820 Documentation of a chlamydia screening test with proper follow-up

G9821 No documentation of a chlamydia screening test with proper follow-up

G9822 Patients who had an endometrial ablation procedure during the 12 months prior to the index date (exclusive of the index date)

G9823 Endometrial sampling or hysteroscopy with biopsy and results documented during the 12 months prior to the index date (exclusive of the index date) of the endometrial ablation

G9824 Endometrial sampling or hysteroscopy with biopsy and results not documented during the 12 months prior to the index date (exclusive of the index date) of the endometrial ablation

G9825 Her-2/neu negative or undocumented/unknown

G9826 Patient transferred to practice after initiation of chemotherapy

G9827 Her2-targeted therapies not administered during the initial course of treatment

G9828 Her2-targeted therapies administered during the initial course of treatment

G9829 Breast adjuvant chemotherapy administered

G9830 Her-2/neu positive

G9831 AJCC stage at breast cancer diagnosis = ii or iii

G9832 AJCC stage at breast cancer diagnosis = I (IA or ib) and t-stage at breast cancer diagnosis does not equal = t1, t1a, t1b

G9833 Patient transfer to practice after initiation of chemotherapy

G9834 Patient has metastatic disease at diagnosis

G9835 Trastuzumab administered within 12 months of diagnosis

G9836 Reason for not administering trastuzumab documented (e.g., patient declined, patient died, patient transferred, contraindication or other clinical exclusion, neoadjuvant chemotherapy or radiation not complete)

G9837 Trastuzumab not administered within 12 months of diagnosis

G9838 Patient has metastatic disease at diagnosis

G9839 Anti-EGFR monoclonal antibody therapy

G9840 Ras (KRAS and NRAS) gene mutation testing performed before initiation of anti-EGFR Moab

G9841 Ras (KRAS and NRAS) gene mutation testing not performed before initiation of anti-EGFR Moab

G9842 Patient has metastatic disease at diagnosis

G9843 Ras (KRAS or NRAS) gene mutation

G9844 Patient did not receive anti-EGFR monoclonal antibody therapy

G9845 Patient received anti-EGFR monoclonal antibody therapy

G9846 Patients who died from cancer

G9847 Patient received systemic cancer-directed therapy in the last 14 days of life

G9848 Patient did not receive systemic cancer-directed therapy in the last 14 days of life

G9849 Patients who died from cancer

G9850 Patient had more than one emergency department visit in the last 30 days of life

G9851 Patient had one or less emergency department visits in the last 30 days of life

(**G9852** Patients who died from cancer
Code deleted effective 12/31/2023, no HCPCS/CPT cross-reference provided.)

(**G9853** Patient admitted to the ICU in the last 30 days of life
Code deleted effective 12/31/2023, no HCPCS/CPT cross-reference provided.)

(**G9854** Patient was not admitted to the ICU in the last 30 days of life
Code deleted effective 12/31/2023, no HCPCS/CPT cross-reference provided.)

G9855 Patients who died from cancer

G9856 Patient was not admitted to hospice

G9857 Patient admitted to hospice

G9858 Patient enrolled in hospice

G9859 Patients who died from cancer

G9860 Patient spent less than three days in hospice care

G9861 Patient spent greater than or equal to three days in hospice care

G9862 Documentation of medical reason(s) for not recommending at least a 10 year follow-up interval (e.g., inadequate prep, familial or personal history of colonic polyps, patient had no adenoma and age is = 66 years old, or life expectancy < 10 years old, other medical reasons)

G9868 Receipt and analysis of remote, asynchronous images for dermatologic and/or ophthalmologic evaluation, for use only in a Medicare-approved cmmi model, less than 10 minutes

G9869 Receipt and analysis of remote, asynchronous images for dermatologic and/or ophthalmologic evaluation, for use only in a Medicare-approved cmmi model, 10-20 minutes

G9870 Receipt and analysis of remote, asynchronous images for dermatologic and/or ophthalmologic evaluation, for use only in a Medicare-approved cmmi model, more than 20 minutes

G9873 First Medicare diabetes prevention program (mdpp) core session was attended by an mdpp beneficiary under the mdpp expanded model (em). a core session is an mdpp service that: (1) is furnished by an mdpp supplier during months 1 through 6 of the mdpp services period; (2) is approximately 1 hour in length; and (3) adheres to a CDC-approved dpp curriculum for core sessions

G9874 Four total Medicare diabetes prevention program (mdpp) core sessions were attended by an mdpp beneficiary under the mdpp expanded model (em). a core session is an mdpp service that: (1) is furnished by an mdpp supplier during months 1 through 6 of the mdpp services period; (2) is approximately 1 hour in length; and (3) adheres to a CDC-approved dpp curriculum for core sessions

G9875 Nine total Medicare diabetes prevention program (mdpp) core sessions were attended by an mdpp beneficiary under the mdpp expanded model (em). a core session is an mdpp service that: (1) is furnished by an mdpp supplier during months 1 through 6 of the mdpp services period; (2) is approximately 1 hour in length; and (3) adheres to a CDC-approved dpp curriculum for core sessions

G9876 Two Medicare diabetes prevention program (mdpp) core maintenance sessions (ms) were attended by an mdpp beneficiary in months (mo) 7-9 under the mdpp expanded model (em). a core maintenance session is an mdpp service that: (1) is furnished by an mdpp supplier during months 7 through 12 of the mdpp services period; (2) is approximately 1 hour in length; and (3) adheres to a CDC-approved dpp curriculum for maintenance sessions. the beneficiary did not achieve at least 5% weight loss (wl) from his/her baseline weight, as measured by at least one in-person weight measurement at a core maintenance session in months 7-9

G9877 Two Medicare diabetes prevention program (mdpp) core maintenance sessions (ms) were attended by an mdpp beneficiary in months (mo) 10-12 under the mdpp expanded model (em). a core maintenance session is an mdpp service that: (1) is furnished by an mdpp supplier during months 7 through 12 of the mdpp services period; (2) is approximately 1 hour in length; and (3) adheres to a CDC-approved dpp curriculum for maintenance sessions. the beneficiary did not achieve at least 5% weight loss (wl) from his/her baseline weight, as measured by at least one in-person weight measurement at a core maintenance session in months 10-12

G9878 Two Medicare diabetes prevention program (mdpp) core maintenance sessions (ms) were attended by an mdpp beneficiary in months (mo) 7-9 under the mdpp expanded model (em). a core maintenance session is an mdpp service that: (1) is furnished by an mdpp supplier during months 7 through 12 of the mdpp services period; (2) is approximately 1 hour in length; and (3) adheres to a CDC-approved dpp curriculum for maintenance sessions. The beneficiary achieved at least 5% weight loss (wl) from his/her baseline weight, as measured by at least one in-person weight measurement at a core maintenance session in months 7-9

G9879 Two Medicare diabetes prevention program (mdpp) core maintenance sessions (ms) were attended by an mdpp beneficiary in months (mo) 10-12 under the mdpp expanded model (em). a core maintenance session is an mdpp service that: (1) is furnished by an mdpp supplier during months 7 through 12 of the mdpp services period; (2) is approximately 1 hour in length; and (3) adheres to a CDC-approved dpp curriculum for maintenance sessions. the beneficiary achieved at least 5% weight loss (wl) from his/her baseline weight, as measured by at least one in-person weight measurement at a core maintenance session in months 10-12

G9880 The mdpp beneficiary achieved at least 5% weight loss (wl) from his/her baseline weight in months 1-12 of the mdpp services period under the mdpp expanded model (em). this is a one-time payment available when a beneficiary first achieves at least 5% weight loss from baseline as measured by an in-person weight measurement at a core session or core maintenance session

G9881 The mdpp beneficiary achieved at least 9% weight loss (wl) from his/her baseline weight in months 1-24 under the mdpp expanded model (em). this is a one-time payment available when a beneficiary first achieves at least 9% weight loss from baseline as measured by an in-person weight measurement at a core session, core maintenance session, or ongoing maintenance session

G9882 Two Medicare diabetes prevention program (mdpp) ongoing maintenance sessions (ms) were attended by an mdpp beneficiary in months (mo) 13-15 under the mdpp expanded model (em). an ongoing maintenance session is an mdpp service that: (1) is furnished by an mdpp supplier during months 13 through 24 of the mdpp services period; (2) is approximately 1 hour in length; and (3) adheres to a CDC-approved dpp curriculum for maintenance sessions. the beneficiary maintained at least 5% weight loss (wl) from his/her baseline weight, as measured by at least one in-person weight measurement at an ongoing maintenance session in months 13-15

G9883 Two Medicare diabetes prevention program (mdpp) ongoing maintenance sessions (ms) were attended by an mdpp beneficiary in months (mo) 16-18 under the mdpp expanded model (em). an ongoing maintenance session is an mdpp service that: (1) is furnished by an mdpp supplier during months 13 through 24 of the mdpp services period; (2) is approximately 1 hour in length; and (3) adheres to a CDC-approved dpp curriculum for maintenance sessions. the beneficiary maintained at least 5% weight loss (wl) from his/her baseline weight, as measured by at least one in-person weight measurement at an ongoing maintenance session in months 16-18

G9884 Two Medicare diabetes prevention program (mdpp) ongoing maintenance sessions (ms) were attended by an mdpp beneficiary in months (mo) 19-21 under the mdpp expanded model (em). an ongoing maintenance session is an mdpp service that: (1) is furnished by an mdpp supplier during months 13 through 24 of the mdpp services period; (2) is approximately 1 hour in length; and (3) adheres to a CDC-approved dpp curriculum for maintenance sessions. the beneficiary maintained at least 5% weight loss (wl) from his/her baseline weight, as measured by at least one in-person weight measurement at an ongoing maintenance session in months 19-21

G9885 Two Medicare diabetes prevention program (mdpp) ongoing maintenance sessions (ms) were attended by an mdpp beneficiary in months (mo) 22-24 under the mdpp expanded model (em). an ongoing maintenance session is an mdpp service that: (1) is furnished by an mdpp supplier during months 13 through 24 of the mdpp services period; (2) is approximately 1 hour in length; and (3) adheres to a CDC-approved dpp curriculum for maintenance sessions. the beneficiary maintained at least 5% weight loss (wl) from his/her baseline weight, as measured by at least one in-person weight measurement at an ongoing maintenance session in months 22-24

G9890 Bridge payment: a one-time payment for the first Medicare diabetes prevention program (mdpp) core session, core maintenance session, or ongoing maintenance session furnished by an mdpp supplier to an mdpp beneficiary during months 1-24 of the mdpp expanded model (em) who has

previously received mdpp services from a different mdpp supplier under the mdpp expanded model. a supplier may only receive one bridge payment per mdpp beneficiary

G9891 Mdpp session reported as a line-item on a claim for a payable mdpp expanded model (em) HCPCS code for a session furnished by the billing supplier under the mdpp expanded model and counting toward achievement of the attendance performance goal for the payable mdpp expanded model HCPCS code (this code is for reporting purposes only)

G9892 Documentation of patient reason(s) for not performing a dilated macular examination

G9893 Dilated macular exam was not performed, reason not otherwise specified

G9894 Androgen deprivation therapy prescribed/administered in combination with external beam radiotherapy to the prostate

G9895 Documentation of medical reason(s) for not prescribing/administering androgen deprivation therapy in combination with external beam radiotherapy to the prostate (e.g., salvage therapy)

G9896 Documentation of patient reason(s) for not prescribing/administering androgen deprivation therapy in combination with external beam radiotherapy to the prostate

G9897 Patients who were not prescribed/administered androgen deprivation therapy in combination with external beam radiotherapy to the prostate, reason not given

G9898 Patients aged 66 or older in institutional special needs plans (SNP) or residing in long-term care with pos code 32, 33, 34, 54, or 56 for more than 90 consecutive days during the measurement period

G9899 Screening, diagnostic, film, digital or digital breast tomosynthesis (3d) mammography results documented and reviewed

G9900 Screening, diagnostic, film, digital or digital breast tomosynthesis (3d) mammography results were not documented and reviewed, reason not otherwise specified

G9901 Patient aged 66 or older in institutional special needs plans (SNP) or residing in long-term care with pos code 32, 33, 34, 54, or 56 for more than 90 consecutive days during the measurement period

G9902 Patient screened for tobacco use and identified as a tobacco user

G9903 Patient screened for tobacco use and identified as a tobacco non-user

(**G9904** Documentation of medical reason(s) for not screening for tobacco use (e.g., limited life expectancy, other medical reason)

Code deleted effective 12/31/2022, no HCPCS/CPT cross-reference provided.)

G9905 Patient not screened for tobacco use

G9906 Patient identified as a tobacco user received tobacco cessation intervention during the measurement period or in the six months prior to the measurement period (counseling and/or pharmacotherapy)

(**G9907** Documentation of medical reason(s) for not providing tobacco cessation intervention on the date of the encounter or within the previous 12 months (e.g., limited life expectancy, other medical reason)

Code deleted effective 12/31/2022, no HCPCS/CPT cross-reference provided.)

G9908 Patient identified as tobacco user did not receive tobacco cessation intervention during the measurement period or in the six months prior to the measurement period (counseling and/or pharmacotherapy)

(**G9909** Documentation of medical reason(s) for not providing tobacco cessation intervention on the date of the encounter or within the previous 12 months if identified as a tobacco user (e.g., limited life

expectancy, other medical reason)
Code deleted effective 12/31/2022, no HCPCS/CPT cross-reference provided.)

G9910 Patients aged 66 or older in institutional special needs plans (SNP) or residing in long-term care with pos code 32, 33, 34, 54 or 56 for more than 90 consecutive days during the measurement period

G9911 Clinically node negative (t1n0m0 or t2n0m0) invasive breast cancer before or after neoadjuvant systemic therapy

G9912 Hepatitis b virus (HBV) status assessed, and results interpreted prior to initiating anti-TNF (tumor necrosis factor) therapy

G9913 Hepatitis b virus (HBV) status not assessed, and results interpreted prior to initiating anti-TNF (tumor necrosis factor) therapy, reason not otherwise specified

▲ **G9914** Patient receiving an anti-TNF agent

G9915 No record of HBV results documented

G9916 Functional status performed once in the last 12 months

G9917 Documentation of advanced stage dementia and caregiver knowledge is limited

G9918 Functional status not performed; reason not otherwise specified

G9919 Screening performed and positive and provision of recommendations

G9920 Screening performed and negative

G9921 No screening performed, partial screening performed or positive screen without recommendations and reason is not given or otherwise specified

G9922 Safety concerns screen provided and if positive then documented mitigation recommendations

G9923 Safety concerns screen provided and negative

G9924 Documentation of medical reason(s) for not providing safety concerns screen or for not providing recommendations, orders or referrals for positive screen (e.g., patient in palliative care, other medical reason)

G9925 Safety concerns screening not provided, reason not otherwise specified

G9926 Safety concerns screening positive screen is without provision of mitigation recommendations, including but not limited to referral to other resources

(**G9927** Documentation of system reason(s) for not prescribing an FDA-approved anticoagulation due to patient being currently enrolled in a clinical trial related to af/atrial flutter treatment
Code deleted effective 12/31/2023, no HCPCS/CPT cross-reference provided.)

G9928 FDA-approved anticoagulant not prescribed; reason not given

G9929 Patient with transient or reversible cause of af (e.g., pneumonia, hyperthyroidism, pregnancy, cardiac surgery)

G9930 Patients who are receiving comfort care only

G9931 Documentation of cha2ds2-vasc risk score of 0 or 1 for men; or 0, 1, or 2 for women

(**G9932** Documentation of patient reason(s) for not having records of negative or managed positive tb screen (e.g., patient does not return for Mantoux (PPD) skin test evaluation)
Code deleted effective 12/31/2022, no HCPCS/CPT cross-reference provided.)

G9933 Adenoma(s) or colorectal cancer detected during screening colonoscopy

G9934 Documentation that neoplasm detected is only diagnosed as traditional serrated adenoma, sessile serrated polyp, or sessile serrated adenoma

G9935 Adenoma(s) or colorectal cancer not detected during screening colonoscopy

G9936 Surveillance colonoscopy - personal history of colonic polyps, colon cancer, or other malignant neoplasm of rectum, rectosigmoid junction, and anus

G9937 Diagnostic colonoscopy

▲ **G9938** Patients aged 66 or older in institutional special needs plans (SNP) or residing in long-term care with pos code 32, 33, 34, 54, or 56 for more than 90 consecutive days during the six months prior to the measurement period through December 31 of the measurement period

G9939 Pathologists/dermatopathologists is the same clinician who performed the biopsy

G9940 Documentation of medical reason(s) for not on a statin (e.g., pregnancy, in vitro fertilization, clomiphene Rx, ESRD, cirrhosis, muscular pain and disease during the measurement period or prior year)

G9941 Back pain was measured by the visual analog scale (vas) within three months preoperatively and at three months (6 - 20 weeks) postoperatively

(**G9942** Patient had any additional spine procedures performed on the same date as the lumbar discectomy/laminectomy

Code deleted effective 12/31/2022, no HCPCS/CPT cross-reference provided.)

G9943 Back pain was not measured by the visual analog scale (vas) or numeric pain scale at three months (6 - 20 weeks) postoperatively

G9944 Back pain was measured by the visual analog scale (vas) within three months preoperatively and at one year (9 to 15 months) postoperatively

G9945 Patient had cancer, acute fracture or infection related to the lumbar spine or patient had neuromuscular, idiopathic or congenital lumbar scoliosis

G9946 Back pain was not measured by the visual analog scale (vas) or numeric pain scale at one year (9 to 15 months) postoperatively

G9947 Leg pain was measured by the visual analog scale (vas) within three months preoperatively and at three months (6 to 20 weeks) postoperatively

(**G9948** Patient had any additional spine procedures performed on the same date as the lumbar discectomy/laminectomy

Code deleted effective 12/31/2022, no HCPCS/CPT cross-reference provided.)

G9949 Leg pain was not measured by the visual analog scale (vas) or numeric pain scale at three months (6 - 20 weeks) postoperatively

G9954 Patient exhibits 2 or more risk factors for post-operative vomiting

G9955 Cases in which an inhalational anesthetic is used only for induction

G9956 Patient received combination therapy consisting of at least two prophylactic pharmacologic anti-emetic agents of different classes preoperatively and/or intraoperatively

G9957 Documentation of medical reason for not receiving combination therapy consisting of at least two prophylactic pharmacologic anti-emetic agents of different classes preoperatively and/or intraoperatively (e.g., intolerance or other medical reason)

G9958 Patient did not receive combination therapy consisting of at least two prophylactic pharmacologic anti-emetic agents of different classes preoperatively and/or intraoperatively

G9959 Systemic antimicrobials not prescribed

G9960 Documentation of medical reason(s) for prescribing systemic antimicrobials

G9961 Systemic antimicrobials prescribed

G9962 Embolization endpoints are documented separately for each embolized vessel and ovarian artery angiography or embolization performed in the presence of variant uterine artery anatomy

G9963 Embolization endpoints are not documented separately for each embolized vessel or ovarian artery angiography or embolization not performed in the presence of variant uterine artery anatomy

G9964 Patient received at least one well-child visit with a PCP during the performance period

G9965 Patient did not receive at least one well-child visit with a PCP during the performance period

G9966 Children who were screened for risk of developmental, behavioral and social delays using a standardized tool with interpretation and report

G9967 Children who were not screened for risk of developmental, behavioral and social delays using a standardized tool with interpretation and report

G9968 Patient was referred to another clinician or specialist during the measurement period

G9969 Clinician who referred the patient to another clinician received a report from the clinician to whom the patient was referred

G9970 Clinician who referred the patient to another clinician did not receive a report from the clinician to whom the patient was referred

G9974 Dilated macular exam performed, including documentation of the presence or absence of macular thickening or geographic atrophy or hemorrhage and the level of macular degeneration severity

G9975 Documentation of medical reason(s) for not performing a dilated macular examination

G9978 Remote in-home visit for the evaluation and management of a new patient for use only in a Medicare-approved bundled payments for care improvement advanced (bpci advanced) model episode of care, which requires these 3 key components: a problem focused history; a problem focused examination; and straightforward medical decision making, furnished in real time using interactive audio and video technology. counseling and coordination of care with other physicians, other qualified health care professionals or agencies are provided consistent with the nature of the problem(s) and the needs of the patient or the family or both. usually, the presenting problem(s) are self limited or minor. typically, 10 minutes are spent with the patient or family or both via real time, audio and video intercommunications technology

G9979 Remote in-home visit for the evaluation and management of a new patient for use only in a Medicare-approved bundled payments for care improvement advanced (bpci advanced) model episode of care, which requires these 3 key components: an expanded problem focused history; an expanded problem focused examination; straightforward medical decision making, furnished in real time using interactive audio and video technology. counseling and coordination of care with other physicians, other qualified health care professionals or agencies are provided consistent with the nature of the problem(s) and the needs of the patient or the family or both. usually, the presenting problem(s) are of low to moderate severity. typically, 20 minutes are spent with the patient or family or both via real time, audio and video intercommunications technology

G9980 Remote in-home visit for the evaluation and management of a new patient for use only in a Medicare-approved bundled payments for care improvement advanced (bpci advanced) model episode of care, which requires these 3 key components: a detailed history; a detailed examination; medical decision making of low complexity, furnished in real time using interactive audio and video technology. counseling and coordination of care with other physicians, other qualified health care professionals or agencies are provided consistent with the nature of the problem(s) and the needs of the patient or the family or both. usually, the presenting problem(s) are of moderate severity. typically, 30 minutes are spent with the patient or family or both via real time, audio and video intercommunications technology

G9981 Remote in-home visit for the evaluation and management of a new patient for use only in a Medicare-approved bundled payments for care improvement advanced (bpci advanced) model episode of care, which requires these 3 key components: a comprehensive history; a comprehensive examination; medical decision making of moderate complexity, furnished in real time using interactive audio and video technology. counseling and coordination of care with other physicians, other qualified health care professionals or agencies are provided consistent with the nature of the problem(s) and the needs of the patient or the family or both. usually, the presenting problem(s) are of moderate to high severity. typically, 45 minutes are spent with the patient or family or both via real time, audio and video intercommunications technology

G9982 Remote in-home visit for the evaluation and management of a new patient for use only in a Medicare-approved bundled payments for care improvement advanced (bpci advanced) model episode of care, which requires these 3 key components: a comprehensive history; a comprehensive examination; medical decision making of high complexity, furnished in real time using interactive audio and video technology. counseling and coordination of care with other physicians, other qualified health care professionals or agencies are provided consistent with the nature of the problem(s) and the needs of the patient or the family or both. usually, the presenting problem(s) are of moderate to high severity. typically, 60 minutes are spent with the patient or family or both via real time, audio and video intercommunications technology

G9983 Remote in-home visit for the evaluation and management of an established patient for use only in a Medicare-approved bundled payments for care improvement advanced (bpci advanced) model episode of care, which requires at least 2 of the following 3 key components: a problem focused history; a problem focused examination; straightforward medical decision making, furnished in real time using interactive audio and video technology. counseling and coordination of care with other physicians, other qualified health care professionals or agencies are provided consistent with the nature of the problem(s) and the needs of the patient or the family or both. usually, the presenting problem(s) are self limited or minor. typically, 10 minutes are spent with the patient or family or both via real time, audio and video intercommunications technology

G9984 Remote in-home visit for the evaluation and management of an established patient for use only in a Medicare-approved bundled payments for care improvement advanced (bpci advanced) model episode of care, which requires at least 2 of the following 3 key components: an expanded problem focused history; an expanded problem focused examination; medical decision making of low complexity, furnished in real time using interactive audio and video technology. counseling and coordination of care with other physicians, other qualified health care professionals or agencies are provided consistent with the nature of the problem(s) and the needs of the patient or the family or both. usually, the presenting problem(s) are of low to moderate severity. typically, 15 minutes are spent with the patient or family or both via real time, audio and video intercommunications technology

G9985 Remote in-home visit for the evaluation and management of an established patient for use only in a Medicare-approved bundled payments for care improvement advanced (bpci advanced) model episode of care, which requires at least 2 of the following 3 key components: a detailed history; a detailed examination; medical decision making of moderate complexity, furnished in real time using interactive audio and video technology. counseling and coordination of care with other physicians, other qualified health care professionals or agencies are provided consistent with the nature of the problem(s) and the needs of the patient or the family or both. usually, the presenting problem(s) are of moderate to high severity. typically, 25 minutes are spent with the patient or family or both via real time, audio and video intercommunications technology

G9986 Remote in-home visit for the evaluation and management of an established patient for use only in a Medicare-approved bundled payments for care improvement advanced (bpci advanced) model episode of care, which requires at least 2 of the following 3 key components: a comprehensive history; a comprehensive examination; medical decision making of high complexity, furnished in real time using interactive audio and video technology. counseling and coordination of care with other physicians, other qualified health care professionals or agencies are provided consistent with the nature of the problem(s) and the needs of the patient or the family or both. usually, the presenting problem(s) are of moderate to high severity. typically, 40 minutes are spent with the patient or family or both via real time, audio and video intercommunications technology

G9987 Bundled payments for care improvement advanced (bpci advanced) model home visit for patient assessment performed by clinical staff for an individual not considered homebound, including, but not necessarily limited to patient assessment of clinical status, safety/fall prevention, functional status/ambulation, medication reconciliation/management, compliance with orders/plan of care, performance of activities of daily living, and ensuring beneficiary connections to community and other services; for use only for a bpci advanced model episode of care; may not be billed for a 30-day period covered by a transitional care management code

G9988 Palliative care services provided to patient any time during the measurement period

(**G9989** Documentation of medical reason(s) for not administering pneumococcal vaccine (e.g., adverse

reaction to vaccine)
Code deleted effective 12/31/2022, no HCPCS/CPT cross-reference provided.)

▲ **G9990** Patient did not receive any pneumococcal conjugate or polysaccharide vaccine on or after their 19th birthday and before the end of the measurement period

▲ **G9991** Patient received any pneumococcal conjugate or polysaccharide vaccine on or after their 19th birthday and before the end of the measurement period

G9992 Palliative care services used by patient any time during the measurement period

G9993 Patient was provided palliative care services any time during the measurement period

G9994 Patient is using palliative care services any time during the measurement period

(**G9995** Patients who use palliative care services any time during the measurement period
Code deleted effective 12/31/2023, no HCPCS/CPT cross-reference provided.)

G9996 Documentation stating the patient has received or is currently receiving palliative or hospice care

G9997 Documentation of patient pregnancy anytime during the measurement period prior to and including the current encounter

▲ **G9998** Documentation of medical reason(s) for an interval of less than 3 years since the last colonoscopy (e.g., last colonoscopy incomplete, last colonoscopy had inadequate prep, piecemeal removal of adenomas, or sessile serrated polyps >= 20 mm in size, last colonoscopy found greater than 10 adenomas, lower gastrointestinal bleeding, or patient at high risk for colon cancer due to underlying medical history ([i.e. Crohn's disease, ulcerative colitis, personal or family history of colon cancer, hereditary colorectal cancer syndromes])

G9999 Documentation of system reason(s) for an interval of less than 3 years since the last colonoscopy (e.g., unable to locate previous colonoscopy report, previous colonoscopy report was incomplete)

Rehabilitative Services

H0001 Alcohol and/or drug assessment

H0002 Behavioral health screening to determine eligibility for admission to treatment program

H0003 Alcohol and/or drug screening; laboratory analysis of specimens for presence of alcohol and/or drugs

H0004 Behavioral health counseling and therapy, per 15 minutes

H0005 Alcohol and/or drug services; group counseling by a clinician

H0006 Alcohol and/or drug services; case management

H0007 Alcohol and/or drug services; crisis intervention (outpatient)

H0008 Alcohol and/or drug services; sub-acute detoxification (hospital inpatient)

H0009 Alcohol and/or drug services; acute detoxification (hospital inpatient)

H0010 Alcohol and/or drug services; sub-acute detoxification (residential addiction program inpatient)

H0011 Alcohol and/or drug services; acute detoxification (residential addiction program inpatient)

H0012 Alcohol and/or drug services; sub-acute detoxification (residential addiction program outpatient)

H0013 Alcohol and/or drug services; acute detoxification (residential addiction program outpatient)

H0014 Alcohol and/or drug services; ambulatory detoxification

H0015 Alcohol and/or drug services; intensive outpatient (treatment program that operates at least 3 hours/day and at least 3 days/week and is based on an individualized treatment plan), including assessment, counseling; crisis intervention, and activity therapies or education

H0016 Alcohol and/or drug services; medical/somatic (medical intervention in ambulatory setting)

H0017 Behavioral health; residential (hospital residential treatment program), without room and board, per diem

H0018 Behavioral health; short-term residential (non-hospital residential treatment program), without room and board, per diem

H0019 Behavioral health; long-term residential (non-medical, non-acute care in a residential treatment program where stay is typically longer than 30 days), without room and board, per diem

H0020 Alcohol and/or drug services; methadone administration and/or service (provision of the drug by a licensed program)

H0021 Alcohol and/or drug training service (for staff and personnel not employed by providers)

H0022 Alcohol and/or drug intervention service (planned facilitation)

H0023 Behavioral health outreach service (planned approach to reach a targeted population)

H0024 Behavioral health prevention information dissemination service (one-way direct or non-direct contact with service audiences to affect knowledge and attitude)

H0025 Behavioral health prevention education service (delivery of services with target population to affect knowledge, attitude and/or behavior)

H0026 Alcohol and/or drug prevention process service, community-based (delivery of services to develop skills of impactors)

H0027 Alcohol and/or drug prevention environmental service (broad range of external activities geared toward modifying systems in order to mainstream prevention through policy and law)

H0028 Alcohol and/or drug prevention problem identification and referral service (e.g., student assistance and employee assistance programs), does not include assessment

H0029	Alcohol and/or drug prevention alternatives service (services for populations that exclude alcohol and other drug use e.g., alcohol free social events)
H0030	Behavioral health hotline service
H0031	Mental health assessment, by non-physician
H0032	Mental health service plan development by non-physician
H0033	Oral medication administration, direct observation
H0034	Medication training and support, per 15 minutes
H0035	Mental health partial hospitalization, treatment, less than 24 hours
H0036	Community psychiatric supportive treatment, face-to-face, per 15 minutes
H0037	Community psychiatric supportive treatment program, per diem
H0038	Self-help/peer services, per 15 minutes
H0039	Assertive community treatment, face-to-face, per 15 minutes
H0040	Assertive community treatment program, per diem
H0041	Foster care, child, non-therapeutic, per diem
H0042	Foster care, child, non-therapeutic, per month
H0043	Supported housing, per diem
H0044	Supported housing, per month
H0045	Respite care services, not in the home, per diem
H0046	Mental health services, not otherwise specified
H0047	Alcohol and/or other drug abuse services, not otherwise specified
H0048	Alcohol and/or other drug testing: collection and handling only, specimens other than blood
H0049	Alcohol and/or drug screening
H0050	Alcohol and/or drug services, brief intervention, per 15 minutes
H1000	Prenatal care, at-risk assessment
H1001	Prenatal care, at-risk enhanced service; antepartum management
H1002	Prenatal care, at risk enhanced service; care coordination
H1003	Prenatal care, at-risk enhanced service; education
H1004	Prenatal care, at-risk enhanced service; follow-up home visit
H1005	Prenatal care, at-risk enhanced service package (includes h1001-h1004)
H1010	Non-medical family planning education, per session
H1011	Family assessment by licensed behavioral health professional for state defined purposes
H2000	Comprehensive multidisciplinary evaluation
H2001	Rehabilitation program, per 1/2 day
H2010	Comprehensive medication services, per 15 minutes
H2011	Crisis intervention service, per 15 minutes
H2012	Behavioral health day treatment, per hour
H2013	Psychiatric health facility service, per diem
H2014	Skills training and development, per 15 minutes
H2015	Comprehensive community support services, per 15 minutes
H2016	Comprehensive community support services, per diem
H2017	Psychosocial rehabilitation services, per 15 minutes

H2018 Psychosocial rehabilitation services, per diem
H2019 Therapeutic behavioral services, per 15 minutes
H2020 Therapeutic behavioral services, per diem
H2021 Community-based wrap-around services, per 15 minutes
H2022 Community-based wrap-around services, per diem
H2023 Supported employment, per 15 minutes
H2024 Supported employment, per diem
H2025 Ongoing support to maintain employment, per 15 minutes
H2026 Ongoing support to maintain employment, per diem
H2027 Psychoeducational service, per 15 minutes
H2028 Sexual offender treatment service, per 15 minutes
H2029 Sexual offender treatment service, per diem
H2030 Mental health clubhouse services, per 15 minutes
H2031 Mental health clubhouse services, per diem
H2032 Activity therapy, per 15 minutes
H2033 Multisystemic therapy for juveniles, per 15 minutes
H2034 Alcohol and/or drug abuse halfway house services, per diem
H2035 Alcohol and/or other drug treatment program, per hour
H2036 Alcohol and/or other drug treatment program, per diem
H2037 Developmental delay prevention activities, dependent child of client, per 15 minutes

DRUGS ADMINISTERED OTHER THAN ORAL METHOD

(EXCEPTION: ORAL IMMUNOSUPPRESSIVE DRUGS)

Guidelines

In addition to the information presented in the INTRODUCTION, several other items unique to this section are defined or identified here:

1. EXCEPTION: Oral immunosuppressive drugs are not included in this section.

2. ROUTE OF ADMINISTRATION: Unless otherwise specified, the drugs listed in this section may be injected either subcutaneously, intramuscularly or intravenously.

3. **SUBSECTION INFORMATION:** Some of the listed subheadings or subsections have special needs or instructions unique to that section. Where these are indicated, special "notes" will be presented preceding or following the listings. Those subsections within the DRUGS ADMINISTERED OTHER THAN ORAL METHOD section that have "notes" are as follows:

Subsection	Code Numbers
Drugs administered other than oral method	J0000-J8999
Immunosuppressive drugs	J7500-J7506
Chemotherapy drugs	J9000-J9999

4. **UNLISTED SERVICE OR PROCEDURE:** A service or procedure may be provided that is not listed in this edition of HCPCS. When reporting such a service, the appropriate "unlisted procedure" code may be used to indicate the service, identifying it by "special report" as defined below. HCPCS terminology is inconsistent in defining unlisted procedures. The procedure definition may include the term(s) "unlisted", "not otherwise classified", "unspecified", "unclassified", "other" and "miscellaneous". Prior to using these codes, try to determine if a Local Level III code or CPT code is available. The "unlisted procedures" and accompanying codes for DRUGS ADMINISTERED OTHER THAN ORAL METHOD are as follows:

   J3490 Unclassified drugs
   J9999 Not otherwise classified, antineoplastic drugs

5. **SPECIAL REPORT:** A service, material or supply that is rarely provided, unusual, variable or new may require a special report in determining medical appropriateness for reimbursement purposes. Pertinent information should include an adequate definition or description of the nature, extent, and need for the service, material or supply.

6. **MODIFIERS:** Listed services may be modified under certain circumstances. When appropriate, the modifying circumstance is identified by adding a modifier to the basic procedure code. CPT and HCPCS National Level II modifiers may be used with CPT and HCPCS National Level II procedure codes. Modifiers commonly used with DRUGS ADMINISTERED OTHER THAN ORAL METHOD are as follows:

   -AA Anesthesia services performed personally by anesthesiologist

   -AD Medical supervision by a physician: more than four concurrent anesthesia procedures.

   -CC Procedure code change (use "CC" when the procedure code submitted was changed either for administrative reasons or because an incorrect code was filed)

-G8 Monitored anesthesia care (MAC) for deep complex, complicated, or markedly invasive surgical procedure

-G9 Monitored anesthesia care (MAC) for patient who has history of severe cardio-pulmonary condition

-TC Technical component. Under certain circumstances, a charge may be made for the technical component alone. Under those circumstances, the technical component charge is identified by adding modifier -TC to the usual procedure code. Technical component charges are institutional charges and are not billed separately by physicians. However, portable x-ray suppliers bill only for the technical component and should use modifier -TC. The charge data from portable x-ray suppliers will then be used to build customary and prevailing profiles.

7. **CPT CODE CROSS-REFERENCE:** Unless otherwise specified, the equivalent CPT codes for all listings in this section fall within the range 90701-90799.

Drugs Administered Other Than Oral Method

The following list of drugs can be injected either subcutaneous, intramuscular, or intravenous. The brand name(s) of the drugs has been included as bold-type in brackets [ ] in some cases.

NOTE: Third party payers may wish to determine a threshold and pay up to a certain dollar limit before developing for the drug. Use procedure code J0110 for processing these cases.

J0120 Injection, tetracycline, up to 250 mg

J0121 Injection, omadacycline, 1 mg

J0122 Injection, eravacycline, 1 mg

J0129 Injection, abatacept, 10 mg (code may be used for Medicare when drug administered under the direct supervision of a physician, not for use when drug is self administered)

J0130 Injection abciximab, 10 mg

J0131 Injection, acetaminophen, not otherwise specified,10 mg

J0132 Injection, acetylcysteine, 100 mg

J0133 Injection, acyclovir, 5 mg

J0134 Injection, acetaminophen (Fresenius kabi) not therapeutically equivalent to J0131, 10 mg

J0135 Injection, adalimumab, 20 mg

J0136 Injection, acetaminophen (b braun) not therapeutically equivalent to J0131, 10 mg

J0150 Injection, adenosine for therapeutic use, 6 mg (not to be used to report any adenosine phosphate compounds, instead use a9270)

J0151 Injection, adenosine for diagnostic use, 1 mg (not to be used to report any adenosine phosphate compounds, instead use a9270)

J0153 Injection, adenosine, 1 mg (not to be used to report any adenosine phosphate compounds)

J0171 Injection, adrenalin, epinephrine, 0.1 mg

J0172 Injection, aducanumab-avwa, 2 mg

J0173 Injection, epinephrine (belcher) not therapeutically equivalent to J0171, 0.1 mg

J0178 Injection, aflibercept, 1 mg

J0179 Injection, brolucizumab-dbll, 1 mg

J0180 Injection, agalsidase beta, 1 mg

• **J0184** Injection, amisulpride, 1 mg

J0185	Injection, aprepitant, 1 mg
J0190	Injection, biperiden lactate, per 5 mg
J0200	Injection, alatrofloxacin mesylate, 100 mg
J0202	Injection, alemtuzumab, 1 mg
J0205	Injection, alglucerase, per 10 units
J0207	Injection, amifostine, 500 mg
J0210	Injection, methyldopate HCl, up to 250 mg
J0215	Injection, alefacept, 0.5 mg
• J0217	Injection, velmanase alfa-tycv, 1 mg
J0219	Injection, avalglucosidase alfa-ngpt, 4 mg
J0220	Injection, alglucosidase alfa, 10 mg, not otherwise specified
J0221	Injection, alglucosidase alfa, (lumizyme), 10 mg
J0222	Injection, patisiran, 0.1 mg
J0223	Injection, givosiran, 0.5 mg
J0224	Injection, lumasiran, 0.5 mg
J0225	Injection, vutrisiran, 1 mg
J0248	Injection, remdesivir, 1 mg
J0256	Injection, alpha 1 proteinase inhibitor (human), not otherwise specified, 10 mg
J0257	Injection, alpha 1 proteinase inhibitor (human), (glassia), 10 mg
J0270	Injection, alprostadil, 1.25 mcg (code may be used for Medicare when drug administered under the direct supervision of a physician, not for use when drug is self administered)
J0275	Alprostadil urethral suppository (code may be used for Medicare when drug administered under the direct supervision of a physician, not for use when drug is self administered)
J0278	Injection, amikacin sulfate, 100 mg
J0280	Injection, aminophyllin, up to 250 mg
J0282	Injection, amiodarone hydrochloride, 30 mg
J0283	Injection, amiodarone hydrochloride (nexterone), 30 mg
J0285	Injection, amphotericin b, 50 mg
J0287	Injection, amphotericin b lipid complex, 10 mg
J0288	Injection, amphotericin b cholesteryl sulfate complex, 10 mg
J0289	Injection, amphotericin b liposome, 10 mg
J0290	Injection, ampicillin sodium, 500 mg
J0291	Injection, plazomicin, 5 mg
J0295	Injection, ampicillin sodium/sulbactam sodium, per 1.5 gm
J0300	Injection, amobarbital, up to 125 mg
J0330	Injection, succinylcholine chloride, up to 20 mg
J0348	Injection, anidulafungin, 1 mg
J0350	Injection, anistreplase, per 30 units
J0360	Injection, hydralazine HCl, up to 20 mg
J0364	Injection, apomorphine hydrochloride, 1 mg
J0365	Injection, aprotonin, 10,000 kiu

J CODES

	J0380	Injection, metaraminol bitartrate, per 10 mg
	J0390	Injection, chloroquine hydrochloride, up to 250 mg
•	**J0391**	Injection, artesunate, 1 mg
	J0395	Injection, arbutamine HCl, 1 mg
	J0400	Injection, aripiprazole, intramuscular, 0.25 mg
	J0401	Injection, aripiprazole, extended release, 1 mg
•	**J0402**	Injection, aripiprazole (abilify asimtufii), 1 mg
	J0456	Injection, azithromycin, 500 mg
	J0461	Injection, atropine sulfate, 0.01 mg
	J0470	Injection, dimercaprol, per 100 mg
	J0475	Injection, baclofen, 10 mg
	J0476	Injection, baclofen, 50 mcg for intrathecal trial
	J0480	Injection, basiliximab, 20 mg
	J0485	Injection, belatacept, 1 mg
	J0490	Injection, belimumab, 10 mg
	J0491	Injection, anifrolumab-fnia, 1 mg
	J0500	Injection, dicyclomine HCl, up to 20 mg
	J0515	Injection, benztropine mesylate, per 1 mg
	J0517	Injection, benralizumab, 1 mg
	J0520	Injection, bethanechol chloride, myotonachol or urecholine, up to 5 mg
	J0558	Injection, penicillin g benzathine and penicillin g procaine, 100,000 units
	J0561	Injection, penicillin g benzathine, 100,000 units
	J0565	Injection, bezlotoxumab, 10 mg
	J0567	Injection, cerliponase alfa, 1 mg
	J0570	Buprenorphine implant, 74.2 mg
	J0571	Buprenorphine, oral, 1 mg
	J0572	Buprenorphine/naloxone, oral, less than or equal to 3 mg buprenorphine
	J0573	Buprenorphine/naloxone, oral, greater than 3 mg, but less than or equal to 6 mg buprenorphine
	J0574	Buprenorphine/naloxone, oral, greater than 6 mg, but less than or equal to 10 mg buprenorphine
	J0575	Buprenorphine/naloxone, oral, greater than 10 mg buprenorphine
•	**J0576**	Injection, buprenorphine extended-release (brixadi), 1 mg
	J0583	Injection, bivalirudin, 1 mg
	J0584	Injection, burosumab-twza 1 mg
	J0585	Injection, onabotulinumtoxina, 1 unit
	J0586	Injection, abobotulinumtoxina, 5 units
	J0587	Injection, rimabotulinumtoxinb, 100 units
	J0588	Injection, incobotulinumtoxin a, 1 unit
	J0591	Injection, deoxycholic acid, 1 mg
	J0592	Injection, buprenorphine hydrochloride, 0.1 mg
	J0593	Injection, lanadelumab-flyo, 1 mg (code may be used for Medicare when drug administered under direct supervision of a physician, not for use when drug is self-administered)

J CODES

J0594	injection, busulfan, 1 mg
J0595	Injection, butorphanol tartrate, 1 mg
J0596	Injection, c1 esterase inhibitor (recombinant), ruconest, 10 units
J0597	Injection, c-1 esterase inhibitor (human), berinert, 10 units
J0598	Injection, c-1 esterase inhibitor (human), cinryze, 10 units
J0599	Injection, c-1 esterase inhibitor (human), (haegarda), 10 units
J0600	Injection, edetate calcium disodium, up to 1000 mg
J0604	Cinacalcet, oral, 1 mg, (for ESRD on dialysis)
J0606	Injection, etelcalcetide, 0.1 mg
J0610	Injection, calcium gluconate (Fresenius kabi), per 10 ml
J0611	Injection, calcium gluconate (wg critical care), per 10 ml
J0620	Injection, calcium glycerophosphate and calcium lactate, per 10 ml
J0630	Injection, calcitonin salmon, up to 400 units
J0636	Injection, calcitriol, 0.1 mcg
J0637	Injection, caspofungin acetate, 5 mg
J0638	Injection, canakinumab, 1 mg
J0640	Injection, leucovorin calcium, per 50 mg
J0641	Injection, levoleucovorin, not otherwise specified, 0.5 mg
J0642	Injection, levoleucovorin (khapzory), 0.5 mg
J0670	Injection, mepivacaine hydrochloride, per 10 ml
• J0688	Injection, cefazolin sodium (hikma), not therapeutically equivalent to j0690, 500 mg
J0689	Injection, cefazolin sodium (Baxter), not therapeutically equivalent to J0690, 500 mg
J0690	Injection, cefazolin sodium, 500 mg
J0691	Injection, lefamulin, 1 mg
J0692	Injection, cefepime hydrochloride, 500 mg
J0693	Injection, cefiderocol, 5 mg
J0694	Injection, cefoxitin sodium, 1 gm
J0695	Injection, ceftolozane 50 mg and tazobactam 25 mg
J0696	Injection, ceftriaxone sodium, per 250 mg
J0697	Injection, sterile cefuroxime sodium, per 750 mg
J0698	Injection, cefotaxime sodium, per gm
J0699	Injection, cefiderocol, 10 mg
J0701	Injection, cefepime hydrochloride (Baxter), not therapeutically equivalent to maxipime, 500 mg
J0702	Injection, betamethasone acetate 3 mg and betamethasone sodium phosphate 3 mg
J0703	Injection, cefepime hydrochloride (b braun), not therapeutically equivalent to maxipime, 500 mg
J0706	Injection, caffeine citrate, 5 mg
J0710	Injection, cephapirin sodium, up to 1 gm
J0712	Injection, ceftaroline fosamil, 10 mg
J0713	Injection, ceftazidime, per 500 mg
J0714	Injection, ceftazidime and avibactam, 0.5 g/0.125 g

	J0715	Injection, ceftizoxime sodium, per 500 mg
	J0716	Injection, centruroides immune f(ab)2, up to 120 milligrams
	J0717	Injection, certolizumab pegol, 1 mg (code may be used for Medicare when drug administered under the direct supervision of a physician, not for use when drug is self administered)
	J0720	Injection, chloramphenicol sodium succinate, up to 1 gm
	J0725	Injection, chorionic gonadotropin, per 1,000 USP units
	J0735	Injection, clonidine hydrochloride, 1 mg
▲	**J0739**	Injection, cabotegravir, 1mg, FDA approved prescription, only for use as HIV pre-exposure prophylaxis (not for use as treatment for HIV)
	J0740	Injection, cidofovir, 375 mg
	J0741	Injection, cabotegravir and rilpivirine, 2mg/3mg
	J0742	Injection, imipenem 4 mg, cilastatin 4 mg and relebactam 2 mg
	J0743	Injection, cilastatin sodium; imipenem, per 250 mg
	J0744	Injection, ciprofloxacin for intravenous infusion, 200 mg
	J0745	Injection, codeine phosphate, per 30 mg
•	**J0750**	Emtricitabine 200mg and tenofovir disoproxil fumarate 300mg, oral, FDA approved prescription, only for use as HIV pre-exposure prophylaxis (not for use as treatment of HIV)
•	**J0751**	Emtricitabine 200mg and tenofovir alafenamide 25mg, oral, FDA approved prescription, only for use as HIV pre-exposure prophylaxis (not for use as treatment of HIV)
	J0760	Injection, colchicine, per 1 mg
	J0770	Injection, colistimethate sodium, up to 150 mg
	J0775	Injection, collagenase, clostridium histolyticum, 0.01 mg
	J0780	Injection, prochlorperazine, up to 10 mg
	J0791	Injection, crizanlizumab-tmca, 5 mg
	J0795	Injection, corticorelin ovine triflutate, 1 microgram
•	**J0799**	FDA approved prescription drug, only for use as HIV pre-exposure prophylaxis (not for use as treatment of HIV), not otherwise classified
	J0800	Injection, corticotropin, up to 40 units
	J0833	Injection, cosyntropin, not otherwise specified, 0.25 mg
	J0834	Injection, cosyntropin, 0.25 mg
	J0840	Injection, Crotalidae polyvalent immune fab (ovine), up to 1 gram
	J0841	Injection, Crotalidae immune f(ab')2 (equine), 120 mg
	J0850	Injection, cytomegalovirus immune globulin intravenous (human), per vial
•	**J0873**	Injection, daptomycin (xellia) not therapeutically equivalent to j0878, 1 mg
	J0875	Injection, dalbavancin, 5 mg
	J0877	Injection, daptomycin (hospira), not therapeutically equivalent to J0878, 1 mg
	J0878	Injection, daptomycin, 1 mg
	J0879	Injection, difelikefalin, 0.1 microgram, (for ESRD on dialysis)
	J0881	Injection, darbepoetin alfa, 1 microgram (non-ESRD use)
	J0882	Injection, darbepoetin alfa, 1 microgram (for ESRD on dialysis)
	J0883	Injection, argatroban, 1 mg (for non-ESRD use)
	J0884	Injection, argatroban, 1 mg (for ESRD on dialysis)

J0885	Injection, epoetin alfa, (for non-ESRD use), 1000 units
J0886	Injection, epoetin alfa, 1000 units (for ESRD on dialysis)
J0887	Injection, epoetin beta, 1 microgram, (for ESRD on dialysis)
J0888	Injection, epoetin beta, 1 microgram, (for non ESRD use)
J0890	Injection, peginesatide, 0.1 mg (for ESRD on dialysis)
J0891	Injection, argatroban (accord), not therapeutically equivalent to J0883, 1 mg (for non-ESRD use)
J0892	Injection, argatroban (accord), not therapeutically equivalent to J0884, 1 mg (for ESRD on dialysis)
J0893	Injection, decitabine (sun pharma) not therapeutically equivalent to J0894, 1 mg
J0894	Injection, decitabine, 1 mg
J0895	Injection, deferoxamine mesylate, 500 mg
J0896	Injection, luspatercept-aamt, 0.25 mg
J0897	Injection, denosumab, 1 mg
J0898	Injection, argatroban (auromedics), not therapeutically equivalent to J0883, 1 mg (for non-ESRD use)
J0899	Injection, argatroban (auromedics), not therapeutically equivalent to J0884, 1 mg (for ESRD on dialysis)
J0900	Injection, testosterone enanthate and estradiol valerate, up to 1 cc
J0945	Injection, brompheniramine maleate, per 10 mg
J1000	Injection, depo-estradiol cypionate, up to 5 mg
J1020	Injection, methylprednisolone acetate, 20 mg
J1030	Injection, methylprednisolone acetate, 40 mg
J1040	Injection, methylprednisolone acetate, 80 mg
J1050	Injection, medroxyprogesterone acetate, 1 mg
J1060	Injection, testosterone cypionate and estradiol cypionate, up to 1 ml
J1070	Injection, testosterone cypionate, up to 100 mg
J1071	Injection, testosterone cypionate, 1 mg
J1080	Injection, testosterone cypionate, 1 cc, 200 mg
J1094	Injection, dexamethasone acetate, 1 mg
J1095	Injection, dexamethasone 9 percent, intraocular, 1 microgram
J1096	Dexamethasone, lacrimal ophthalmic insert, 0.1 mg
J1097	Phenylephrine 10.16 mg/ml and ketorolac 2.88 mg/ml ophthalmic irrigation solution, 1 ml
J1100	Injection, dexamethasone sodium phosphate, 1 mg
• J1105	Dexmedetomidine, oral, 1 mcg
J1110	Injection, dihydroergotamine mesylate, per 1 mg
J1120	Injection, acetazolamide sodium, up to 500 mg
J1130	Injection, diclofenac sodium, 0.5 mg
J1160	Injection, digoxin, up to 0.5 mg
J1162	Injection, digoxin immune fab (ovine), per vial
J1165	Injection, phenytoin sodium, per 50 mg
J1170	Injection, hydromorphone, up to 4 mg

J CODES

Not payable by Medicare | Non-covered by Medicare | Special coverage instructions | Carrier judgement

	J1180	Injection, dyphylline, up to 500 mg
	J1190	Injection, dexrazoxane hydrochloride, per 250 mg
	J1200	Injection, diphenhydramine HCl, up to 50 mg
	J1201	Injection, cetirizine hydrochloride, 0.5 mg
	J1205	Injection, chlorothiazide sodium, per 500 mg
	J1212	Injection, DMSO, dimethyl sulfoxide, 50%, 50 ml
	J1230	Injection, methadone HCl, up to 10 mg
	J1240	Injection, dimenhydrinate, up to 50 mg
	J1245	Injection, dipyridamole, per 10 mg
•	J1246	Injection, dinutuximab, 0.1 mg
	J1250	Injection, dobutamine hydrochloride, per 250 mg
	J1260	Injection, dolasetron mesylate, 10 mg
	J1265	Injection, dopamine HCl, 40 mg
	J1267	Injection, doripenem, 10 mg
	J1270	Injection, doxercalciferol, 1 mcg
	J1290	Injection, ecallantide, 1 mg
	J1300	Injection, eculizumab, 10 mg
	J1301	Injection, edaravone, 1 mg
	J1302	Injection, sutimlimab-jome, 10 mg
	J1303	Injection, ravulizumab-cwvz, 10 mg
•	J1304	Injection, tofersen, 1 mg
	J1305	Injection, evinacumab-dgnb, 5mg
	J1306	Injection, inclisiran, 1 mg
	J1320	Injection, amitriptyline HCl, up to 20 mg
	J1322	Injection, elosulfase alfa, 1 mg
	J1324	Injection, enfuvirtide, 1 mg
	J1325	Injection, epoprostenol, 0.5 mg
	J1327	Injection, eptifibatide, 5 mg
	J1330	Injection, ergonovine maleate, up to 0.2 mg
	J1335	Injection, ertapenem sodium, 500 mg
	J1364	Injection, erythromycin lactobionate, per 500 mg
	J1380	Injection, estradiol valerate, up to 10 mg
	J1410	Injection, estrogen conjugated, per 25 mg
•	J1412	Injection, valoctocogene roxaparvovec-rvox, per ml, containing nominal 2 x 10^13 vector genomes
•	J1413	Injection, delandistrogene moxeparvovec-rokl, per therapeutic dose
	J1426	Injection, casimersen, 10 mg
	J1427	Injection, viltolarsen, 10 mg
	J1428	Injection, eteplirsen, 10 mg
	J1429	Injection, golodirsen, 10 mg
	J1430	Injection, ethanolamine oleate, 100 mg

J1435	Injection, estrone, per 1 mg
J1436	Injection, etidronate disodium, per 300 mg
J1437	Injection, ferric derisomaltose, 10 mg
J1438	Injection, etanercept, 25 mg (code may be used for Medicare when drug administered under the direct supervision of a physician, not for use when drug is self administered)
J1439	Injection, ferric carboxymaltose, 1 mg
J1442	Injection, filgrastim (g-csf), excludes biosimilars, 1 microgram
J1443	Injection, ferric pyrophosphate citrate solution (triferic), 0.1 mg of iron
J1444	Injection, ferric pyrophosphate citrate powder, 0.1 mg of iron
J1445	Injection, ferric pyrophosphate citrate solution (triferic avnu), 0.1 mg of iron
J1446	Injection, tbo-filgrastim, 5 micrograms
J1447	Injection, tbo-filgrastim, 1 microgram
J1448	Injection, trilaciclib, 1mg
J1450	Injection fluconazole, 200 mg
J1451	Injection, fomepizole, 15 mg
J1452	Injection, fomivirsen sodium, intraocular, 1.65 mg
J1453	Injection, fosaprepitant, 1 mg
J1454	Injection, fosnetupitant 235 mg and palonosetron 0.25 mg
J1455	Injection, foscarnet sodium, per 1000 mg
J1456	Injection, fosaprepitant (teva), not therapeutically equivalent to J1453, 1 mg
J1457	Injection, gallium nitrate, 1 mg
J1458	Injection, galsulfase, 1 mg
J1459	Injection, immune globulin (privigen), intravenous, non-lyophilized (e.g., liquid), 500 mg
J1460	Injection, gamma globulin, intramuscular, 1 cc
J1551	Injection, immune globulin (cutaquig), 100 mg
J1554	Injection, immune globulin (asceniv), 500 mg
J1555	Injection, immune globulin (cuvitru), 100 mg
J1556	Injection, immune globulin (bivigam), 500 mg
J1557	Injection, immune globulin, (gammaplex), intravenous, non-lyophilized (e.g., liquid), 500 mg
J1558	Injection, immune globulin (xembify), 100 mg
J1559	Injection, immune globulin (hizentra), 100 mg
J1560	Injection, gamma globulin, intramuscular, over 10 cc
J1561	Injection, immune globulin, (gamunex-c/gammaked), non-lyophilized (e.g., liquid), 500 mg
J1562	Injection, immune globulin (vivaglobin), 100 mg
J1566	Injection, immune globulin, intravenous, lyophilized (e.g., powder), not otherwise specified, 500 mg
J1568	Injection, immune globulin, (Octagam), intravenous, non-lyophilized (e.g., liquid), 500 mg
J1569	Injection, immune globulin, (gammagard liquid), non-lyophilized, (e.g., liquid), 500 mg
J1570	Injection, ganciclovir sodium, 500 mg
J1571	Injection, hepatitis b immune globulin (HepaGam b), intramuscular, 0.5 ml

J CODES

	J1572	Injection, immune globulin, (flebogamma/flebogamma dif), intravenous, non-lyophilized (e.g., liquid), 500 mg
	J1573	Injection, hepatitis b immune globulin (HepaGam b), intravenous, 0.5 ml
	J1574	Injection, ganciclovir sodium (exela) not therapeutically equivalent to J1570, 500 mg
	J1575	Injection, immune globulin/hyaluronidase, (hyqvia), 100 mg immune globulin
	J1580	Injection, garamycin, gentamicin, up to 80 mg
	J1590	Injection, gatifloxacin, 10 mg
	J1595	Injection, glatiramer acetate, 20 mg
●	J1596	Injection, glycopyrrolate, 0.1 mg
	J1599	Injection, immune globulin, intravenous, non-lyophilized (e.g., liquid), not otherwise specified, 500 mg
	J1600	Injection, gold sodium thiomalate, up to 50 mg
	J1602	Injection, golimumab, 1 mg, for intravenous use
	J1610	Injection, glucagon hydrochloride, per 1 mg
	J1611	Injection, glucagon hydrochloride (Fresenius kabi), not therapeutically equivalent to J1610, per 1 mg
	J1620	Injection, gonadorelin hydrochloride, per 100 mcg
	J1626	Injection, granisetron hydrochloride, 100 mcg
	J1627	Injection, granisetron, extended-release, 0.1 mg
	J1628	Injection, guselkumab, 1 mg
	J1630	Injection, haloperidol, up to 5 mg
	J1631	Injection, haloperidol decanoate, per 50 mg
	J1632	Injection, brexanolone, 1 mg
	J1640	Injection, hemin, 1 mg
	J1642	Injection, heparin sodium, (heparin lock flush), per 10 units
	J1643	Injection, heparin sodium (Pfizer), not therapeutically equivalent to J1644, per 1000 units
	J1644	Injection, heparin sodium, per 1000 units
	J1645	Injection, dalteparin sodium, per 2500 iu
	J1650	Injection, enoxaparin sodium, 10 mg
	J1652	Injection, fondaparinux sodium, 0.5 mg
	J1655	Injection, tinzaparin sodium, 1000 iu
	J1670	Injection, tetanus immune globulin, human, up to 250 units
	J1675	Injection, histrelin acetate, 10 micrograms
	J1700	Injection, hydrocortisone acetate, up to 25 mg
	J1710	Injection, hydrocortisone sodium phosphate, up to 50 mg
	J1720	Injection, hydrocortisone sodium succinate, up to 100 mg
	J1725	Injection, hydroxyprogesterone caproate, 1 mg
	J1726	Injection, hydroxyprogesterone caproate, (Makena), 10 mg
	J1729	Injection, hydroxyprogesterone caproate, not otherwise specified, 10 mg
	J1730	Injection, diazoxide, up to 300 mg
	J1738	Injection, meloxicam, 1 mg

J1740	Injection, ibandronate sodium, 1 mg
J1741	Injection, ibuprofen, 100 mg
J1742	Injection, ibutilide fumarate, 1 mg
J1743	Injection, idursulfase, 1 mg
J1744	Injection, icatibant, 1 mg
J1745	Injection, infliximab, excludes biosimilar, 10 mg
J1746	Injection, ibalizumab-uiyk, 10 mg
J1750	Injection, iron dextran, 50 mg
J1756	Injection, iron sucrose, 1 mg
J1786	Injection, imiglucerase, 10 units
J1790	Injection, droperidol, up to 5 mg
J1800	Injection, propranolol HCl, up to 1 mg
J1810	Injection, droperidol and fentanyl citrate, up to 2 ml ampule
J1815	Injection, insulin, per 5 units
J1817	Insulin for administration through dme (i.e., insulin pump) per 50 units
J1823	Injection, inebilizumab-cdon, 1 mg
J1826	Injection, interferon beta-1a, 30 mcg
J1830	Injection, interferon beta-1b, 0.25 mg (code may be used for Medicare when drug administered under the direct supervision of a physician, not for use when drug is self administered)
J1833	Injection, isavuconazonium, 1 mg
J1835	Injection, itraconazole, 50 mg
J1840	Injection, kanamycin sulfate, up to 500 mg
J1850	Injection, kanamycin sulfate, up to 75 mg
J1885	Injection, ketorolac tromethamine, per 15 mg
J1890	Injection, cephalothin sodium, up to 1 gram
J1930	Injection, lanreotide, 1 mg
J1931	Injection, laronidase, 0.1 mg
J1932	Injection, lanreotide, (cipla), 1 mg
• J1939	Injection, bumetanide, 0.5 mg
J1940	Injection, furosemide, up to 20 mg
J1942	Injection, aripiprazole lauroxil, 1 mg
J1943	Injection, aripiprazole lauroxil, (aristada initio), 1 mg
J1944	Injection, aripiprazole lauroxil, (aristada), 1 mg
J1945	Injection, lepirudin, 50 mg
J1950	Injection, leuprolide acetate (for depot suspension), per 3.75 mg
J1951	Injection, leuprolide acetate for depot suspension (fensolvi), 0.25 mg
J1952	Leuprolide injectable, camcevi, 1 mg
J1953	Injection, levetiracetam, 10 mg
J1955	Injection, levocarnitine, per 1 gm
J1956	Injection, levofloxacin, 250 mg
J1960	Injection, levorphanol tartrate, up to 2 mg

J1980	Injection, hyoscyamine sulfate, up to 0.25 mg
J1990	Injection, chlordiazepoxide HCl, up to 100 mg
J2001	Injection, lidocaine HCl for intravenous infusion, 10 mg
J2010	Injection, lincomycin HCl, up to 300 mg
J2020	Injection, linezolid, 200 mg
J2021	Injection, linezolid (hospira) not therapeutically equivalent to J2020, 200 mg
J2060	Injection, lorazepam, 2 mg
J2062	Loxapine for inhalation, 1 mg
J2150	Injection, mannitol, 25% in 50 ml
J2170	Injection, mecasermin, 1 mg
J2175	Injection, meperidine hydrochloride, per 100 mg
J2180	Injection, meperidine and promethazine HCl, up to 50 mg
J2182	Injection, mepolizumab, 1 mg
J2184	Injection, meropenem (b. braun) not therapeutically equivalent to J2185, 100 mg
J2185	Injection, meropenem, 100 mg
J2186	Injection, meropenem and vaborbactam, 10mg/10mg (20mg)
J2210	Injection, methylergonovine maleate, up to 0.2 mg
J2212	Injection, methylnaltrexone, 0.1 mg
J2247	Injection, micafungin sodium (par pharm) not therapeutically equivalent to J2248, 1 mg
J2248	Injection, micafungin sodium, 1 mg
J2250	Injection, midazolam hydrochloride, per 1 mg
J2251	Injection, midazolam hydrochloride (wg critical care) not therapeutically equivalent to J2250, per 1 mg
J2260	Injection, milrinone lactate, 5 mg
J2265	Injection, minocycline hydrochloride, 1 mg
J2270	Injection, morphine sulfate, up to 10 mg
J2271	Injection, morphine sulfate, 100mg
J2272	Injection, morphine sulfate (Fresenius kabi) not therapeutically equivalent to J2270, up to 10 mg
J2274	Injection, morphine sulfate, preservative-free for epidural or intrathecal use, 10 mg
J2275	Injection, morphine sulfate (preservative-free sterile solution), per 10 mg
J2278	Injection, ziconotide, 1 microgram
J2280	Injection, moxifloxacin, 100 mg
J2281	Injection, moxifloxacin (Fresenius kabi) not therapeutically equivalent to J2280, 100 mg
J2300	Injection, nalbuphine hydrochloride, per 10 mg
J2310	Injection, naloxone hydrochloride, per 1 mg
J2311	Injection, naloxone hydrochloride (zimhi), 1 mg
J2315	Injection, naltrexone, depot form, 1 mg
J2320	Injection, nandrolone decanoate, up to 50 mg
J2323	Injection, natalizumab, 1 mg
J2325	Injection, nesiritide, 0.1 mg
J2326	Injection, nusinersen, 0.1 mg

J2327	Injection, risankizumab-rzaa, intravenous, 1 mg
J2350	Injection, ocrelizumab, 1 mg
J2353	Injection, octreotide, depot form for intramuscular injection, 1 mg
J2354	Injection, octreotide, non-depot form for subcutaneous or intravenous injection, 25 mcg
J2355	Injection, oprelvekin, 5 mg
J2356	Injection, tezepelumab-ekko, 1 mg
J2357	Injection, omalizumab, 5 mg
J2358	Injection, olanzapine, long-acting, 1 mg
J2360	Injection, orphenadrine citrate, up to 60 mg
J2370	Injection, phenylephrine HCl, up to 1 ml
(J2400	Injection, chloroprocaine hydrochloride, per 30 ml Code deleted effective 12/31/2022, no HCPCS/CPT cross-reference provided.)
J2401	Injection, chloroprocaine hydrochloride, per 1 mg
J2402	Injection, chloroprocaine hydrochloride (clorotekal), per 1 mg
• J2404	Injection, nicardipine, 0.1 mg
J2405	Injection, ondansetron hydrochloride, per 1 mg
J2406	Injection, oritavancin (kimyrsa), 10 mg
J2407	Injection, oritavancin (orbactiv), 10 mg
J2410	Injection, oxymorphone HCl, up to 1 mg
J2425	Injection, palifermin, 50 micrograms
J2426	Injection, paliperidone palmitate extended release, 1 mg
J2430	Injection, pamidronate disodium, per 30 mg
J2440	Injection, papaverine HCl, up to 60 mg
J2460	Injection, oxytetracycline HCl, up to 50 mg
J2469	Injection, palonosetron HCl, 25 mcg
J2501	Injection, paricalcitol, 1 mcg
J2502	Injection, pasireotide long acting, 1 mg
J2503	Injection, pegaptanib sodium, 0.3 mg
J2504	Injection, pegademase bovine, 25 iu
J2505	Injection, pegfilgrastim, 6 mg
J2506	Injection, pegfilgrastim, excludes biosimilar, 0.5 mg
J2507	Injection, pegloticase, 1 mg
• J2508	Injection, pegunigalsidase alfa-iwxj, 1 mg
J2510	Injection, penicillin g procaine, aqueous, up to 600,000 units
J2513	Injection, pentastarch, 10% solution, 100 ml
J2515	Injection, pentobarbital sodium, per 50 mg
J2540	Injection, penicillin g potassium, up to 600,000 units
J2543	Injection, piperacillin sodium/tazobactam sodium, 1 gram/0.125 grams (1.125 grams)
J2545	Pentamidine isethionate, inhalation solution, FDA-approved final product, non-compounded, administered through dme, unit dose form, per 300 mg
J2547	Injection, peramivir, 1 mg

J CODES

J2550	Injection, promethazine HCl, up to 50 mg
J2560	Injection, phenobarbital sodium, up to 120 mg
J2562	Injection, plerixafor, 1 mg
J2590	Injection, oxytocin, up to 10 units
J2597	Injection, desmopressin acetate, per 1 mcg
J2650	Injection, prednisolone acetate, up to 1 ml
J2670	Injection, tolazoline HCl, up to 25 mg
J2675	Injection, progesterone, per 50 mg
● J2679	Injection, fluphenazine hcl, 1.25 mg
J2680	Injection, fluphenazine decanoate, up to 25 mg
J2690	Injection, procainamide HCl, up to 1 gm
J2700	Injection, oxacillin sodium, up to 250 mg
J2704	Injection, propofol, 10 mg
J2710	Injection, neostigmine methylsulfate, up to 0.5 mg
J2720	Injection, protamine sulfate, per 10 mg
J2724	Injection, protein c concentrate, intravenous, human, 10 iu
J2725	Injection, protirelin, per 250 mcg
J2730	Injection, pralidoxime chloride, up to 1 gm
J2760	Injection, phentolamine mesylate, up to 5 mg
J2765	Injection, metoclopramide HCl, up to 10 mg
J2770	Injection, quinupristin/dalfopristin, 500 mg (150/350)
J2777	Injection, faricimab-svoa, 0.1 mg
J2778	Injection, ranibizumab, 0.1 mg
J2779	Injection, ranibizumab, via intravitreal implant (susvimo), 0.1 mg
J2780	Injection, ranitidine hydrochloride, 25 mg
J2783	Injection, rasburicase, 0.5 mg
J2785	Injection, regadenoson, 0.1 mg
J2786	Injection, reslizumab, 1 mg
J2787	Riboflavin 5'-phosphate, ophthalmic solution, up to 3 ml
J2788	Injection, rho d immune globulin, human, minidose, 50 micrograms (250 i.u.)
J2790	Injection, rho d immune globulin, human, full dose, 300 micrograms (1500 i.u.)
J2791	Injection, rho(d) immune globulin (human), (rhophylac), intramuscular or intravenous, 100 iu
J2792	Injection, rho d immune globulin, intravenous, human, solvent detergent, 100 iu
J2793	Injection, rilonacept, 1 mg
J2794	Injection, risperidone (risperdal consta), 0.5 mg
J2795	Injection, ropivacaine hydrochloride, 1 mg
J2796	Injection, romiplostim, 10 micrograms
J2797	Injection, rolapitant, 0.5 mg
J2798	Injection, risperidone, (perseris), 0.5 mg
● J2799	Injection, risperidone (uzedy), 1 mg

J2800	Injection, methocarbamol, up to 10 ml
J2805	Injection, sincalide, 5 micrograms
J2810	Injection, theophylline, per 40 mg
J2820	Injection, sargramostim (gm-csf), 50 mcg
J2840	Injection, sebelipase alfa, 1 mg
J2850	Injection, secretin, synthetic, human, 1 microgram
J2860	Injection, siltuximab, 10 mg
J2910	Injection, aurothioglucose, up to 50 mg
J2916	Injection, sodium ferric gluconate complex in sucrose injection, 12.5 mg
J2920	Injection, methylprednisolone sodium succinate, up to 40 mg
J2930	Injection, methylprednisolone sodium succinate, up to 125 mg
J2940	Injection, somatrem, 1 mg
J2941	Injection, somatropin, 1 mg
J2950	Injection, promazine HCl, up to 25 mg
J2993	Injection, reteplase, 18.1 mg
J2995	Injection, streptokinase, per 250,000 iu
J2997	Injection, alteplase recombinant, 1 mg
J2998	Injection, plasminogen, human-tvmh, 1 mg
J3000	Injection, streptomycin, up to 1 gm
J3010	Injection, fentanyl citrate, 0.1 mg
J3030	Injection, sumatriptan succinate, 6 mg (code may be used for Medicare when drug administered under the direct supervision of a physician, not for use when drug is self administered)
J3031	Injection, fremanezumab-vfrm, 1 mg (code may be used for Medicare when drug administered under the direct supervision of a physician, not for use when drug is self-administered)
J3032	Injection, eptinezumab-jjmr, 1 mg
J3060	Injection, taliglucerase alfa, 10 units
J3070	Injection, pentazocine, 30 mg
J3090	Injection, tedizolid phosphate, 1 mg
J3095	Injection, telavancin, 10 mg
J3101	Injection, tenecteplase, 1 mg
J3105	Injection, terbutaline sulfate, up to 1 mg
J3110	Injection, teriparatide, 10 mcg
J3111	Injection, romosozumab-aqqg, 1 mg
J3120	Injection, testosterone enanthate, up to 100 mg
J3121	Injection, testosterone enanthate, 1 mg
J3130	Injection, testosterone enanthate, up to 200 mg
J3140	Injection, testosterone suspension, up to 50 mg
J3145	Injection, testosterone undecanoate, 1 mg
J3150	Injection, testosterone propionate, up to 100 mg
J3230	Injection, chlorpromazine HCl, up to 50 mg
J3240	Injection, thyrotropin alpha, 0.9 mg, provided in 1.1 mg vial

J CODES

J3241	Injection, teprotumumab-trbw, 10 mg
J3243	Injection, tigecycline, 1 mg
J3244	Injection, tigecycline (accord) not therapeutically equivalent to J3243, 1 mg
J3245	Injection, tildrakizumab, 1 mg
J3246	Injection, tirofiban HCl, 0.25 mg
J3250	Injection, trimethobenzamide HCl, up to 200 mg
J3260	Injection, tobramycin sulfate, up to 80 mg
J3262	Injection, tocilizumab, 1 mg
J3265	Injection, torsemide, 10 mg/ml
J3280	Injection, thiethylperazine maleate, up to 10 mg
J3285	Injection, treprostinil, 1 mg
J3299	Injection, triamcinolone acetonide (xipere), 1 mg
J3300	Injection, triamcinolone acetonide, preservative free, 1 mg
J3301	Injection, triamcinolone acetonide, not otherwise specified, 10 mg
J3302	Injection, triamcinolone diacetate, per 5 mg
J3303	Injection, triamcinolone hexacetonide, per 5 mg
J3304	Injection, triamcinolone acetonide, preservative-free, extended-release, microsphere formulation, 1 mg
J3305	Injection, trimetrexate glucuronate, per 25 mg
J3310	Injection, perphenazine, up to 5 mg
J3315	Injection, triptorelin pamoate, 3.75 mg
J3316	Injection, triptorelin, extended-release, 3.75 mg
J3320	Injection, spectinomycin dihydrochloride, up to 2 gm
J3350	Injection, urea, up to 40 gm
J3355	Injection, urofollitropin, 75 iu
J3357	Ustekinumab, for subcutaneous injection, 1 mg
J3358	Ustekinumab, for intravenous injection, 1 mg
J3360	Injection, diazepam, up to 5 mg
J3364	Injection, urokinase, 5000 iu vial
J3365	Injection, iv, urokinase, 250,000 i.u. vial
J3370	Injection, vancomycin HCl, 500 mg
J3371	Injection, vancomycin HCl (mylan) not therapeutically equivalent to J3370, 500 mg
J3372	Injection, vancomycin HCl (xellia) not therapeutically equivalent to J3370, 500 mg
J3380	Injection, vedolizumab, 1 mg
J3385	Injection, velaglucerase alfa, 100 units
J3396	Injection, verteporfin, 0.1 mg
J3397	Injection, vestronidase alfa-vjbk, 1 mg
J3398	Injection, voretigene neparvovec-rzyl, 1 billion vector genomes
J3399	Injection, onasemnogene abeparvovec-xioi, per treatment, up to 5x10^15 vector genomes
J3400	Injection, triflupromazine HCl, up to 20 mg

•	J3401	Beremagene geperpavec-svdt for topical administration, containing nominal 5 x 10^9 pfu/ml vector genomes, per 0.1 ml
	J3410	Injection, hydroxyzine HCl, up to 25 mg
	J3411	Injection, thiamine HCl, 100 mg
	J3415	Injection, pyridoxine HCl, 100 mg
	J3420	Injection, vitamin b-12 cyanocobalamin, up to 1000 mcg
•	J3425	Injection, hydroxocobalamin, 10 mcg
	J3430	Injection, phytonadione (vitamin k), per 1 mg
	J3465	Injection, voriconazole, 10 mg
	J3470	Injection, hyaluronidase, up to 150 units
	J3471	Injection, hyaluronidase, ovine, preservative free, per 1 USP unit (up to 999 USP units)
	J3472	Injection, hyaluronidase, ovine, preservative free, per 1000 USP units
	J3473	Injection, hyaluronidase, recombinant, 1 USP unit
	J3475	Injection, magnesium sulfate, per 500 mg
	J3480	Injection, potassium chloride, per 2 meq
	J3485	Injection, zidovudine, 10 mg
	J3486	Injection, ziprasidone mesylate, 10 mg
	J3489	Injection, zoledronic acid, 1 mg
	J3490	Unclassified drugs
	J3520	Edetate disodium, per 150 mg
	J3530	Nasal vaccine inhalation
	J3535	Drug administered through a metered dose inhaler
	J3570	Laetrile, amygdalin, vitamin b17
	J3590	Unclassified biologics
	J3591	Unclassified drug or biological used for ESRD on dialysis
	J7030	Infusion, normal saline solution , 1000 cc
	J7040	Infusion, normal saline solution, sterile (500 ml = 1 unit)
	J7042	5% dextrose/normal saline (500 ml = 1 unit)
	J7050	Infusion, normal saline solution, 250 cc
	J7060	5% dextrose/water (500 ml = 1 unit)
	J7070	Infusion, d5w, 1000 cc
	J7100	Infusion, dextran 40, 500 ml
	J7110	Infusion, dextran 75, 500 ml
	J7120	Ringers lactate infusion, up to 1000 cc
	J7121	5% dextrose in lactated ringers infusion, up to 1000 cc
	J7131	Hypertonic saline solution, 1 ml
	J7168	Prothrombin complex concentrate (human), kcentra, per i.u. of factor ix activity
	J7169	Injection, coagulation factor xa (recombinant), inactivated-zhzo (andexxa), 10 mg
	J7170	Injection, emicizumab-kxwh, 0.5 mg
	J7175	Injection, factor x, (human), 1 i.u.
	J7177	Injection, human fibrinogen concentrate (fibryga), 1 mg

J CODES

J7178	Injection, human fibrinogen concentrate, not otherwise specified, 1 mg
J7179	Injection, von willebrand factor (recombinant), (vonvendi), 1 i.u. vwf:rco
J7180	Injection, factor xiii (antihemophilic factor, human), 1 i.u.
J7181	Injection, factor xiii a-subunit, (recombinant), per iu
J7182	Injection, factor viii, (antihemophilic factor, recombinant), (novoeight), per iu
J7183	Injection, von willebrand factor complex (human), wilate, 1 i.u. vwf:rco
J7185	Injection, factor viii (antihemophilic factor, recombinant) (xyntha), per i.u.
J7186	Injection, antihemophilic factor viii/von willebrand factor complex (human), per factor viii i.u.
J7187	Injection, von willebrand factor complex (humate-p), per iu vwf:rco
J7188	Injection, factor viii (antihemophilic factor, recombinant), (obizur), per i.u.
J7189	Factor viia (antihemophilic factor, recombinant), (novoseven rt), 1 microgram
J7190	Factor viii (antihemophilic factor, human) per i.u.
J7191	Factor viii (antihemophilic factor (porcine)), per i.u.
J7192	Factor viii (antihemophilic factor, recombinant) per i.u., not otherwise specified
J7193	Factor ix (antihemophilic factor, purified, non-recombinant) per i.u.
J7194	Factor ix, complex, per i.u.
J7195	Injection, factor ix (antihemophilic factor, recombinant) per iu, not otherwise specified
J7196	Injection, antithrombin recombinant, 50 i.u.
J7197	Antithrombin iii (human), per i.u.
J7198	Anti-inhibitor, per i.u.
J7199	Hemophilia clotting factor, not otherwise classified
J7200	Injection, factor ix, (antihemophilic factor, recombinant), rixubis, per iu
J7201	Injection, factor ix, fc fusion protein, (recombinant), alprolix, 1 i.u.
J7202	Injection, factor ix, albumin fusion protein, (recombinant), idelvion, 1 i.u.
J7203	Injection factor ix, (antihemophilic factor, recombinant), glycopegylated, (rebinyn), 1 iu
J7204	Injection, factor viii, antihemophilic factor (recombinant), (esperoct), glycopegylated-exei, per iu
J7205	Injection, factor viii fc fusion protein (recombinant), per iu
J7207	Injection, factor viii, (antihemophilic factor, recombinant), pegylated, 1 i.u.
J7208	Injection, factor viii, (antihemophilic factor, recombinant), pegylated-aucl, (jivi), 1 i.u.
J7209	Injection, factor viii, (antihemophilic factor, recombinant), (nuwiq), 1 i.u.
J7210	Injection, factor viii, (antihemophilic factor, recombinant), (afstyla), 1 i.u.
J7211	Injection, factor viii, (antihemophilic factor, recombinant), (kovaltry), 1 i.u.
J7212	Factor viia (antihemophilic factor, recombinant)-jncw (sevenfact), 1 microgram
J7294	Segesterone acetate and ethinyl estradiol 0.15mg, 0.013mg per 24 hours; yearly vaginal system, each
J7295	Ethinyl estradiol and etonogestrel 0.015mg, 0.12mg per 24 hours; monthly vaginal ring, each
J7296	Levonorgestrel-releasing intrauterine contraceptive system, (kyleena), 19.5 mg
J7297	Levonorgestrel-releasing intrauterine contraceptive system (liletta), 52 mg
J7298	Levonorgestrel-releasing intrauterine contraceptive system (mirena), 52 mg
J7300	Intrauterine copper contraceptive
J7301	Levonorgestrel-releasing intrauterine contraceptive system (skyla), 13.5 mg

J7302	Levonorgestrel-releasing intrauterine contraceptive system, 52 mg
J7303	Contraceptive supply, hormone containing vaginal ring, each
J7304	Contraceptive supply, hormone containing patch, each
J7306	Levonorgestrel (contraceptive) implant system, including implants and supplies
J7307	Etonogestrel (contraceptive) implant system, including implant and supplies
J7308	Aminolevulinic acid HCl for topical administration, 20%, single unit dosage form (354 mg)
J7309	Methyl aminolevulinate (mal) for topical administration, 16.8%, 1 gram
J7310	Ganciclovir, 4.5 mg, long-acting implant
J7311	Injection, fluocinolone acetonide, intravitreal implant (retisert), 0.01 mg
J7312	Injection, dexamethasone, intravitreal implant, 0.1 mg
J7313	Injection, fluocinolone acetonide, intravitreal implant (iluvien), 0.01 mg
J7314	Injection, fluocinolone acetonide, intravitreal implant (yutiq), 0.01 mg
J7315	Mitomycin, ophthalmic, 0.2 mg
J7316	Injection, ocriplasmin, 0.125 mg
J7318	Hyaluronan or derivative, durolane, for intra-articular injection, 1 mg
J7320	Hyaluronan or derivative, genvisc 850, for intra-articular injection, 1 mg
J7321	Hyaluronan or derivative, Hyalgan, Supartz or visco-3, for intra-articular injection, per dose
J7322	Hyaluronan or derivative, hymovis, for intra-articular injection, 1 mg
J7323	Hyaluronan or derivative, Euflexxa, for intra-articular injection, per dose
J7324	Hyaluronan or derivative, Orthovisc, for intra-articular injection, per dose
J7325	Hyaluronan or derivative, Synvisc or Synvisc-one, for intra-articular injection, 1 mg
J7326	Hyaluronan or derivative, gel-one, for intra-articular injection, per dose
J7327	Hyaluronan or derivative, monovisc, for intra-articular injection, per dose
J7328	Hyaluronan or derivative, gelsyn-3, for intra-articular injection, 0.1 mg
J7329	Hyaluronan or derivative, trivisc, for intra-articular injection, 1 mg
J7330	Autologous cultured chondrocytes, implant
J7331	Hyaluronan or derivative, synojoynt, for intra-articular injection, 1 mg
J7332	Hyaluronan or derivative, triluron, for intra-articular injection, 1 mg
J7333	Hyaluronan or derivative, visco-3, for intra-articular injection, per dose
J7335	Capsaicin 8% patch, per 10 square centimeters
J7336	Capsaicin 8% patch, per square centimeter
J7340	Carbidopa 5 mg/levodopa 20 mg enteral suspension, 100 ml
J7342	Instillation, ciprofloxacin otic suspension, 6 mg
J7345	Aminolevulinic acid HCl for topical administration, 10% gel, 10 mg
J7351	Injection, bimatoprost, intracameral implant, 1 microgram
J7352	Afamelanotide implant, 1 mg
J7401	Mometasone furoate sinus implant, 10 micrograms
J7402	Mometasone furoate sinus implant, (sinuva), 10 micrograms

Immunosuppressive Drugs (Includes Non-Injectables)

J7500	Azathioprine, oral, 50 mg

J7501	Azathioprine, parenteral, 100 mg
J7502	Cyclosporine, oral, 100 mg
J7503	Tacrolimus, extended release, (Envarsus xr), oral, 0.25 mg
J7504	Lymphocyte immune globulin, antithymocyte globulin, equine, parenteral, 250 mg
J7505	Muromonab-cd3, parenteral, 5 mg
J7506	Prednisone, oral, per 5 mg
J7507	Tacrolimus, immediate release, oral, 1 mg
J7508	Tacrolimus, extended release, (astagraf xl), oral, 0.1 mg
J7509	Methylprednisolone oral, per 4 mg
J7510	Prednisolone oral, per 5 mg
J7511	Lymphocyte immune globulin, antithymocyte globulin, rabbit, parenteral, 25 mg
J7512	Prednisone, immediate release or delayed release, oral, 1 mg
J7513	Daclizumab, parenteral, 25 mg
J7515	Cyclosporine, oral, 25 mg
J7516	Cyclosporin, parenteral, 250 mg
J7517	Mycophenolate mofetil, oral, 250 mg
J7518	Mycophenolic acid, oral, 180 mg
J7520	Sirolimus, oral, 1 mg
J7525	Tacrolimus, parenteral, 5 mg
J7527	Everolimus, oral, 0.25 mg
J7599	Immunosuppressive drug, not otherwise classified
J7604	Acetylcysteine, inhalation solution, compounded product, administered through dme, unit dose form, per gram
J7605	Arformoterol, inhalation solution, FDA approved final product, non-compounded, administered through dme, unit dose form, 15 micrograms
J7606	Formoterol fumarate, inhalation solution, FDA approved final product, non-compounded, administered through dme, unit dose form, 20 micrograms
J7607	Levalbuterol, inhalation solution, compounded product, administered through dme, concentrated form, 0.5 mg
J7608	Acetylcysteine, inhalation solution, FDA-approved final product, non-compounded, administered through dme, unit dose form, per gram
J7609	Albuterol, inhalation solution, compounded product, administered through dme, unit dose, 1 mg
J7610	Albuterol, inhalation solution, compounded product, administered through dme, concentrated form, 1 mg
J7611	Albuterol, inhalation solution, FDA-approved final product, non-compounded, administered through dme, concentrated form, 1 mg
J7612	Levalbuterol, inhalation solution, FDA-approved final product, non-compounded, administered through dme, concentrated form, 0.5 mg
J7613	Albuterol, inhalation solution, FDA-approved final product, non-compounded, administered through dme, unit dose, 1 mg
J7614	Levalbuterol, inhalation solution, FDA-approved final product, non-compounded, administered through dme, unit dose, 0.5 mg
J7615	Levalbuterol, inhalation solution, compounded product, administered through dme, unit dose, 0.5 mg

J7620 Albuterol, up to 2.5 mg and ipratropium bromide, up to 0.5 mg, FDA-approved final product, non-compounded, administered through dme

J7622 Beclomethasone, inhalation solution, compounded product, administered through dme, unit dose form, per milligram

J7624 Betamethasone, inhalation solution, compounded product, administered through dme, unit dose form, per milligram

J7626 Budesonide, inhalation solution, FDA-approved final product, non-compounded, administered through dme, unit dose form, up to 0.5 mg

J7627 Budesonide, inhalation solution, compounded product, administered through dme, unit dose form, up to 0.5 mg

J7628 Bitolterol mesylate, inhalation solution, compounded product, administered through dme, concentrated form, per milligram

J7629 Bitolterol mesylate, inhalation solution, compounded product, administered through dme, unit dose form, per milligram

J7631 Cromolyn sodium, inhalation solution, FDA-approved final product, non-compounded, administered through dme, unit dose form, per 10 milligrams

J7632 Cromolyn sodium, inhalation solution, compounded product, administered through dme, unit dose form, per 10 milligrams

J7633 Budesonide, inhalation solution, FDA-approved final product, non-compounded, administered through dme, concentrated form, per 0.25 milligram

J7634 Budesonide, inhalation solution, compounded product, administered through dme, concentrated form, per 0.25 milligram

J7635 Atropine, inhalation solution, compounded product, administered through dme, concentrated form, per milligram

J7636 Atropine, inhalation solution, compounded product, administered through dme, unit dose form, per milligram

J7637 Dexamethasone, inhalation solution, compounded product, administered through dme, concentrated form, per milligram

J7638 Dexamethasone, inhalation solution, compounded product, administered through dme, unit dose form, per milligram

J7639 Dornase alfa, inhalation solution, FDA-approved final product, non-compounded, administered through dme, unit dose form, per milligram

J7640 Formoterol, inhalation solution, compounded product, administered through dme, unit dose form, 12 micrograms

J7641 Flunisolide, inhalation solution, compounded product, administered through dme, unit dose, per milligram

J7642 Glycopyrrolate, inhalation solution, compounded product, administered through dme, concentrated form, per milligram

J7643 Glycopyrrolate, inhalation solution, compounded product, administered through dme, unit dose form, per milligram

J7644 Ipratropium bromide, inhalation solution, FDA-approved final product, non-compounded, administered through dme, unit dose form, per milligram

J7645 Ipratropium bromide, inhalation solution, compounded product, administered through dme, unit dose form, per milligram

J7647 Isoetharine HCl, inhalation solution, compounded product, administered through dme, concentrated form, per milligram

J7648 Isoetharine HCl, inhalation solution, FDA-approved final product, non-compounded, administered through dme, concentrated form, per milligram

J7649 Isoetharine HCl, inhalation solution, FDA-approved final product, non-compounded, administered through dme, unit dose form, per milligram

J7650 Isoetharine HCl, inhalation solution, compounded product, administered through dme, unit dose form, per milligram

J7657 Isoproterenol HCl, inhalation solution, compounded product, administered through dme, concentrated form, per milligram

J7658 Isoproterenol HCl, inhalation solution, FDA-approved final product, non-compounded, administered through dme, concentrated form, per milligram

J7659 Isoproterenol HCl, inhalation solution, FDA-approved final product, non-compounded, administered through dme, unit dose form, per milligram

J7660 Isoproterenol HCl, inhalation solution, compounded product, administered through dme, unit dose form, per milligram

J7665 Mannitol, administered through an inhaler, 5 mg

J7667 Metaproterenol sulfate, inhalation solution, compounded product, concentrated form, per 10 milligrams

J7668 Metaproterenol sulfate, inhalation solution, FDA-approved final product, non-compounded, administered through dme, concentrated form, per 10 milligrams

J7669 Metaproterenol sulfate, inhalation solution, FDA-approved final product, non-compounded, administered through dme, unit dose form, per 10 milligrams

J7670 Metaproterenol sulfate, inhalation solution, compounded product, administered through dme, unit dose form, per 10 milligrams

J7674 Methacholine chloride administered as inhalation solution through a nebulizer, per 1 mg

J7676 Pentamidine isethionate, inhalation solution, compounded product, administered through dme, unit dose form, per 300 mg

J7677 Revefenacin inhalation solution, FDA-approved final product, non-compounded, administered through dme, 1 microgram

J7680 Terbutaline sulfate, inhalation solution, compounded product, administered through dme, concentrated form, per milligram

J7681 Terbutaline sulfate, inhalation solution, compounded product, administered through dme, unit dose form, per milligram

J7682 Tobramycin, inhalation solution, FDA-approved final product, non-compounded, unit dose form, administered through dme, per 300 milligrams

J7683 Triamcinolone, inhalation solution, compounded product, administered through dme, concentrated form, per milligram

J7684 Triamcinolone, inhalation solution, compounded product, administered through dme, unit dose form, per milligram

J7685 Tobramycin, inhalation solution, compounded product, administered through dme, unit dose form, per 300 milligrams

J7686 Treprostinil, inhalation solution, FDA-approved final product, non-compounded, administered through dme, unit dose form, 1.74 mg

J7699 Noc drugs, inhalation solution administered through dme

J7799 Noc drugs, other than inhalation drugs, administered through dme

J7999 Compounded drug, not otherwise classified

J8498 Antiemetic drug, rectal/suppository, not otherwise specified

J8499	Prescription drug, oral, non chemotherapeutic, nos
J8501	Aprepitant, oral, 5 mg
J8510	Busulfan; oral, 2 mg
J8515	Cabergoline, oral, 0.25 mg
J8520	Capecitabine, oral, 150 mg
J8521	Capecitabine, oral, 500 mg
J8530	Cyclophosphamide; oral, 25 mg
J8540	Dexamethasone, oral, 0.25 mg
J8560	Etoposide; oral, 50 mg
J8562	Fludarabine phosphate, oral, 10 mg
J8565	Gefitinib, oral, 250 mg
J8597	Antiemetic drug, oral, not otherwise specified
J8600	Melphalan; oral, 2 mg
J8610	Methotrexate; oral, 2.5 mg
J8650	Nabilone, oral, 1 mg
J8655	Netupitant 300 mg and palonosetron 0.5 mg, oral
J8670	Rolapitant, oral, 1 mg
J8700	Temozolomide, oral, 5 mg
J8705	Topotecan, oral, 0.25 mg
J8999	Prescription drug, oral, chemotherapeutic, nos

CHEMOTHERAPY DRUGS

Guidelines

In addition to the information presented in the INTRODUCTION, several other items unique to this section are defined or identified here:

1. **EXCEPTION:** Oral immunosuppressive drugs are not included in this section.

2. **ROUTE OF ADMINISTRATION:** Unless otherwise specified, the drugs listed in this section may be injected either subcutaneously, intramuscularly or intravenously.

3. **DRUG COST ONLY:** The codes listed in this section include the cost of the chemotherapy drug only and do not include the administration of the drug.

4. **SUBSECTION INFORMATION:** Some of the listed subheadings or subsections have special needs or instructions unique to that section. Where these are indicated, special "notes" will be presented preceding or following the listings. Those subsections within the CHEMOTHERAPY DRUGS section that have "notes" are as follows:

Subsection	Code Numbers
Chemotherapy drugs	J9000–J9999

5. **UNLISTED SERVICE OR PROCEDURE:** A service or procedure may be provided that is not listed in this edition of HCPCS. When reporting such a service, the appropriate "unlisted procedure" code may be used to indicate the service, identifying it by "special report" as defined below. HCPCS terminology is inconsistent in defining unlisted procedures. The procedure definition may include the term(s) "unlisted", "not otherwise classified", "unspecified", "unclassified", "other" and "miscellaneous". Prior to using these codes, try to determine if a Local Level III code or CPT code is available. The "unlisted procedures" and accompanying codes for CHEMOTHERAPY DRUGS are as follows:

   J9999 Not otherwise classified, antineoplastic drugs

6. **SPECIAL REPORT:** A service, material or supply that is rarely provided, unusual, variable or new may require a special report in determining medical appropriateness for reimbursement purposes. Pertinent information should include an adequate definition or description of the nature, extent, and need for the service, material or supply.

7. **MODIFIERS:** Listed services may be modified under certain circumstances. When appropriate, the modifying circumstance is identified by adding a modifier to the basic procedure code. CPT and HCPCS National Level II modifiers may be used with CPT and HCPCS National Level II procedure codes. Modifiers commonly used with CHEMOTHERAPY DRUGS are as follows:

   -CC Procedure code change (used when the procedure code submitted was changed either for administrative reasons or because an incorrect code was filed)

   -TC Technical component. Under certain circumstances, a charge may be made for the technical component alone. Under these circumstances, the technical component charge is identified by adding the modifier -TC to the usual procedure code. Technical component charges are institutional charges and are not billed separately by physicians. Portable x-ray suppliers bill only for the technical component however and should use modifier -TC.

8. **CPT CODE CROSS-REFERENCE:** Unless otherwise specified, the equivalent CPT code for all listings in this section is 96545.

Chemotherapy Drugs

J9000 Injection, doxorubicin hydrochloride, 10 mg
J9010 Injection, alemtuzumab, 10 mg
J9015 Injection, aldesleukin, per single use vial
J9017 Injection, arsenic trioxide, 1 mg
J9019 Injection, asparaginase (erwinaze), 1,000 iu
J9020 Injection, asparaginase, not otherwise specified, 10,000 units
J9021 Injection, asparaginase, recombinant, (rylaze), 0.1 mg
J9022 Injection, atezolizumab, 10 mg
J9023 Injection, avelumab, 10 mg
J9025 Injection, azacitidine, 1 mg
J9027 Injection, clofarabine, 1 mg
J9030 BCG live intravesical instillation, 1 mg
J9031 BCG (intravesical) per instillation
J9032 Injection, belinostat, 10 mg
J9033 Injection, bendamustine HCl (treanda), 1 mg
J9034 Injection, bendamustine HCl (bendeka), 1 mg
J9035 Injection, bevacizumab, 10 mg
J9036 Injection, bendamustine hydrochloride, (belrapzo/bendamustine), 1 mg
J9037 Injection, belantamab mafodotin-blmf, 0.5 mg
J9039 Injection, blinatumomab, 1 microgram
J9040 Injection, bleomycin sulfate, 15 units
J9041 Injection, bortezomib, 0.1 mg
J9042 Injection, brentuximab vedotin, 1 mg
J9043 Injection, cabazitaxel, 1 mg
(J9044 Injection, bortezomib, not otherwise specified, 0.1 mg
Code deleted effective 12/31/2022, no HCPCS/CPT cross-reference provided.)
J9045 Injection, carboplatin, 50 mg
J9046 Injection, bortezomib, (dr. Reddy's), not therapeutically equivalent to j9041, 0.1 mg
J9047 Injection, carfilzomib, 1 mg
J9048 Injection, bortezomib (Fresenius kabi), not therapeutically equivalent to j9041, 0.1 mg
J9049 Injection, bortezomib (hospira), not therapeutically equivalent to j9041, 0.1 mg
J9050 Injection, carmustine, 100 mg
• J9052 Injection, carmustine (accord), not therapeutically equivalent to j9050, 100 mg
J9055 Injection, cetuximab, 10 mg
J9057 Injection, copanlisib, 1 mg
J9060 Injection, cisplatin, powder or solution, 10 mg
J9061 Injection, amivantamab-vmjw, 2 mg
J9065 Injection, cladribine, per 1 mg
J9070 Cyclophosphamide, 100 mg

	J9071	Injection, cyclophosphamide, (auromedics), 5 mg
•	J9072	Injection, cyclophosphamide, (Dr. Reddy's), 5 mg
	J9098	Injection, cytarabine liposome, 10 mg
	J9100	Injection, cytarabine, 100 mg
	J9118	Injection, calaspargase pegol-mknl, 10 units
	J9119	Injection, cemiplimab-rwlc, 1 mg
	J9120	Injection, dactinomycin, 0.5 mg
	J9130	Dacarbazine, 100 mg
	J9144	Injection, daratumumab, 10 mg and hyaluronidase-fihj
	J9145	Injection, daratumumab, 10 mg
	J9150	Injection, daunorubicin, 10 mg
	J9151	Injection, daunorubicin citrate, liposomal formulation, 10 mg
	J9153	Injection, liposomal, 1 mg daunorubicin and 2.27 mg cytarabine
	J9155	Injection, degarelix, 1 mg
(	J9160	Injection, denileukin diftitox, 300 micrograms Code deleted effective 12/31/2023, no HCPCS/CPT cross-reference provided.)
	J9165	Injection, diethylstilbestrol diphosphate, 250 mg
	J9171	Injection, docetaxel, 1 mg
•	J9172	Injection, docetaxel (ingenus) not therapeutically equivalent to j9171, 1 mg
	J9173	Injection, durvalumab, 10 mg
	J9175	Injection, Elliott's' b solution, 1 ml
	J9176	Injection, elotuzumab, 1 mg
	J9177	Injection, enfortumab vedotin-ejfv, 0.25 mg
	J9178	Injection, epirubicin HCl, 2 mg
	J9179	Injection, eribulin mesylate, 0.1 mg
	J9181	Injection, etoposide, 10 mg
	J9185	Injection, fludarabine phosphate, 50 mg
	J9190	Injection, fluorouracil, 500 mg
	J9198	Injection, gemcitabine hydrochloride, (infugem), 100 mg
	J9199	Injection, gemcitabine hydrochloride (infugem), 200 mg
	J9200	Injection, floxuridine, 500 mg
	J9201	Injection, gemcitabine hydrochloride, not otherwise specified, 200 mg
	J9202	Goserelin acetate implant, per 3.6 mg
	J9203	Injection, gemtuzumab ozogamicin, 0.1 mg
	J9204	Injection, mogamulizumab-kpkc, 1 mg
	J9205	Injection, irinotecan liposome, 1 mg
	J9206	Injection, irinotecan, 20 mg
	J9207	Injection, ixabepilone, 1 mg
	J9208	Injection, ifosfamide, 1 gram
	J9209	Injection, mesna, 200 mg

J CODES

J9210	Injection, emapalumab-lzsg, 1 mg
J9211	Injection, idarubicin hydrochloride, 5 mg
J9212	Injection, interferon alfacon-1, recombinant, 1 microgram
J9213	Injection, interferon, alfa-2a, recombinant, 3 million units
J9214	Injection, interferon, alfa-2b, recombinant, 1 million units
J9215	Injection, interferon, alfa-n3, (human leukocyte derived), 250,000 iu
J9216	Injection, interferon, gamma 1-b, 3 million units
J9217	Leuprolide acetate (for depot suspension), 7.5 mg
J9218	Leuprolide acetate, per 1 mg
J9219	Leuprolide acetate implant, 65 mg
J9223	Injection, lurbinectedin, 0.1 mg
J9225	Histrelin implant (vantas), 50 mg
J9226	Histrelin implant (supprelin la), 50 mg
J9227	Injection, isatuximab-irfc, 10 mg
J9228	Injection, ipilimumab, 1 mg
J9229	Injection, inotuzumab ozogamicin, 0.1 mg
J9230	Injection, mechlorethamine hydrochloride, (nitrogen mustard), 10 mg
J9245	Injection, melphalan hydrochloride, not otherwise specified, 50 mg
J9246	Injection, melphalan (evomela), 1 mg
J9247	Injection, melphalan flufenamide, 1mg
J9250	Methotrexate sodium, 5 mg
• J9255	Injection, methotrexate (accord) not therapeutically equivalent to j9250 and j9260, 50 mg
• J9258	Injection, paclitaxel protein-bound particles (teva) not therapeutically equivalent to j9264, 1 mg
J9260	Methotrexate sodium, 50 mg
J9261	Injection, nelarabine, 50 mg
J9262	Injection, omacetaxine mepesuccinate, 0.01 mg
J9263	Injection, oxaliplatin, 0.5 mg
J9264	Injection, paclitaxel protein-bound particles, 1 mg
J9265	Injection, paclitaxel, 30 mg
J9266	Injection, pegaspargase, per single dose vial
J9267	Injection, paclitaxel, 1 mg
J9268	Injection, pentostatin, 10 mg
J9269	Injection, tagraxofusp-erzs, 10 micrograms
J9270	Injection, plicamycin, 2.5 mg
J9271	Injection, pembrolizumab, 1 mg
J9272	Injection, dostarlimab-gxly, 10 mg
J9273	Injection, tisotumab vedotin-tftv, 1 mg
J9274	Injection, tebentafusp-tebn, 1 microgram
J9280	Injection, mitomycin, 5 mg
J9281	Mitomycin pyelocalyceal instillation, 1 mg

	J9285	Injection, olaratumab, 10 mg
•	J9286	Injection, glofitamab-gxbm, 2.5 mg
	J9293	Injection, mitoxantrone hydrochloride, per 5 mg
	J9295	Injection, necitumumab, 1 mg
	J9298	Injection, nivolumab and relatlimab-rmbw, 3 mg/1 mg
	J9299	Injection, nivolumab, 1 mg
	J9300	Injection, gemtuzumab ozogamicin, 5 mg
	J9301	Injection, obinutuzumab, 10 mg
	J9302	Injection, ofatumumab, 10 mg
	J9303	Injection, panitumumab, 10 mg
	J9304	Injection, pemetrexed (pemfexy), 10 mg
	J9305	Injection, pemetrexed, not otherwise specified, 10 mg
	J9306	Injection, pertuzumab, 1 mg
	J9307	Injection, pralatrexate, 1 mg
	J9308	Injection, ramucirumab, 5 mg
	J9309	Injection, polatuzumab vedotin-piiq, 1 mg
	J9310	Injection, rituximab, 100 mg
	J9311	Injection, rituximab 10 mg and hyaluronidase
	J9312	Injection, rituximab, 10 mg
	J9313	Injection, moxetumomab pasudotox-tdfk, 0.01 mg
	J9315	Injection, romidepsin, 1 mg
•	J9321	Injection, epcoritamab-bysp, 0.16 mg
•	J9324	Injection, pemetrexed (pemrydi rtu), 10 mg
•	J9333	Injection, rozanolixizumab-noli, 1 mg
•	J9334	Injection, efgartigimod alfa, 2 mg and hyaluronidase-qvfc

K CODES: FOR DME-MACs USE ONLY

Guidelines

In addition to the information presented in the INTRODUCTION, several other items unique to this section are defined or identified here:

1. **EXCLUSIVE USE BY DME-MACs:** The codes listed in this section are assigned by CMS on a temporary basis and are for the exclusive use of the Durable Medical Equipment Medicare Administrative Contractors (DME-MACs). These codes are not to be used by providers for reporting purposes unless specifically instructed to do so by the local carrier.

2. **UNLISTED SERVICE OR PROCEDURE:** A service or procedure may be provided that is not listed in this edition of HCPCS. When reporting such a service, the appropriate "unlisted procedure" code may be used to indicate the service, identifying it by "special report" as defined below. HCPCS terminology is inconsistent in defining unlisted procedures. The procedure definition may include the term(s) "unlisted", "not otherwise classified", "unspecified", "unclassified", "other" and "miscellaneous". Prior to using these codes, try to determine if a Local Level III code or CPT code is available.

3. **SPECIAL REPORT:** A service, material or supply that is rarely provided, unusual, variable or new may require a special report in determining medical appropriateness for reimbursement purposes. Pertinent information should include an adequate definition or description of the nature, extent, and need for the service, material or supply.

4. **CPT CODE CROSS-REFERENCE:** Unless otherwise specified, the equivalent CPT code for all listings in this section is 99070.

Temporary Codes for DMERCS

K0001 Standard wheelchair

K0002 Standard hemi (low seat) wheelchair

K0003 Lightweight wheelchair

K0004 High strength, lightweight wheelchair

K0005 Ultralightweight wheelchair

K0006 Heavy duty wheelchair

K0007 Extra heavy duty wheelchair

K0008 Custom manual wheelchair/base

K0009 Other manual wheelchair/base

K0010 Standard - weight frame motorized/power wheelchair

K0011 Standard - weight frame motorized/power wheelchair with programmable control parameters for speed adjustment, tremor dampening, acceleration control and braking

K0012 Lightweight portable motorized/power wheelchair

K0013 Custom motorized/power wheelchair base

K0014 Other motorized/power wheelchair base

K0015 Detachable, non-adjustable height armrest, replacement only, each

K0017 Detachable, adjustable height armrest, base, replacement only, each

K0018 Detachable, adjustable height armrest, upper portion, replacement only, each

K0019 Arm pad, replacement only, each

K0020 Fixed, adjustable height armrest, pair

K0037 High mount flip-up footrest, each

K0038 Leg strap, each

K0039 Leg strap, h style, each

K0040 Adjustable angle footplate, each

K0041 Large size footplate, each

K0042 Standard size footplate, replacement only, each

K0043 Footrest, lower extension tube, replacement only, each

K0044 Footrest, upper hanger bracket, replacement only, each

K0045 Footrest, complete assembly, replacement only, each

K0046 Elevating leg rest, lower extension tube, replacement only, each

K0047 Elevating leg rest, upper hanger bracket, replacement only, each

K0050 Ratchet assembly, replacement only

K0051 Cam release assembly, footrest or leg rest, replacement only, each

K0052 Swing away, detachable footrests, replacement only, each

K0053 Elevating footrests, articulating (telescoping), each

K0056 Seat height less than 17" or equal to or greater than 21" for a high strength, lightweight, or ultralightweight wheelchair

K0065 Spoke protectors, each

K0069 Rear wheel assembly, complete, with solid tire, spokes or molded, replacement only, each

K0070 Rear wheel assembly, complete, with pneumatic tire, spokes or molded, replacement only, each

K0071 Front caster assembly, complete, with pneumatic tire, replacement only, each

K0072 Front caster assembly, complete, with semi-pneumatic tire, replacement only, each

K0073 Caster pin lock, each

K0077 Front caster assembly, complete, with solid tire, replacement only, each

K0098 Drive belt for power wheelchair, replacement only

K0105 IV hanger, each

K0108 Wheelchair component or accessory, not otherwise specified

K0195 Elevating leg rests, pair (for use with capped rental wheelchair base)

K0455 Infusion pump used for uninterrupted parenteral administration of medication, (e.g., epoprostenol or treprostinil)

K0462 Temporary replacement for patient owned equipment being repaired, any type

K0552 Supplies for external non-insulin drug infusion pump, syringe type cartridge, sterile, each

(**K0553** Supply allowance for therapeutic continuous glucose monitor (cgm), includes all supplies and accessories, 1 month supply = 1 unit of service
Code deleted effective 12/31/2022, no HCPCS/CPT cross-reference provided.)

(**K0554** Receiver (monitor), dedicated, for use with therapeutic glucose continuous monitor system
Code deleted effective 12/31/2022, no HCPCS/CPT cross-reference provided.)

K0601 Replacement battery for external infusion pump owned by patient, silver oxide, 1.5 volt, each

K0602 Replacement battery for external infusion pump owned by patient, silver oxide, 3 volt, each

K0603	Replacement battery for external infusion pump owned by patient, alkaline, 1.5 volt, each
K0604	Replacement battery for external infusion pump owned by patient, lithium, 3.6 volt, each
K0605	Replacement battery for external infusion pump owned by patient, lithium, 4.5 volt, each
K0606	Automatic external defibrillator, with integrated electrocardiogram analysis, garment type
K0607	Replacement battery for automated external defibrillator, garment type only, each
K0608	Replacement garment for use with automated external defibrillator, each
K0609	Replacement electrodes for use with automated external defibrillator, garment type only, each
K0669	Wheelchair accessory, wheelchair seat or back cushion, does not meet specific code criteria or no written coding verification from dme pdac
K0672	Addition to lower extremity orthosis, removable soft interface, all components, replacement only, each
K0730	Controlled dose inhalation drug delivery system
K0733	Power wheelchair accessory, 12 to 24 amp hour sealed lead acid battery, each (e.g., gel cell, absorbed glass mat)
K0738	Portable gaseous oxygen system, rental; home compressor used to fill portable oxygen cylinders; includes portable containers, regulator, flowmeter, humidifier, cannula or mask, and tubing
K0739	Repair or nonroutine service for durable medical equipment other than oxygen equipment requiring the skill of a technician, labor component, per 15 minutes
K0740	Repair or nonroutine service for oxygen equipment requiring the skill of a technician, labor component, per 15 minutes
K0743	Suction pump, home model, portable, for use on wounds
K0744	Absorptive wound dressing for use with suction pump, home model, portable, pad size 16 square inches or less
K0745	Absorptive wound dressing for use with suction pump, home model, portable, pad size more than 16 square inches but less than or equal to 48 square inches
K0746	Absorptive wound dressing for use with suction pump, home model, portable, pad size greater than 48 square inches
K0800	Power operated vehicle, group 1 standard, patient weight capacity up to and including 300 pounds
K0801	Power operated vehicle, group 1 heavy duty, patient weight capacity 301 to 450 pounds
K0802	Power operated vehicle, group 1 very heavy duty, patient weight capacity 451 to 600 pounds
K0806	Power operated vehicle, group 2 standard, patient weight capacity up to and including 300 pounds
K0807	Power operated vehicle, group 2 heavy duty, patient weight capacity 301 to 450 pounds
K0808	Power operated vehicle, group 2 very heavy duty, patient weight capacity 451 to 600 pounds
K0812	Power operated vehicle, not otherwise classified
K0813	Power wheelchair, group 1 standard, portable, sling/solid seat and back, patient weight capacity up to and including 300 pounds
K0814	Power wheelchair, group 1 standard, portable, captains chair, patient weight capacity up to and including 300 pounds
K0815	Power wheelchair, group 1 standard, sling/solid seat and back, patient weight capacity up to and including 300 pounds
K0816	Power wheelchair, group 1 standard, captains chair, patient weight capacity up to and including 300 pounds
K0820	Power wheelchair, group 2 standard, portable, sling/solid seat/back, patient weight capacity up to and including 300 pounds
K0821	Power wheelchair, group 2 standard, portable, captains chair, patient weight capacity up to and including 300 pounds

K0822 Power wheelchair, group 2 standard, sling/solid seat/back, patient weight capacity up to and including 300 pounds

K0823 Power wheelchair, group 2 standard, captains chair, patient weight capacity up to and including 300 pounds

K0824 Power wheelchair, group 2 heavy duty, sling/solid seat/back, patient weight capacity 301 to 450 pounds

K0825 Power wheelchair, group 2 heavy duty, captains chair, patient weight capacity 301 to 450 pounds

K0826 Power wheelchair, group 2 very heavy duty, sling/solid seat/back, patient weight capacity 451 to 600 pounds

K0827 Power wheelchair, group 2 very heavy duty, captains chair, patient weight capacity 451 to 600 pounds

K0828 Power wheelchair, group 2 extra heavy duty, sling/solid seat/back, patient weight capacity 601 pounds or more

K0829 Power wheelchair, group 2 extra heavy duty, captains chair, patient weight 601 pounds or more

K0830 Power wheelchair, group 2 standard, seat elevator, sling/solid seat/back, patient weight capacity up to and including 300 pounds

K0831 Power wheelchair, group 2 standard, seat elevator, captains chair, patient weight capacity up to and including 300 pounds

K0835 Power wheelchair, group 2 standard, single power option, sling/solid seat/back, patient weight capacity up to and including 300 pounds

K0836 Power wheelchair, group 2 standard, single power option, captains chair, patient weight capacity up to and including 300 pounds

K0837 Power wheelchair, group 2 heavy duty, single power option, sling/solid seat/back, patient weight capacity 301 to 450 pounds

K0838 Power wheelchair, group 2 heavy duty, single power option, captains chair, patient weight capacity 301 to 450 pounds

K0839 Power wheelchair, group 2 very heavy duty, single power option, sling/solid seat/back, patient weight capacity 451 to 600 pounds

K0840 Power wheelchair, group 2 extra heavy duty, single power option, sling/solid seat/back, patient weight capacity 601 pounds or more

K0841 Power wheelchair, group 2 standard, multiple power option, sling/solid seat/back, patient weight capacity up to and including 300 pounds

K0842 Power wheelchair, group 2 standard, multiple power option, captains chair, patient weight capacity up to and including 300 pounds

K0843 Power wheelchair, group 2 heavy duty, multiple power option, sling/solid seat/back, patient weight capacity 301 to 450 pounds

K0848 Power wheelchair, group 3 standard, sling/solid seat/back, patient weight capacity up to and including 300 pounds

K0849 Power wheelchair, group 3 standard, captains chair, patient weight capacity up to and including 300 pounds

K0850 Power wheelchair, group 3 heavy duty, sling/solid seat/back, patient weight capacity 301 to 450 pounds

K0851 Power wheelchair, group 3 heavy duty, captains chair, patient weight capacity 301 to 450 pounds

K0852 Power wheelchair, group 3 very heavy duty, sling/solid seat/back, patient weight capacity 451 to 600 pounds

K0853 Power wheelchair, group 3 very heavy duty, captains chair, patient weight capacity 451 to 600 pounds

K0854 Power wheelchair, group 3 extra heavy duty, sling/solid seat/back, patient weight capacity 601 pounds or more

K0855 Power wheelchair, group 3 extra heavy duty, captains chair, patient weight capacity 601 pounds or more

K0856 Power wheelchair, group 3 standard, single power option, sling/solid seat/back, patient weight capacity up to and including 300 pounds

K0857 Power wheelchair, group 3 standard, single power option, captains chair, patient weight capacity up to and including 300 pounds

K0858 Power wheelchair, group 3 heavy duty, single power option, sling/solid seat/back, patient weight 301 to 450 pounds

K0859 Power wheelchair, group 3 heavy duty, single power option, captains chair, patient weight capacity 301 to 450 pounds

K0860 Power wheelchair, group 3 very heavy duty, single power option, sling/solid seat/back, patient weight capacity 451 to 600 pounds

K0861 Power wheelchair, group 3 standard, multiple power option, sling/solid seat/back, patient weight capacity up to and including 300 pounds

K0862 Power wheelchair, group 3 heavy duty, multiple power option, sling/solid seat/back, patient weight capacity 301 to 450 pounds

K0863 Power wheelchair, group 3 very heavy duty, multiple power option, sling/solid seat/back, patient weight capacity 451 to 600 pounds

K0864 Power wheelchair, group 3 extra heavy duty, multiple power option, sling/solid seat/back, patient weight capacity 601 pounds or more

K0868 Power wheelchair, group 4 standard, sling/solid seat/back, patient weight capacity up to and including 300 pounds

K0869 Power wheelchair, group 4 standard, captains chair, patient weight capacity up to and including 300 pounds

K0870 Power wheelchair, group 4 heavy duty, sling/solid seat/back, patient weight capacity 301 to 450 pounds

K0871 Power wheelchair, group 4 very heavy duty, sling/solid seat/back, patient weight capacity 451 to 600 pounds

K0877 Power wheelchair, group 4 standard, single power option, sling/solid seat/back, patient weight capacity up to and including 300 pounds

K0878 Power wheelchair, group 4 standard, single power option, captains chair, patient weight capacity up to and including 300 pounds

K0879 Power wheelchair, group 4 heavy duty, single power option, sling/solid seat/back, patient weight capacity 301 to 450 pounds

K0880 Power wheelchair, group 4 very heavy duty, single power option, sling/solid seat/back, patient weight 451 to 600 pounds

K0884 Power wheelchair, group 4 standard, multiple power option, sling/solid seat/back, patient weight capacity up to and including 300 pounds

K0885 Power wheelchair, group 4 standard, multiple power option, captains chair, patient weight capacity up to and including 300 pounds

K0886 Power wheelchair, group 4 heavy duty, multiple power option, sling/solid seat/back, patient weight capacity 301 to 450 pounds

K0890 Power wheelchair, group 5 pediatric, single power option, sling/solid seat/back, patient weight capacity up to and including 125 pounds

K0891 Power wheelchair, group 5 pediatric, multiple power option, sling/solid seat/back, patient weight capacity up to and including 125 pounds

K0898 Power wheelchair, not otherwise classified

K0899 Power mobility device, not coded by dme pdac or does not meet criteria

K0900 Customized durable medical equipment, other than wheelchair

K0901 Knee orthosis (ko), single upright, thigh and calf, with adjustable flexion and extension joint (unicentric or polycentric), medial-lateral and rotation control, with or without varus/valgus adjustment, prefabricated, off-the-shelf

K0902 Knee orthosis (ko), double upright, thigh and calf, with adjustable flexion and extension joint (unicentric or polycentric), medial-lateral and rotation control, with or without varus/valgus adjustment, prefabricated, off-the-shelf

K0903 For diabetics only, multiple density insert, made by direct carving with cam technology from a rectified cad model created from a digitized scan of the patient, total contact with patient's foot, including arch, base layer minimum of 3/16 inch material of shore a 35 durometer (or higher), includes arch filler and other shaping material, custom fabricated, each

(**K1001** Electronic positional obstructive sleep apnea treatment, with sensor, includes all components and accessories, any type
Code deleted effective 12/31/2023, no HCPCS/CPT cross-reference provided.)

(**K1002** Cranial electrotherapy stimulation (CES) system, any type
Code deleted effective 12/31/2023, no HCPCS/CPT cross-reference provided.)

(**K1003** Whirlpool tub, walk-in, portable
Code deleted effective 12/31/2023, no HCPCS/CPT cross-reference provided.)

K1004 Low frequency ultrasonic diathermy treatment device for home use, includes all components and accessories

(**K1005** Disposable collection and storage bag for breast milk, any size, any type, each
Code deleted effective 12/31/2023, no HCPCS/CPT cross-reference provided.)

(**K1006** Suction pump, home model, portable or stationary, electric, any type, for use with external urine management system
Code deleted effective 12/31/2023, no HCPCS/CPT cross-reference provided.)

K1007 Bilateral hip, knee, ankle, foot device, powered, includes pelvic component, single or double upright(s), knee joints any type, with or without ankle joints any type, includes all components and accessories, motors, microprocessors, sensors

(**K1009** Speech volume modulation system, any type, including all components and accessories
Code deleted effective 12/31/2023, no HCPCS/CPT cross-reference provided.)

K1010 Indwelling intraurethral drainage device with valve, patient inserted, replacement only, each

K1011 Activation device for intraurethral drainage device with valve, replacement only, each

K1012 Charger and base station for intraurethral activation device, replacement only

(**K1013** Enema tube, with or without adapter, any type, replacement only, each
Code deleted effective 12/31/2023, no HCPCS/CPT cross-reference provided.)

(**K1014** Addition, endoskeletal knee-shin system, 4 bar linkage or multiaxial, fluid swing and stance phase control
Code deleted effective 12/31/2023, no HCPCS/CPT cross-reference provided.)

(**K1015** Foot, adductus positioning device, adjustable
Code deleted effective 12/31/2023, no HCPCS/CPT cross-reference provided.)

(**K1016** Transcutaneous electrical nerve stimulator for electrical stimulation of the trigeminal nerve
Code deleted effective 12/31/2023, no HCPCS/CPT cross-reference provided.)

(**K1017** Monthly supplies for use of device coded at k1016
Code deleted effective 12/31/2023, no HCPCS/CPT cross-reference provided.)

(**K1018** External upper limb tremor stimulator of the peripheral nerves of the wrist
Code deleted effective 12/31/2023, no HCPCS/CPT cross-reference provided.)

(**K1019** Replacement supplies and accessories for external upper limb tremor stimulator of the peripheral nerves of the wrist
Code deleted effective 12/31/2023, no HCPCS/CPT cross-reference provided.)

(**K1020** Non-invasive vagus nerve stimulator
Code deleted effective 12/31/2023, no HCPCS/CPT cross-reference provided.)

(**K1021** Exsufflation belt, includes all supplies and accessories
Code deleted effective 12/31/2023, no HCPCS/CPT cross-reference provided.)

(**K1022** Addition to lower extremity prosthesis, endoskeletal, knee disarticulation, above knee, hip disarticulation, positional rotation unit, any type
Code deleted effective 12/31/2023, no HCPCS/CPT cross-reference provided.)

(**K1023** Distal transcutaneous electrical nerve stimulator, stimulates peripheral nerves of the upper arm
Code deleted effective 12/31/2023, no HCPCS/CPT cross-reference provided.)

(**K1024** Non-pneumatic compression controller with sequential calibrated gradient pressure
Code deleted effective 12/31/2023, no HCPCS/CPT cross-reference provided.)

(**K1025** Non-pneumatic sequential compression garment, full arm
Code deleted effective 12/31/2023, no HCPCS/CPT cross-reference provided.)

(**K1026** Mechanical allergen particle barrier/inhalation filter, cream, nasal, topical
Code deleted effective 12/31/2023, no HCPCS/CPT cross-reference provided.)

K1027 Oral device/appliance used to reduce upper airway collapsibility, without fixed mechanical hinge, custom fabricated, includes fitting and adjustment

(**K1028** Power source and control electronics unit for oral device/appliance for neuromuscular electrical stimulation of the tongue muscle for the reduction of snoring and obstructive sleep apnea, controlled by phone application
Code deleted effective 12/31/2023, no HCPCS/CPT cross-reference provided.)

(**K1029** Oral device/appliance for neuromuscular electrical stimulation of the tongue muscle, used in conjunction with the power source and control electronics unit, controlled by phone application, 90-day supply
Code deleted effective 12/31/2023, no HCPCS/CPT cross-reference provided.)

K1030 External recharging system for battery (internal) for use with implanted cardiac contractility modulation generator, replacement only

(**K1031** Non-pneumatic compression controller without calibrated gradient pressure
Code deleted effective 12/31/2023, no HCPCS/CPT cross-reference provided.)

(**K1032** Non-pneumatic sequential compression garment, full leg
Code deleted effective 12/31/2023, no HCPCS/CPT cross-reference provided.)

(**K1033** Non-pneumatic sequential compression garment, half leg
Code deleted effective 12/31/2023, no HCPCS/CPT cross-reference provided.)

K1034 Provision of covid-19 test, nonprescription self-administered and self-collected use, FDA approved, authorized or cleared, one test count
Code deleted effective 12/31/2023, no HCPCS/CPT cross-reference provided.)

ORTHOTIC PROCEDURES

Guidelines

In addition to the information presented in the INTRODUCTION, several other items unique to this section are defined or identified here:

1. **SUBSECTION INFORMATION:** Some of the listed subheadings or subsections have special needs or instructions unique to that section. Where these are indicated, special "notes" will be presented preceding or following the listings. Those subsections within the ORTHOTIC PROCEDURES section that have "notes" are as follows:

Subsection	Code Numbers
Scoliosis procedures	L1000–L1499
Orthotic devices-lower limb	L1600–L2999
Lower limb-hip-knee-angle-foot (or any combination)	L2000–L2199
Orthotic devices-upper limb	L3650–L3999

2. **UNLISTED SERVICE OR PROCEDURE:** A service or procedure may be provided that is not listed in this edition of HCPCS. When reporting such a service, the appropriate "unlisted procedure" code may be used to indicate the service, identifying it by "special report" as defined below. HCPCS terminology is inconsistent in defining unlisted procedures. The procedure definition may include the term(s) "unlisted", "not otherwise classified", "unspecified", "unclassified", "other" and "miscellaneous". Prior to using these codes, try to determine if a Local Level III code or CPT code is available. The "unlisted procedures" and accompanying codes for ORTHOTIC PROCEDURES are as follows:

   L0999 Addition to spinal orthosis, not otherwise specified
   L1499 Spinal orthosis, not otherwise specified
   L2999 Lower extremity orthosis, not otherwise specified
   L3649 Orthopedic shoe, modification, addition or transfer, not otherwise specified
   L3999 Upper limb orthosis, not otherwise specified

3. **SPECIAL REPORT:** A service, material or supply that is rarely provided, unusual, variable or new may require a special report in determining medical appropriateness for reimbursement purposes. Pertinent information should include an adequate definition or description of the nature, extent, and need for the service, material or supply.

4. **MODIFIERS:** Listed services may be modified under certain circumstances. When appropriate, the modifying circumstance is identified by adding a modifier to the basic procedure code. CPT and HCPCS National Level II modifiers may be used with CPT and HCPCS National Level II procedure codes. Modifiers commonly used with ORTHOTIC PROCEDURES are as follows:

   -CC Procedure code change (use "CC" when the procedure code submitted was changed either for administrative reasons or because an incorrect code was filed)

   -LT Left side (used to identify procedures performed on the left side of the body)

   -RT Right side (used to identify procedures performed on the right side of the body)

   -TC Technical component. Under certain circumstances, a charge may be made for the technical component alone. Under those circumstances, the technical component charge is identified by adding modifier -TC to the usual procedure number. Technical component charges are institutional charges and are not billed separately by physicians. However, portable x-ray suppliers bill only for the technical component and should use modifier -TC. The change data from portable x-ray suppliers will then be used to build customary and prevailing profiles.

5. **CPT CODE CROSS-REFERENCE:** Unless otherwise specified, the equivalent CPT code for all listings in this section is 99070.

6. **DURABLE MEDICAL EQUIPMENT REGIONAL CARRIERS (DMERCS):** Effective October 1, 1993, claims orthotics must be billed to one of four regional carriers depending upon the residence of the beneficiary. The transition dates for DMERC claims is from November 1, 1993 to March 1, 1994, depending upon the state you practice in. See the Introduction for a complete discussion of DMERCs.

Orthotic Devices Spinal – Cervical

L0112 Cranial cervical orthosis, congenital torticollis type, with or without soft interface material, adjustable range of motion joint, custom fabricated

L0113 Cranial cervical orthosis, torticollis type, with or without joint, with or without soft interface material, prefabricated, includes fitting and adjustment

L0120 Cervical, flexible, non-adjustable, prefabricated, off-the-shelf (foam collar)

L0130 Cervical, flexible, thermoplastic collar, molded to patient

L0140 Cervical, semi-rigid, adjustable (plastic collar)

L0150 Cervical, semi-rigid, adjustable molded chin cup (plastic collar with mandibular/occipital piece)

L0160 Cervical, semi-rigid, wire frame occipital/mandibular support, prefabricated, off-the-shelf

L0170 Cervical, collar, molded to patient model

L0172 Cervical, collar, semi-rigid thermoplastic foam, two-piece, prefabricated, off-the-shelf

L0174 Cervical, collar, semi-rigid, thermoplastic foam, two piece with thoracic extension, prefabricated, off-the-shelf

L0180 Cervical, multiple post collar, occipital/mandibular supports, adjustable

L0190 Cervical, multiple post collar, occipital/mandibular supports, adjustable cervical bars (SOMI, Guilford, Taylor types)

L0200 Cervical, multiple post collar, occipital/mandibular supports, adjustable cervical bars, and thoracic extension

Spinal - Thoracic-Lumbar-Sacral

L0220 Thoracic, rib belt, custom fabricated

L0450 TLSO, flexible, provides trunk support, upper thoracic region, produces intracavitary pressure to reduce load on the intervertebral disks with rigid stays or panel(s), includes shoulder straps and closures, prefabricated, off-the-shelf

L0452 TLSO, flexible, provides trunk support, upper thoracic region, produces intracavitary pressure to reduce load on the intervertebral disks with rigid stays or panel(s), includes shoulder straps and closures, custom fabricated

L0454 TLSO flexible, provides trunk support, extends from sacrococcygeal junction to above T-9 vertebra, restricts gross trunk motion in the sagittal plane, produces intracavitary pressure to reduce load on the intervertebral disks with rigid stays or panel(s), includes shoulder straps and closures, prefabricated item that has been trimmed, bent, molded, assembled, or otherwise customized to fit a specific patient by an individual with expertise

L0455 TLSO, flexible, provides trunk support, extends from sacrococcygeal junction to above T-9 vertebra, restricts gross trunk motion in the sagittal plane, produces intracavitary pressure to reduce load on the intervertebral disks with rigid stays or panel(s), includes shoulder straps and closures, prefabricated, off-the-shelf

L0456 TLSO, flexible, provides trunk support, thoracic region, rigid posterior panel and soft anterior apron, extends from the sacrococcygeal junction and terminates just inferior to the scapular spine, restricts gross trunk motion in the sagittal plane, produces intracavitary pressure to reduce load on the intervertebral disks, includes straps and closures, prefabricated item that has been trimmed, bent, molded, assembled, or otherwise customized to fit a specific patient by an individual with expertise

L0457 TLSO, flexible, provides trunk support, thoracic region, rigid posterior panel and soft anterior apron, extends from the sacrococcygeal junction and terminates just inferior to the scapular spine, restricts gross trunk motion in the sagittal plane, produces intracavitary pressure to reduce load on the intervertebral disks, includes straps and closures, prefabricated, off-the-shelf

L0458 TLSO, triplanar control, modular segmented spinal system, two rigid plastic shells, posterior extends from the sacrococcygeal junction and terminates just inferior to the scapular spine, anterior extends from the symphysis pubis to the xiphoid, soft liner, restricts gross trunk motion in the sagittal, coronal, and transverse planes, lateral strength is provided by overlapping plastic and stabilizing closures, includes straps and closures, prefabricated, includes fitting and adjustment

L0460 TLSO, triplanar control, modular segmented spinal system, two rigid plastic shells, posterior extends from the sacrococcygeal junction and terminates just inferior to the scapular spine, anterior extends from the symphysis pubis to the sternal notch, soft liner, restricts gross trunk motion in the sagittal, coronal, and transverse planes, lateral strength is provided by overlapping plastic and stabilizing closures, includes straps and closures, prefabricated item that has been trimmed, bent, molded, assembled, or otherwise customized to fit a specific patient by an individual with expertise

L0462 TLSO, triplanar control, modular segmented spinal system, three rigid plastic shells, posterior extends from the sacrococcygeal junction and terminates just inferior to the scapular spine, anterior extends from the symphysis pubis to the sternal notch, soft liner, restricts gross trunk motion in the sagittal, coronal, and transverse planes, lateral strength is provided by overlapping plastic and stabilizing closures, includes straps and closures, prefabricated, includes fitting and adjustment

L0464 TLSO, triplanar control, modular segmented spinal system, four rigid plastic shells, posterior extends from sacrococcygeal junction and terminates just inferior to scapular spine, anterior extends from symphysis pubis to the sternal notch, soft liner, restricts gross trunk motion in sagittal, coronal, and transverse planes, lateral strength is provided by overlapping plastic and stabilizing closures, includes straps and closures, prefabricated, includes fitting and adjustment

L0466 TLSO, sagittal control, rigid posterior frame and flexible soft anterior apron with straps, closures and padding, restricts gross trunk motion in sagittal plane, produces intracavitary pressure to reduce load on intervertebral disks, prefabricated item that has been trimmed, bent, molded, assembled, or otherwise customized to fit a specific patient by an individual with expertise

L0467 TLSO, sagittal control, rigid posterior frame and flexible soft anterior apron with straps, closures and padding, restricts gross trunk motion in sagittal plane, produces intracavitary pressure to reduce load on intervertebral disks, prefabricated, off-the-shelf

L0468 TLSO, sagittal-coronal control, rigid posterior frame and flexible soft anterior apron with straps, closures and padding, extends from sacrococcygeal junction over scapulae, lateral strength provided by pelvic, thoracic, and lateral frame pieces, restricts gross trunk motion in sagittal, and coronal planes, produces intracavitary pressure to reduce load on intervertebral disks, prefabricated item that has been trimmed, bent, molded, assembled, or otherwise customized to fit a specific patient by an individual with expertise

L0469 TLSO, sagittal-coronal control, rigid posterior frame and flexible soft anterior apron with straps, closures and padding, extends from sacrococcygeal junction over scapulae, lateral strength provided by pelvic, thoracic, and lateral frame pieces, restricts gross trunk motion in sagittal and coronal planes, produces intracavitary pressure to reduce load on intervertebral disks, prefabricated, off-the-shelf

L0470 TLSO, triplanar control, rigid posterior frame and flexible soft anterior apron with straps, closures and padding, extends from sacrococcygeal junction to scapula, lateral strength provided by pelvic, thoracic, and lateral frame pieces, rotational strength provided by subclavicular extensions, restricts gross trunk motion in sagittal, coronal, and transverse planes, provides intracavitary pressure to reduce load on the intervertebral disks, includes fitting and shaping the frame, prefabricated, includes fitting and adjustment

L0472 TLSO, triplanar control, hyperextension, rigid anterior and lateral frame extends from symphysis pubis to sternal notch with two anterior components (one pubic and one sternal), posterior and lateral pads with straps and closures, limits spinal flexion, restricts gross trunk motion in sagittal, coronal, and transverse planes, includes fitting and shaping the frame, prefabricated, includes fitting and adjustment

L0480 TLSO, triplanar control, one piece rigid plastic shell without interface liner, with multiple straps and closures, posterior extends from sacrococcygeal junction and terminates just inferior to scapular spine, anterior extends from symphysis pubis to sternal notch, anterior or posterior opening, restricts gross trunk motion in sagittal, coronal, and transverse planes, includes a carved plaster or cad-cam model, custom fabricated

L0482 TLSO, triplanar control, one piece rigid plastic shell with interface liner, multiple straps and closures, posterior extends from sacrococcygeal junction and terminates just inferior to scapular spine, anterior extends from symphysis pubis to sternal notch, anterior or posterior opening, restricts gross trunk motion in sagittal, coronal, and transverse planes, includes a carved plaster or cad-cam model, custom fabricated

L0484 TLSO, triplanar control, two piece rigid plastic shell without interface liner, with multiple straps and closures, posterior extends from sacrococcygeal junction and terminates just inferior to scapular spine, anterior extends from symphysis pubis to sternal notch, lateral strength is enhanced by overlapping plastic, restricts gross trunk motion in the sagittal, coronal, and transverse planes, includes a carved plaster or cad-cam model, custom fabricated

L0486 TLSO, triplanar control, two piece rigid plastic shell with interface liner, multiple straps and closures, posterior extends from sacrococcygeal junction and terminates just inferior to scapular spine, anterior extends from symphysis pubis to sternal notch, lateral strength is enhanced by overlapping plastic, restricts gross trunk motion in the sagittal, coronal, and transverse planes, includes a carved plaster or cad-cam model, custom fabricated

L0488 TLSO, triplanar control, one piece rigid plastic shell with interface liner, multiple straps and closures, posterior extends from sacrococcygeal junction and terminates just inferior to scapular spine, anterior extends from symphysis pubis to sternal notch, anterior or posterior opening, restricts gross trunk motion in sagittal, coronal, and transverse planes, prefabricated, includes fitting and adjustment

L0490 TLSO, sagittal-coronal control, one piece rigid plastic shell, with overlapping reinforced anterior, with multiple straps and closures, posterior extends from sacrococcygeal junction and terminates at or before the T-9 vertebra, anterior extends from symphysis pubis to xiphoid, anterior opening, restricts gross trunk motion in sagittal and coronal planes, prefabricated, includes fitting and adjustment

L0491 TLSO, sagittal-coronal control, modular segmented spinal system, two rigid plastic shells, posterior extends from the sacrococcygeal junction and terminates just inferior to the scapular spine, anterior extends from the symphysis pubis to the xiphoid, soft liner, restricts gross trunk motion in the sagittal and coronal planes, lateral strength is provided by overlapping plastic and stabilizing closures, includes straps and closures, prefabricated, includes fitting and adjustment

L0492 TLSO, sagittal-coronal control, modular segmented spinal system, three rigid plastic shells, posterior extends from the sacrococcygeal junction and terminates just inferior to the scapular spine, anterior extends from the symphysis pubis to the xiphoid, soft liner, restricts gross trunk motion in the sagittal and coronal planes, lateral strength is provided by overlapping plastic and stabilizing closures, includes straps and closures, prefabricated, includes fitting and adjustment

Spinal - Sacroiliac Semi-Rigid

L0621 Sacroiliac orthosis, flexible, provides pelvic-sacral support, reduces motion about the sacroiliac joint, includes straps, closures, may include pendulous abdomen design, prefabricated, off-the-shelf

L0622 Sacroiliac orthosis, flexible, provides pelvic-sacral support, reduces motion about the sacroiliac joint, includes straps, closures, may include pendulous abdomen design, custom fabricated

L0623 Sacroiliac orthosis, provides pelvic-sacral support, with rigid or semi-rigid panels over the sacrum and abdomen, reduces motion about the sacroiliac joint, includes straps, closures, may include pendulous abdomen design, prefabricated, off-the-shelf

L0624 Sacroiliac orthosis, provides pelvic-sacral support, with rigid or semi-rigid panels placed over the sacrum and abdomen, reduces motion about the sacroiliac joint, includes straps, closures, may include pendulous abdomen design, custom fabricated

L0625 Lumbar orthosis, flexible, provides lumbar support, posterior extends from L-1 to below L-5 vertebra, produces intracavitary pressure to reduce load on the intervertebral discs, includes straps, closures, may include pendulous abdomen design, shoulder straps, stays, prefabricated, off-the-shelf

L0626 Lumbar orthosis, sagittal control, with rigid posterior panel(s), posterior extends from L-1 to below L-5 vertebra, produces intracavitary pressure to reduce load on the intervertebral discs, includes straps, closures, may include padding, stays, shoulder straps, pendulous abdomen design, prefabricated item that has been trimmed, bent, molded, assembled, or otherwise customized to fit a specific patient by an individual with expertise

L0627 Lumbar orthosis, sagittal control, with rigid anterior and posterior panels, posterior extends from L-1 to below L-5 vertebra, produces intracavitary pressure to reduce load on the intervertebral discs, includes straps, closures, may include padding, shoulder straps, pendulous abdomen design, prefabricated item that has been trimmed, bent, molded, assembled, or otherwise customized to fit a specific patient by an individual with expertise

L0628 Lumbar-sacral orthosis, flexible, provides lumbo-sacral support, posterior extends from sacrococcygeal junction to T-9 vertebra, produces intracavitary pressure to reduce load on the intervertebral discs, includes straps, closures, may include stays, shoulder straps, pendulous abdomen design, prefabricated, off-the-shelf

L0629 Lumbar-sacral orthosis, flexible, provides lumbo-sacral support, posterior extends from sacrococcygeal junction to T-9 vertebra, produces intracavitary pressure to reduce load on the intervertebral discs, includes straps, closures, may include stays, shoulder straps, pendulous abdomen design, custom fabricated

L0630 Lumbar-sacral orthosis, sagittal control, with rigid posterior panel(s), posterior extends from sacrococcygeal junction to T-9 vertebra, produces intracavitary pressure to reduce load on the intervertebral discs, includes straps, closures, may include padding, stays, shoulder straps, pendulous abdomen design, prefabricated item that has been trimmed, bent, molded, assembled, or otherwise customized to fit a specific patient by an individual with expertise

L0631 Lumbar-sacral orthosis, sagittal control, with rigid anterior and posterior panels, posterior extends from sacrococcygeal junction to T-9 vertebra, produces intracavitary pressure to reduce load on the intervertebral discs, includes straps, closures, may include padding, shoulder straps, pendulous abdomen design, prefabricated item that has been trimmed, bent, molded, assembled, or otherwise customized to fit a specific patient by an individual with expertise

L0632 Lumbar-sacral orthosis, sagittal control, with rigid anterior and posterior panels, posterior extends from sacrococcygeal junction to T-9 vertebra, produces intracavitary pressure to reduce load on the intervertebral discs, includes straps, closures, may include padding, shoulder straps, pendulous abdomen design, custom fabricated

L0633 Lumbar-sacral orthosis, sagittal-coronal control, with rigid posterior frame/panel(s), posterior extends from sacrococcygeal junction to T-9 vertebra, lateral strength provided by rigid lateral frame/panels, produces intracavitary pressure to reduce load on intervertebral discs, includes straps, closures, may include padding, stays, shoulder straps, pendulous abdomen design, prefabricated item that has been trimmed, bent, molded, assembled, or otherwise customized to fit a specific patient by an individual with expertise

L0634 Lumbar-sacral orthosis, sagittal-coronal control, with rigid posterior frame/panel(s), posterior extends from sacrococcygeal junction to T-9 vertebra, lateral strength provided by rigid lateral frame/panel(s), produces intracavitary pressure to reduce load on intervertebral discs, includes straps, closures, may include padding, stays, shoulder straps, pendulous abdomen design, custom fabricated

L0635 Lumbar-sacral orthosis, sagittal-coronal control, lumbar flexion, rigid posterior frame/panel(s), lateral articulating design to flex the lumbar spine, posterior extends from sacrococcygeal junction to T-9 vertebra, lateral strength provided by rigid lateral frame/panel(s), produces intracavitary pressure to reduce load on intervertebral discs, includes straps, closures, may include padding, anterior panel, pendulous abdomen design, prefabricated, includes fitting and adjustment

L0636 Lumbar sacral orthosis, sagittal-coronal control, lumbar flexion, rigid posterior frame/panels, lateral articulating design to flex the lumbar spine, posterior extends from sacrococcygeal junction to T-9 vertebra, lateral strength provided by rigid lateral frame/panels, produces intracavitary pressure to reduce load on intervertebral discs, includes straps, closures, may include padding, anterior panel, pendulous abdomen design, custom fabricated

L0637 Lumbar-sacral orthosis, sagittal-coronal control, with rigid anterior and posterior frame/panels, posterior extends from sacrococcygeal junction to T-9 vertebra, lateral strength provided by rigid lateral frame/panels, produces intracavitary pressure to reduce load on intervertebral discs, includes straps, closures, may include padding, shoulder straps, pendulous abdomen design, prefabricated item that has been trimmed, bent, molded, assembled, or otherwise customized to fit a specific patient by an individual with expertise

L0638 Lumbar-sacral orthosis, sagittal-coronal control, with rigid anterior and posterior frame/panels, posterior extends from sacrococcygeal junction to T-9 vertebra, lateral strength provided by rigid lateral frame/panels, produces intracavitary pressure to reduce load on intervertebral discs, includes straps, closures, may include padding, shoulder straps, pendulous abdomen design, custom fabricated

L0639 Lumbar-sacral orthosis, sagittal-coronal control, rigid shell(s)/panel(s), posterior extends from sacrococcygeal junction to T-9 vertebra, anterior extends from symphysis pubis to xyphoid, produces intracavitary pressure to reduce load on the intervertebral discs, overall strength is provided by overlapping rigid material and stabilizing closures, includes straps, closures, may include soft interface, pendulous abdomen design, prefabricated item that has been trimmed, bent, molded, assembled, or otherwise customized to fit a specific patient by an individual with expertise

L0640 Lumbar-sacral orthosis, sagittal-coronal control, rigid shell(s)/panel(s), posterior extends from sacrococcygeal junction to T-9 vertebra, anterior extends from symphysis pubis to xyphoid, produces intracavitary pressure to reduce load on the intervertebral discs, overall strength is provided by overlapping rigid material and stabilizing closures, includes straps, closures, may include soft interface, pendulous abdomen design, custom fabricated

L0641 Lumbar orthosis, sagittal control, with rigid posterior panel(s), posterior extends from L-1 to below L-5 vertebra, produces intracavitary pressure to reduce load on the intervertebral discs, includes straps, closures, may include padding, stays, shoulder straps, pendulous abdomen design, prefabricated, off-the-shelf

L0642 Lumbar orthosis, sagittal control, with rigid anterior and posterior panels, posterior extends from L-1 to below L-5 vertebra, produces intracavitary pressure to reduce load on the intervertebral discs, includes straps, closures, may include padding, shoulder straps, pendulous abdomen design, prefabricated, off-the-shelf

L0643 Lumbar-sacral orthosis, sagittal control, with rigid posterior panel(s), posterior extends from sacrococcygeal junction to T-9 vertebra, produces intracavitary pressure to reduce load on the intervertebral discs, includes straps, closures, may include padding, stays, shoulder straps, pendulous abdomen design, prefabricated, off-the-shelf

L0648 Lumbar-sacral orthosis, sagittal control, with rigid anterior and posterior panels, posterior extends from sacrococcygeal junction to T-9 vertebra, produces intracavitary pressure to reduce load on the intervertebral discs, includes straps, closures, may include padding, shoulder straps, pendulous abdomen design, prefabricated, off-the-shelf

L0649 Lumbar-sacral orthosis, sagittal-coronal control, with rigid posterior frame/panel(s), posterior extends from sacrococcygeal junction to T-9 vertebra, lateral strength provided by rigid lateral frame/panels, produces intracavitary pressure to reduce load on intervertebral discs, includes straps, closures, may include padding, stays, shoulder straps, pendulous abdomen design, prefabricated, off-the-shelf

L0650 Lumbar-sacral orthosis, sagittal-coronal control, with rigid anterior and posterior frame/panel(s), posterior extends from sacrococcygeal junction to T-9 vertebra, lateral strength provided by rigid lateral frame/panel(s), produces intracavitary pressure to reduce load on intervertebral discs, includes straps, closures, may include padding, shoulder straps, pendulous abdomen design, prefabricated, off-the-shelf

L0651 Lumbar-sacral orthosis, sagittal-coronal control, rigid shell(s)/panel(s), posterior extends from sacrococcygeal junction to T-9 vertebra, anterior extends from symphysis pubis to xyphoid, produces intracavitary pressure to reduce load on the intervertebral discs, overall strength is provided by overlapping rigid material and stabilizing closures, includes straps, closures, may include soft interface, pendulous abdomen design, prefabricated, off-the-shelf

Spinal - Cervical-Thoracic-Lumbar-Sacral – Halo Procedure

L0700 Cervical-thoracic-lumbar-sacral-orthoses (CTLSO), anterior-posterior-lateral control, molded to patient model, (Minerva type)

L0710 CTLSO, anterior-posterior-lateral-control, molded to patient model, with interface material, (Minerva type)

L0810 Halo procedure, cervical halo incorporated into jacket vest

L0820 Halo procedure, cervical halo incorporated into plaster body jacket

L0830 Halo procedure, cervical halo incorporated into Milwaukee type orthosis

Additions to Spinal Orthoses

L0859 Addition to halo procedure, magnetic resonance image compatible systems, rings and pins, any material

L0861 Addition to halo procedure, replacement liner/interface material

L0970 TLSO, corset front

L0972 LSO, corset front

L0974 TLSO, full corset

L0976 LSO, full corset

L0978 Axillary crutch extension

L0980 Peroneal straps, prefabricated, off-the-shelf, pair

L0982 Stocking supporter grips, prefabricated, off-the-shelf, set of four (4)

L0984 Protective body sock, prefabricated, off-the-shelf, each

L0999 Addition to spinal orthosis, not otherwise specified

Orthotic Devices - Scoliosis Procedures

NOTE: The orthotic care of scoliosis differs from other orthotic care in that the treatment is more dynamic in nature and utilizes ongoing, continual modification of the orthosis to the patient's changing condition. This coding structure uses the proper names or eponyms of the procedures because they have historic and universal acceptance in the profession. It should be recognized that variations to the basic procedures described by the founders/developers are accepted in various medical and orthotic practices throughout the country. All procedures include a model of patient when indicated.

L1000	Cervical-thoracic-lumbar-sacral orthosis (CTLSO) (Milwaukee), inclusive of furnishing initial orthosis, including model
L1001	Cervical thoracic lumbar sacral orthosis, immobilizer, infant size, prefabricated, includes fitting and adjustment
L1005	Tension based scoliosis orthosis and accessory pads, includes fitting and adjustment
L1010	Addition to cervical-thoracic-lumbar-sacral orthosis (CTLSO) or scoliosis orthosis, axilla sling
L1020	Addition to CTLSO or scoliosis orthosis, kyphosis pad
L1025	Addition to CTLSO or scoliosis orthosis, kyphosis pad, floating
L1030	Addition to CTLSO or scoliosis orthosis, lumbar bolster pad
L1040	Addition to CTLSO or scoliosis orthosis, lumbar or lumbar rib pad
L1050	Addition to CTLSO or scoliosis orthosis, sternal pad
L1060	Addition to CTLSO or scoliosis orthosis, thoracic pad
L1070	Addition to CTLSO or scoliosis orthosis, trapezius sling
L1080	Addition to CTLSO or scoliosis orthosis, outrigger
L1085	Addition to CTLSO or scoliosis orthosis, outrigger, bilateral with vertical extensions
L1090	Addition to CTLSO or scoliosis orthosis, lumbar sling
L1100	Addition to CTLSO or scoliosis orthosis, ring flange, plastic or leather
L1110	Addition to CTLSO or scoliosis orthosis, ring flange, plastic or leather, molded to patient model
L1120	Addition to CTLSO, scoliosis orthosis, cover for upright, each
L1200	Thoracic-lumbar-sacral-orthosis (TLSO), inclusive of furnishing initial orthosis only
L1210	Addition to TLSO, (low profile), lateral thoracic extension
L1220	Addition to TLSO, (low profile), anterior thoracic extension
L1230	Addition to TLSO, (low profile), Milwaukee type superstructure
L1240	Addition to TLSO, (low profile), lumbar derotation pad
L1250	Addition to TLSO, (low profile), anterior ASIS pad
L1260	Addition to TLSO, (low profile), anterior thoracic derotation pad
L1270	Addition to TLSO, (low profile), abdominal pad
L1280	Addition to TLSO, (low profile), rib gusset (elastic), each
L1290	Addition to TLSO, (low profile), lateral trochanteric pad
L1300	Other scoliosis procedure, body jacket molded to patient model
L1310	Other scoliosis procedure, post-operative body jacket
L1499	Spinal orthosis, not otherwise specified

Orthotic Devices - Lower Limb

NOTE: The procedures L1600-L2999 are considered as "base" or the "basic procedures" and may be modified by listing other procedures from the "additions" (L2200-L2999) section and adding them to the base procedure.

L1600 Hip orthosis, abduction control of hip joints, flexible, Frejka type with cover, prefabricated item that has been trimmed, bent, molded, assembled, or otherwise customized to fit a specific patient by an individual with expertise

L1610 Hip orthosis, abduction control of hip joints, flexible, (Frejka cover only), prefabricated item that has been trimmed, bent, molded, assembled, or otherwise customized to fit a specific patient by an individual with expertise

L1620 Hip orthosis, abduction control of hip joints, flexible, (Pavlik harness), prefabricated item that has been trimmed, bent, molded, assembled, or otherwise customized to fit a specific patient by an individual with expertise

L1630 Hip orthosis, abduction control of hip joints, semi-flexible (von Rosen type), custom fabricated

L1640 Hip orthosis, abduction control of hip joints, static, pelvic band or spreader bar, thigh cuffs, custom fabricated

L1650 Hip orthosis, abduction control of hip joints, static, adjustable, (Ilfeld type), prefabricated, includes fitting and adjustment

L1652 Hip orthosis, bilateral thigh cuffs with adjustable abductor spreader bar, adult size, prefabricated, includes fitting and adjustment, any type

L1660 Hip orthosis, abduction control of hip joints, static, plastic, prefabricated, includes fitting and adjustment

L1680 Hip orthosis, abduction control of hip joints, dynamic, pelvic control, adjustable hip motion control, thigh cuffs (rancho hip action type), custom fabricated

L1685 Hip orthosis, abduction control of hip joint, postoperative hip abduction type, custom fabricated

L1686 Hip orthosis, abduction control of hip joint, postoperative hip abduction type, prefabricated, includes fitting and adjustment

L1690 Combination, bilateral, lumbo-sacral, hip, femur orthosis providing adduction and internal rotation control, prefabricated, includes fitting and adjustment

L1700 Legg Perthes orthosis, (Toronto type), custom fabricated

L1710 Legg Perthes orthosis, (Newington type), custom fabricated

L1720 Legg Perthes orthosis, trilateral, (Tachdjian type), custom fabricated

L1730 Legg Perthes orthosis, (Scottish rite type), custom fabricated

L1755 Legg Perthes orthosis, (patten bottom type), custom fabricated

L1810 Knee orthosis, elastic with joints, prefabricated item that has been trimmed, bent, molded, assembled, or otherwise customized to fit a specific patient by an individual with expertise

L1812 Knee orthosis, elastic with joints, prefabricated, off-the-shelf

L1820 Knee orthosis, elastic with condylar pads and joints, with or without patellar control, prefabricated, includes fitting and adjustment

L1830 Knee orthosis, immobilizer, canvas longitudinal, prefabricated, off-the-shelf

L1831 Knee orthosis, locking knee joint(s), positional orthosis, prefabricated, includes fitting and adjustment

L1832 Knee orthosis, adjustable knee joints (unicentric or polycentric), positional orthosis, rigid support, prefabricated item that has been trimmed, bent, molded, assembled, or otherwise customized to fit a specific patient by an individual with expertise

L1833 Knee orthosis, adjustable knee joints (unicentric or polycentric), positional orthosis, rigid support, prefabricated, off-the shelf

L1834 Knee orthosis, without knee joint, rigid, custom fabricated

L1836 Knee orthosis, rigid, without joint(s), includes soft interface material, prefabricated, off-the-shelf

L1840 Knee orthosis, derotation, medial-lateral, anterior cruciate ligament, custom fabricated

L1843 Knee orthosis, single upright, thigh and calf, with adjustable flexion and extension joint (unicentric or polycentric), medial-lateral and rotation control, with or without varus/valgus adjustment, prefabricated item that has been trimmed, bent, molded, assembled, or otherwise customized to fit a specific patient by an individual with expertise

L1844 Knee orthosis, single upright, thigh and calf, with adjustable flexion and extension joint (unicentric or polycentric), medial-lateral and rotation control, with or without varus/valgus adjustment, custom fabricated

L1845 Knee orthosis, double upright, thigh and calf, with adjustable flexion and extension joint (unicentric or polycentric), medial-lateral and rotation control, with or without varus/valgus adjustment, prefabricated item that has been trimmed, bent, molded, assembled, or otherwise customized to fit a specific patient by an individual with expertise

L1846 Knee orthosis, double upright, thigh and calf, with adjustable flexion and extension joint (unicentric or polycentric), medial-lateral and rotation control, with or without varus/valgus adjustment, custom fabricated

L1847 Knee orthosis, double upright with adjustable joint, with inflatable air support chamber(s), prefabricated item that has been trimmed, bent, molded, assembled, or otherwise customized to fit a specific patient by an individual with expertise

L1848 Knee orthosis, double upright with adjustable joint, with inflatable air support chamber(s), prefabricated, off-the-shelf

L1850 Knee orthosis, Swedish type, prefabricated, off-the-shelf

L1851 Knee orthosis (KO), single upright, thigh and calf, with adjustable flexion and extension joint (unicentric or polycentric), medial-lateral and rotation control, with or without varus/valgus adjustment, prefabricated, off-the-shelf

L1852 Knee orthosis (KO), double upright, thigh and calf, with adjustable flexion and extension joint (unicentric or polycentric), medial-lateral and rotation control, with or without varus/valgus adjustment, prefabricated, off-the-shelf

L1860 Knee orthosis, modification of supracondylar prosthetic socket, custom fabricated (sk)

L1900 Ankle foot orthosis, spring wire, dorsiflexion assist calf band, custom fabricated

L1902 Ankle orthosis, ankle gauntlet or similar, with or without joints, prefabricated, off-the-shelf

L1904 Ankle foot orthosis, multiligamentous ankle support, prefabricated, off-the-shelf

L1906 Ankle foot orthosis, multiligamentous ankle support, prefabricated, off-the-shelf

L1907 Ankle orthosis, supramalleolar with straps, with or without interface/pads, custom fabricated

L1910 Ankle foot orthosis, posterior, single bar, clasp attachment to shoe counter, prefabricated, includes fitting and adjustment

L1920 Ankle foot orthosis, single upright with static or adjustable stop (Phelps or Perlstein type), custom fabricated

L1932 AFO, rigid anterior tibial section, total carbon fiber or equal material, prefabricated, includes fitting and adjustment

L1940 Ankle foot orthosis, plastic or other material, custom fabricated

L1945 Ankle foot orthosis, plastic, rigid anterior tibial section (floor reaction), custom fabricated

L1950 Ankle foot orthosis, spiral, (institute of rehabilitative medicine type), plastic, custom fabricated

L1951 Ankle foot orthosis, spiral, (institute of rehabilitative medicine type), plastic or other material, prefabricated, includes fitting and adjustment

L1960 Ankle foot orthosis, posterior solid ankle, plastic, custom fabricated

L1970 Ankle foot orthosis, plastic with ankle joint, custom fabricated

L1971 Ankle foot orthosis, plastic or other material with ankle joint, prefabricated, includes fitting and adjustment

L1980 Ankle foot orthosis, single upright free plantar dorsiflexion, solid stirrup, calf band/cuff (single bar 'BK' orthosis), custom fabricated

L1990 Ankle foot orthosis, double upright free plantar dorsiflexion, solid stirrup, calf band/cuff (double bar 'BK' orthosis), custom fabricated

L2000 Knee ankle foot orthosis, single upright, free knee, free ankle, solid stirrup, thigh and calf bands/cuffs (single bar 'AK' orthosis), custom fabricated

L2005 Knee ankle foot orthosis, any material, single or double upright, stance control, automatic lock and swing phase release, any type of activation, includes ankle joint, any type, custom fabricated

L2010 Knee ankle foot orthosis, single upright, free ankle, solid stirrup, thigh and calf bands/cuffs (single bar 'AK' orthosis), without knee joint, custom fabricated

L2006 Knee ankle foot device, any material, single or double upright, swing and/or stance phase microprocessor control with adjustability, includes all components (e.g., sensors, batteries, charger), any type of activation, with or without ankle joint(s), custom fabricated

L2020 Knee ankle foot orthosis, double upright, free ankle, solid stirrup, thigh and calf bands/cuffs (double bar 'AK' orthosis), custom fabricated

L2030 Knee ankle foot orthosis, double upright, free ankle, solid stirrup, thigh and calf bands/cuffs, (double bar 'AK' orthosis), without knee joint, custom fabricated

L2034 Knee ankle foot orthosis, full plastic, single upright, with or without free motion knee, medial lateral rotation control, with or without free motion ankle, custom fabricated

L2035 Knee ankle foot orthosis, full plastic, static (pediatric size), without free motion ankle, prefabricated, includes fitting and adjustment

L2036 Knee ankle foot orthosis, full plastic, double upright, with or without free motion knee, with or without free motion ankle, custom fabricated

L2037 Knee ankle foot orthosis, full plastic, single upright, with or without free motion knee, with or without free motion ankle, custom fabricated

L2038 Knee ankle foot orthosis, full plastic, with or without free motion knee, multi-axis ankle, custom fabricated

Torsion Control

L2040 Hip knee ankle foot orthosis, torsion control, bilateral rotation straps, pelvic band/belt, custom fabricated

Not payable by Medicare | Non-covered by Medicare | Special coverage instructions | Carrier judgement

L2050 Hip knee ankle foot orthosis, torsion control, bilateral torsion cables, hip joint, pelvic band/belt, custom fabricated

L2060 Hip knee ankle foot orthosis, torsion control, bilateral torsion cables, ball bearing hip joint, pelvic band/ belt, custom fabricated

L2070 Hip knee ankle foot orthosis, torsion control, unilateral rotation straps, pelvic band/belt, custom fabricated

L2080 Hip knee ankle foot orthosis, torsion control, unilateral torsion cable, hip joint, pelvic band/belt, custom fabricated

L2090 Hip knee ankle foot orthosis, torsion control, unilateral torsion cable, ball bearing hip joint, pelvic band/ belt, custom fabricated

Fracture Orthoses and Additions

L2106 Ankle foot orthosis, fracture orthosis, tibial fracture cast orthosis, thermoplastic type casting material, custom fabricated

L2108 Ankle foot orthosis, fracture orthosis, tibial fracture cast orthosis, custom fabricated

L2112 Ankle foot orthosis, fracture orthosis, tibial fracture orthosis, soft, prefabricated, includes fitting and adjustment

L2114 Ankle foot orthosis, fracture orthosis, tibial fracture orthosis, semi-rigid, prefabricated, includes fitting and adjustment

L2116 Ankle foot orthosis, fracture orthosis, tibial fracture orthosis, rigid, prefabricated, includes fitting and adjustment

L2126 Knee ankle foot orthosis, fracture orthosis, femoral fracture cast orthosis, thermoplastic type casting material, custom fabricated

L2128 Knee ankle foot orthosis, fracture orthosis, femoral fracture cast orthosis, custom fabricated

L2132 KAFO, fracture orthosis, femoral fracture cast orthosis, soft, prefabricated, includes fitting and adjustment

L2134 KAFO, fracture orthosis, femoral fracture cast orthosis, semi-rigid, prefabricated, includes fitting and adjustment

L2136 KAFO, fracture orthosis, femoral fracture cast orthosis, rigid, prefabricated, includes fitting and adjustment

L2180 Addition to lower extremity fracture orthosis, plastic shoe insert with ankle joints

L2182 Addition to lower extremity fracture orthosis, drop lock knee joint

L2184 Addition to lower extremity fracture orthosis, limited motion knee joint

L2186 Addition to lower extremity fracture orthosis, adjustable motion knee joint, Lerman type

L2188 Addition to lower extremity fracture orthosis, quadrilateral brim

L2190 Addition to lower extremity fracture orthosis, waist belt

L2192 Addition to lower extremity fracture orthosis, hip joint, pelvic band, thigh flange, and pelvic belt

Additions To Lower Extremity Orthosis

L2200 Addition to lower extremity, limited ankle motion, each joint

L2210 Addition to lower extremity, dorsiflexion assist (plantar flexion resist), each joint

L2220 Addition to lower extremity, dorsiflexion and plantar flexion assist/resist, each joint

L2230 Addition to lower extremity, split flat caliper stirrups and plate attachment

L2232 Addition to lower extremity orthosis, rocker bottom for total contact ankle foot orthosis, for custom fabricated orthosis only

L2240 Addition to lower extremity, round caliper and plate attachment

L2250 Addition to lower extremity, foot plate, molded to patient model, stirrup attachment

L2260 Addition to lower extremity, reinforced solid stirrup (Scott-Craig type)

L2265 Addition to lower extremity, long tongue stirrup

L2270 Addition to lower extremity, varus/valgus correction ('t') strap, padded/lined or malleolus pad

L2275 Addition to lower extremity, varus/valgus correction, plastic modification, padded/lined

L2280 Addition to lower extremity, molded inner boot

L2300 Addition to lower extremity, abduction bar (bilateral hip involvement), jointed, adjustable

L2310 Addition to lower extremity, abduction bar-straight

L2320 Addition to lower extremity, non-molded lacer, for custom fabricated orthosis only

L2330 Addition to lower extremity, lacer molded to patient model, for custom fabricated orthosis only

L2335 Addition to lower extremity, anterior swing band

L2340 Addition to lower extremity, pre-tibial shell, molded to patient model

L2350 Addition to lower extremity, prosthetic type, (BK) socket, molded to patient model, (used for 'PTB' 'AFO' orthoses)

L2360 Addition to lower extremity, extended steel shank

L2370 Addition to lower extremity, patten bottom

L2375 Addition to lower extremity, torsion control, ankle joint and half solid stirrup

L2380 Addition to lower extremity, torsion control, straight knee joint, each joint

L2385 Addition to lower extremity, straight knee joint, heavy duty, each joint

L2387 Addition to lower extremity, polycentric knee joint, for custom fabricated knee ankle foot orthosis, each joint

L2390 Addition to lower extremity, offset knee joint, each joint

L2395 Addition to lower extremity, offset knee joint, heavy duty, each joint

L2397 Addition to lower extremity orthosis, suspension sleeve

Additions to Knee Joints

L2405 Addition to knee joint, drop lock, each

L2415 Addition to knee lock with integrated release mechanism (bail, cable, or equal), any material, each joint

L2425 Addition to knee joint, disc or dial lock for adjustable knee flexion, each joint

L2430 Addition to knee joint, ratchet lock for active and progressive knee extension, each joint

L2492 Addition to knee joint, lift loop for drop lock ring

Addition to Lower Extremity

L2500 Addition to lower extremity, thigh/weight bearing, gluteal/ ischial weight bearing, ring

L2510 Addition to lower extremity, thigh/weight bearing, quadri- lateral brim, molded to patient model

L2520 Addition to lower extremity, thigh/weight bearing, quadri- lateral brim, custom fitted

L2525 Addition to lower extremity, thigh/weight bearing, ischial containment/narrow m-l brim molded to patient model

L2526 Addition to lower extremity, thigh/weight bearing, ischial containment/narrow m-l brim, custom fitted

L2530 Addition to lower extremity, thigh-weight bearing, lacer, non-molded

L2540 Addition to lower extremity, thigh/weight bearing, lacer, molded to patient model

L2550 Addition to lower extremity, thigh/weight bearing, high roll cuff

L2570 Addition to lower extremity, pelvic control, hip joint, clevis type two position joint, each

L2580 Addition to lower extremity, pelvic control, pelvic sling

L2600 Addition to lower extremity, pelvic control, hip joint, clevis type, or thrust bearing, free, each

L2610 Addition to lower extremity, pelvic control, hip joint, clevis or thrust bearing, lock, each

L2620 Addition to lower extremity, pelvic control, hip joint, heavy duty, each

L2622 Addition to lower extremity, pelvic control, hip joint, adjustable flexion, each

L2624 Addition to lower extremity, pelvic control, hip joint, adjustable flexion, extension, abduction control, each

L2627 Addition to lower extremity, pelvic control, plastic, molded to patient model, reciprocating hip joint and cables

L2628 Addition to lower extremity, pelvic control, metal frame, reciprocating hip joint and cables

L2630 Addition to lower extremity, pelvic control, band and belt, unilateral

L2640 Addition to lower extremity, pelvic control, band and belt, bilateral

L2650 Addition to lower extremity, pelvic and thoracic control, gluteal pad, each

L2660 Addition to lower extremity, thoracic control, thoracic band

L2670 Addition to lower extremity, thoracic control, paraspinal uprights

L2680 Addition to lower extremity, thoracic control, lateral support uprights

L2750 Addition to lower extremity orthosis, plating chrome or nickel, per bar

L2755 Addition to lower extremity orthosis, high strength, lightweight material, all hybrid lamination/prepreg composite, per segment, for custom fabricated orthosis only

L2760 Addition to lower extremity orthosis, extension, per extension, per bar (for lineal adjustment for growth)

L2768 Orthotic side bar disconnect device, per bar

L2780 Addition to lower extremity orthosis, non-corrosive finish, per bar

L2785 Addition to lower extremity orthosis, drop lock retainer, each

L2795 Addition to lower extremity orthosis, knee control, full kneecap

L2800 Addition to lower extremity orthosis, knee control, knee cap, medial or lateral pull, for use with custom fabricated orthosis only

L2810 Addition to lower extremity orthosis, knee control, condylar pad

L2820 Addition to lower extremity orthosis, soft interface for molded plastic, below knee section

L2830 Addition to lower extremity orthosis, soft interface for molded plastic, above knee section

L2840 Addition to lower extremity orthosis, tibial length sock, fracture or equal, each

L2850 Addition to lower extremity orthosis, femoral length sock, fracture or equal, each

L2861 Addition to lower extremity joint, knee or ankle, concentric adjustable torsion style mechanism for custom fabricated orthotics only, each

L2999 Lower extremity orthoses, not otherwise specified

Foot- Insert and Arch Support

L3000 Foot, insert, removable, molded to patient model, 'UCB' type, Berkeley shell, each

L3001 Foot, insert, removable, molded to patient model, Spenco, each

L3002 Foot, insert, removable, molded to patient model, Plastazote or equal, each

L3003 Foot, insert, removable, molded to patient model, silicone gel, each

L3010 Foot, insert, removable, molded to patient model, longitudinal arch support, each

L3020 Foot, insert, removable, molded to patient model, longitudinal/ metatarsal support, each

L3030 Foot, insert, removable, formed to patient foot, each

L3031 Foot, insert/plate, removable, addition to lower extremity orthosis, high strength, lightweight material, all hybrid lamination/prepreg composite, each

L3040 Foot, arch support, removable, pre molded, longitudinal, each

L3050 Foot, arch support, removable, pre molded, metatarsal, each

L3060 Foot, arch support, removable, pre molded, longitudinal/ metatarsal, each

L3070 Foot, arch support, non-removable attached to shoe, longitudinal, each

L3080 Foot, arch support, non-removable attached to shoe, metatarsal, each

L3090 Foot, arch support, non-removable attached to shoe, longitudinal/metatarsal, each

L3100 Hallus-valgus night dynamic splint, prefabricated, off-the-shelf

L3140 Foot, abduction rotation bar, including shoes

L3150 Foot, abduction rotation bar, without shoes

L3160 Foot, adjustable shoe-styled positioning device

• **L3161** Foot, adductus positioning device, adjustable

L3170 Foot, plastic, silicone or equal, heel stabilizer, prefabricated, off-the-shelf, each

Orthopedic Footwear

L3201 Orthopedic shoe, oxford with supinator or pronator, infant

L3202 Orthopedic shoe, oxford with supinator or pronator, child

L3203 Orthopedic shoe, oxford with supinator or pronator, junior

L3204	Orthopedic shoe, High-top with supinator or pronator, infant
L3206	Orthopedic shoe, High-top with supinator or pronator, child
L3207	Orthopedic shoe, High-top with supinator or pronator, junior
L3208	Surgical boot, each, infant
L3209	Surgical boot, each, child
L3211	Surgical boot, each, junior
L3212	Benesch boot, pair, infant
L3213	Benesch boot, pair, child
L3214	Benesch boot, pair, junior
L3215	Orthopedic footwear, ladies shoe, oxford, each
L3216	Orthopedic footwear, ladies shoe, depth inlay, each
L3217	Orthopedic footwear, ladies shoe, High-top, depth inlay, each
L3219	Orthopedic footwear, mens shoe, oxford, each
L3221	Orthopedic footwear, mens shoe, depth inlay, each
L3222	Orthopedic footwear, mens shoe, High-top, depth inlay, each
L3224	Orthopedic footwear, woman's shoe, oxford, used as an integral part of a brace (orthosis)
L3225	Orthopedic footwear, man's shoe, oxford, used as an integral part of a brace (orthosis)
L3230	Orthopedic footwear, custom shoe, depth inlay, each
L3250	Orthopedic footwear, custom molded shoe, removable inner mold, prosthetic shoe, each
L3251	Foot, shoe molded to patient model, silicone shoe, each
L3252	Foot, shoe molded to patient model, Plastazote (or similar), custom fabricated, each
L3253	Foot, molded shoe Plastazote (or similar) custom fitted, each
L3254	Non-standard size or width
L3255	Non-standard size or length
L3257	Orthopedic footwear, additional charge for split size
L3260	Surgical boot/shoe, each
L3265	Plastazote sandal, each

Shoe Modification Lifts

L3300	Lift, elevation, heel, tapered to metatarsals, per inch
L3310	Lift, elevation, heel and sole, neoprene, per inch
L3320	Lift, elevation, heel and sole, cork, per inch
L3330	Lift, elevation, metal extension (skate)
L3332	Lift, elevation, inside shoe, tapered, up to one-half inch
L3334	Lift, elevation, heel, per inch

Wedges

L3340	Heel wedge, SACH

L3350 Heel wedge

L3360 Sole wedge, outside sole

L3370 Sole wedge, between sole

L3380 Clubfoot wedge

L3390 Outflare wedge

L3400 Metatarsal bar wedge, rocker

L3410 Metatarsal bar wedge, between sole

L3420 Full sole and heel wedge, between sole

Heels

L3430 Heel, counter, plastic reinforced

L3440 Heel, counter, leather reinforced

L3450 Heel, SACH cushion type

L3455 Heel, new leather, standard

L3460 Heel, new rubber, standard

L3465 Heel, Thomas with wedge

L3470 Heel, Thomas extended to ball

L3480 Heel, pad and depression for spur

L3485 Heel, pad, removable for spur

Orthopedic Shoe Additions

L3500 Orthopedic shoe addition, insole, leather

L3510 Orthopedic shoe addition, insole, rubber

L3520 Orthopedic shoe addition, insole, felt covered with leather

L3530 Orthopedic shoe addition, sole, half

L3540 Orthopedic shoe addition, sole, full

L3550 Orthopedic shoe addition, toe tap standard

L3560 Orthopedic shoe addition, toe tap, horseshoe

L3570 Orthopedic shoe addition, special extension to instep (leather with eyelets)

L3580 Orthopedic shoe addition, convert instep to Velcro closure

L3590 Orthopedic shoe addition, convert firm shoe counter to soft counter

L3595 Orthopedic shoe addition, march bar

Transfer or Replacement

L3600 Transfer of an orthosis from one shoe to another, caliper plate, existing

L3610 Transfer of an orthosis from one shoe to another, caliper plate, new

L3620 Transfer of an orthosis from one shoe to another, solid stirrup, existing

L3630 Transfer of an orthosis from one shoe to another, solid stirrup, new

L3640 Transfer of an orthosis from one shoe to another, Dennis Browne splint (Riveton), both shoes

L3649 Orthopedic shoe, modification, addition or transfer, not otherwise specified

Orthotic Devices – Upper Limb

L3650 Shoulder orthosis, figure of eight design abduction restrainer, prefabricated, off-the-shelf

L3660 Shoulder orthosis, figure of eight design abduction restrainer, canvas and webbing, prefabricated, off-the-shelf

L3670 Shoulder orthosis, acromio/clavicular (canvas and webbing type), prefabricated, off-the-shelf

L3671 Shoulder orthosis, shoulder joint design, without joints, may include soft interface, straps, custom fabricated, includes fitting and adjustment

L3674 Shoulder orthosis, abduction positioning (airplane design), thoracic component and support bar, with or without nontorsion joint/turnbuckle, may include soft interface, straps, custom fabricated, includes fitting and adjustment

L3675 Shoulder orthosis, vest type abduction restrainer, canvas webbing type or equal, prefabricated, off-the-shelf

L3677 Shoulder orthosis, shoulder joint design, without joints, may include soft interface, straps, prefabricated item that has been trimmed, bent, molded, assembled, or otherwise customized to fit a specific patient by an individual with expertise

L3678 Shoulder orthosis, shoulder joint design, without joints, may include soft interface, straps, prefabricated, off-the-shelf

L3702 Elbow orthosis, without joints, may include soft interface, straps, custom fabricated, includes fitting and adjustment

L3710 Elbow orthosis, elastic with metal joints, prefabricated, off-the-shelf

L3720 Elbow orthosis, double upright with forearm/arm cuffs, free motion, custom fabricated

L3730 Elbow orthosis, double upright with forearm/arm cuffs, extension/ flexion assist, custom fabricated

L3740 Elbow orthosis, double upright with forearm/arm cuffs, adjustable position lock with active control, custom fabricated

L3760 Elbow orthosis (EO), with adjustable position locking joint(s), prefabricated, item that has been trimmed, bent, molded, assembled, or otherwise customized to fit a specific patient by an individual with expertise

L3761 Elbow orthosis (EO), with adjustable position locking joint(s), prefabricated, off-the-shelf

L3762 Elbow orthosis, rigid, without joints, includes soft interface material, prefabricated, off-the-shelf

L3763 Elbow wrist hand orthosis, rigid, without joints, may include soft interface, straps, custom fabricated, includes fitting and adjustment

L3764 Elbow wrist hand orthosis, includes one or more nontorsion joints, elastic bands, turnbuckles, may include soft interface, straps, custom fabricated, includes fitting and adjustment

L3765 Elbow wrist hand finger orthosis, rigid, without joints, may include soft interface, straps, custom fabricated, includes fitting and adjustment

L3766 Elbow wrist hand finger orthosis, includes one or more nontorsion joints, elastic bands, turnbuckles, may include soft interface, straps, custom fabricated, includes fitting and adjustment

L3806 Wrist hand finger orthosis, includes one or more nontorsion joint(s), turnbuckles, elastic bands/springs, may include soft interface material, straps, custom fabricated, includes fitting and adjustment

L3807 Wrist hand finger orthosis, without joint(s), prefabricated item that has been trimmed, bent, molded, assembled, or otherwise customized to fit a specific patient by an individual with expertise

L3808 Wrist hand finger orthosis, rigid without joints, may include soft interface material; straps, custom fabricated, includes fitting and adjustment

L3809 Wrist hand finger orthosis, without joint(s), prefabricated, off-the-shelf, any type

L3891 Addition to upper extremity joint, wrist or elbow, concentric adjustable torsion style mechanism for custom fabricated orthotics only, each

Wrist-Hand-Finger Orthoses

L3900 Wrist hand finger orthosis, dynamic flexor hinge, reciprocal wrist extension/ flexion, finger flexion/extension, wrist or finger driven, custom fabricated

L3901 Wrist hand finger orthosis, dynamic flexor hinge, reciprocal wrist extension/ flexion, finger flexion/extension, cable driven, custom fabricated

L3904 Wrist hand finger orthosis, external powered, electric, custom fabricated

L3905 Wrist hand orthosis, includes one or more nontorsion joints, elastic bands, turnbuckles, may include soft interface, straps, custom fabricated, includes fitting and adjustment

L3906 Wrist hand orthosis, without joints, may include soft interface, straps, custom fabricated, includes fitting and adjustment

L3908 Wrist hand orthosis, wrist extension control cock-up, non-molded, prefabricated, off-the-shelf

L3912 Hand finger orthosis (HFO), flexion glove with elastic finger control, prefabricated, off-the-shelf

L3913 Hand finger orthosis, without joints, may include soft interface, straps, custom fabricated, includes fitting and adjustment

L3915 Wrist hand orthosis, includes one or more nontorsion joint(s), elastic bands, turnbuckles, may include soft interface, straps, prefabricated item that has been trimmed, bent, molded, assembled, or otherwise customized to fit a specific patient by an individual with expertise

L3916 Wrist hand orthosis, includes one or more nontorsion joint(s), elastic bands, turnbuckles, may include soft interface, straps, prefabricated, off-the-shelf

L3917 Hand orthosis, metacarpal fracture orthosis, prefabricated item that has been trimmed, bent, molded, assembled, or otherwise customized to fit a specific patient by an individual with expertise

L3918 Hand orthosis, metacarpal fracture orthosis, prefabricated, off-the-shelf

L3919 Hand orthosis, without joints, may include soft interface, straps, custom fabricated, includes fitting and adjustment

L3921 Hand finger orthosis, includes one or more nontorsion joints, elastic bands, turnbuckles, may include soft interface, straps, custom fabricated, includes fitting and adjustment

L3923 Hand finger orthosis, without joints, may include soft interface, straps, prefabricated item that has been trimmed, bent, molded, assembled, or otherwise customized to fit a specific patient by an individual with expertise

L3924 Hand finger orthosis, without joints, may include soft interface, straps, prefabricated, off-the-shelf

L3925 Finger orthosis, proximal interphalangeal (pip)/distal interphalangeal (dip), non-torsion joint/spring, extension/flexion, may include soft interface material, prefabricated, off-the-shelf

L3927 Finger orthosis, proximal interphalangeal (pip)/distal interphalangeal (dip), without joint/spring, extension/flexion (e.g., static or ring type), may include soft interface material, prefabricated, off-the-shelf

L3929 Hand finger orthosis, includes one or more nontorsion joint(s), turnbuckles, elastic bands/springs, may include soft interface material, straps, prefabricated item that has been trimmed, bent, molded, assembled, or otherwise customized to fit a specific patient by an individual with expertise

L3930 Hand finger orthosis, includes one or more nontorsion joint(s), turnbuckles, elastic bands/springs, may include soft interface material, straps, prefabricated, off-the-shelf

L3931 Wrist hand finger orthosis, includes one or more nontorsion joint(s), turnbuckles, elastic bands/springs, may include soft interface material, straps, prefabricated, includes fitting and adjustment

L3933 Finger orthosis, without joints, may include soft interface, custom fabricated, includes fitting and adjustment

L3935 Finger orthosis, nontorsion joint, may include soft interface, custom fabricated, includes fitting and adjustment

L3956 Addition of joint to upper extremity orthosis, any material; per joint

Shoulder-Elbow-Wrist-Hand Orthoses (SEWHO)

L3960 Shoulder elbow wrist hand orthosis, abduction positioning, airplane design, prefabricated, includes fitting and adjustment

L3961 Shoulder elbow wrist hand orthosis, shoulder cap design, without joints, may include soft interface, straps, custom fabricated, includes fitting and adjustment

L3962 Shoulder elbow wrist hand orthosis, abduction positioning, Erb's palsy design, prefabricated, includes fitting and adjustment

L3967 Shoulder elbow wrist hand orthosis, abduction positioning (airplane design), thoracic component and support bar, without joints, may include soft interface, straps, custom fabricated, includes fitting and adjustment

L3971 Shoulder elbow wrist hand orthosis, shoulder cap design, includes one or more nontorsion joints, elastic bands, turnbuckles, may include soft interface, straps, custom fabricated, includes fitting and adjustment

L3973 Shoulder elbow wrist hand orthosis, abduction positioning (airplane design), thoracic component and support bar, includes one or more nontorsion joints, elastic bands, turnbuckles, may include soft interface, straps, custom fabricated, includes fitting and adjustment

L3975 Shoulder elbow wrist hand finger orthosis, shoulder cap design, without joints, may include soft interface, straps, custom fabricated, includes fitting and adjustment

L3976 Shoulder elbow wrist hand finger orthosis, abduction positioning (airplane design), thoracic component and support bar, without joints, may include soft interface, straps, custom fabricated, includes fitting and adjustment

L3977 Shoulder elbow wrist hand finger orthosis, shoulder cap design, includes one or more nontorsion joints, elastic bands, turnbuckles, may include soft interface, straps, custom fabricated, includes fitting and adjustment

L3978 Shoulder elbow wrist hand finger orthosis, abduction positioning (airplane design), thoracic component and support bar, includes one or more nontorsion joints, elastic bands, turnbuckles, may include soft interface, straps, custom fabricated, includes fitting and adjustment

Upper Limb – Fracture Orthoses

L3980 Upper extremity fracture orthosis, humeral, prefabricated, includes fitting and adjustment

L3981 Upper extremity fracture orthosis, humeral, prefabricated, includes shoulder cap design, with or without joints, forearm section, may include soft interface, straps, includes fitting and adjustments

L3982 Upper extremity fracture orthosis, radius/ulnar, prefabricated, includes fitting and adjustment

L3984 Upper extremity fracture orthosis, wrist, prefabricated, includes fitting and adjustment

L3995 Addition to upper extremity orthosis, sock, fracture or equal, each

L3999 Upper limb orthosis, not otherwise specified

Specific Repair

L4000 Replace girdle for spinal orthosis (CTLSO or so)

L4002 Replacement strap, any orthosis, includes all components, any length, any type

L4010 Replace trilateral socket brim

L4020 Replace quadrilateral socket brim, molded to patient model

L4030 Replace quadrilateral socket brim, custom fitted

L4040 Replace molded thigh lacer, for custom fabricated orthosis only

L4045 Replace non-molded thigh lacer, for custom fabricated orthosis only

L4050 Replace molded calf lacer, for custom fabricated orthosis only

L4055 Replace non-molded calf lacer, for custom fabricated orthosis only

L4060 Replace high roll cuff

L4070 Replace proximal and distal upright for KAFO

L4080 Replace metal bands KAFO, proximal thigh

L4090 Replace metal bands KAFO-AFO, calf or distal thigh

L4100 Replace leather cuff KAFO, proximal thigh

L4110 Replace leather cuff KAFO-AFO, calf or distal thigh

L4130 Replace pretibial shell

L4205 Repair of orthotic device, labor component, per 15 minutes

L4210 Repair of orthotic device, repair or replace minor parts

Ancillary Orthotic Services

L4350 Ankle control orthosis, stirrup style, rigid, includes any type of interface (e.g., pneumatic, gel), prefabricated, off-the-shelf

L4360 Walking boot, pneumatic and/or vacuum, with or without joints, with or without interface material, prefabricated item that has been trimmed, bent, molded, assembled, or otherwise customized to fit a specific patient by an individual with expertise

L4361 Walking boot, pneumatic and/or vacuum, with or without joints, with or without interface material, prefabricated, off-the-shelf

L4370 Pneumatic full leg splint, prefabricated, off-the-shelf

L4386 Walking boot, non-pneumatic, with or without joints, with or without interface material, prefabricated item that has been trimmed, bent, molded, assembled, or otherwise customized to fit a specific patient by an individual with expertise

L4387 Walking boot, non-pneumatic, with or without joints, with or without interface material, prefabricated, off-the-shelf

L4392 Replacement, soft interface material, static AFO

L4394 Replace soft interface material, foot drop splint

L4396 Static or dynamic ankle foot orthosis, including soft interface material, adjustable for fit, for positioning, may be used for minimal ambulation, prefabricated item that has been trimmed, bent, molded, assembled, or otherwise customized to fit a specific patient by an individual with expertise

L4397 Static or dynamic ankle foot orthosis, including soft interface material, adjustable for fit, for positioning, may be used for minimal ambulation, prefabricated, off-the-shelf

L4398 Foot drop splint, recumbent positioning device, prefabricated, off-the-shelf

L4631 Ankle foot orthosis, walking boot type, varus/valgus correction, rocker bottom, anterior tibial shell, soft interface, custom arch support, plastic or other material, includes straps and closures, custom fabricated

PROSTHETIC PROCEDURES

Guidelines

In addition to the information presented in the INTRODUCTION, several other items unique to this section are defined or identified here:

1. **PROSTHETIC DEVICES:** Prosthetic devices (other than dental) which replace all or part of an internal body organ (including contiguous tissue) or replace all or part of the function of a permanently inoperative or malfunctioning internal body organ, are covered when furnished upon a physician's order. This does not require a determination that there is no possibility that the patient's condition may improve in the future. If the medical record and the judgement of the attending physician indicate that the condition is of long and indefinite duration, the test of permanence is met. The device(s) may also be covered as a supply item when furnished incident to a physician's service.

2. **SUBSECTION INFORMATION:** Some of the listed subheadings or subsections have special needs or instructions unique to that section. Where these are indicated, special "notes" will be presented preceding or following the listings. Those subsections within the PROSTHETIC PROCEDURES section that have "notes" are as follows:

Subsection	Code Numbers
Prosthetic procedures-lower limb	L5000–L5999
Upper limb	L6000–L6590
Additions-upper limb	L6600–L6999

3. **UNLISTED SERVICE OR PROCEDURE:** A service or procedure may be provided that is not listed in this edition of HCPCS. When reporting such a service, the appropriate "unlisted procedure" code may be used to indicate the service, identifying it by "special report" as defined below. HCPCS terminology is inconsistent in defining unlisted procedures. The procedure definition may include the term(s) "unlisted", "not otherwise classified", "unspecified", "unclassified", "other" and "miscellaneous". Prior to using these codes, try to determine if a Local Level III code or CPT code is available. The "unlisted procedures" and accompanying codes for PROSTHETIC PROCEDURES are as follows:

   L5999 Lower extremity prosthesis, not otherwise specified
   L7499 Upper extremity prosthesis, not otherwise specified
   L8039 Breast prosthesis, not otherwise specified
   L8239 Gradient compression stocking, not otherwise specified
   L8499 Unlisted procedure for miscellaneous prosthetic services
   L8699 Prosthetic implant, not otherwise specified

4. **SPECIAL REPORT:** A service, material or supply that is rarely provided, unusual, variable or new may require a special report in determining medical appropriateness for reimbursement purposes. Pertinent information should include an adequate definition or description of the nature, extent, and need for the service, material or supply.

5. **MODIFIERS:** Listed services may be modified under certain circumstances. When appropriate, the modifying circumstance is identified by adding a modifier to the basic procedure code. CPT and HCPCS National Level II modifiers may be used with CPT and HCPCS National Level II procedure codes. Modifiers commonly used with PROSTHETIC PROCEDURES are as follows:

   -CC Procedure code change (use "CC" when the procedure code submitted was changed either for administrative reasons or because an incorrect code was filed)

   -LT Left side (used to identify procedures performed on the left side of the body)
   -RT Right side (used to identify procedures performed on the right side of the body)

-TC Technical component. Under certain circumstances, a charge may be made for the technical component alone. Under those circumstances, the technical component charge is identified by adding modifier -TC to the usual procedure number. Technical component charges are institutional charges and are not billed separately by physicians. However, portable x-ray suppliers bill only for the technical component and should use modifier -TC. The charge data from portable x-ray suppliers will then be used to build customary and prevailing profiles.

6. **CPT CODE CROSS-REFERENCE:** Unless otherwise specified, the equivalent CPT code for all listings in this section is 99070.

7. **DURABLE MEDICAL EQUIPMENT REGIONAL CARRIERS (DMERCS):** Effective October 1, 1993 claims for prosthetics must be billed to one of four regional carriers depending upon the residence of the beneficiary. The transition dates for DMERC claims is from November 1, 1993 to March 1, 1994, depending upon the state you practice in. See the Introduction for a complete discussion of DMERCs.

Lower Limb

NOTE: The procedures in this section are considered as "base" or "basic" procedures, and they may be modified by listing items, procedures or special materials from the "additions" section and adding them to the base procedure.

L5000 Partial foot, shoe insert with longitudinal arch, toe filler

L5010 Partial foot, molded socket, ankle height, with toe filler

L5020 Partial foot, molded socket, tibial tubercle height, with toe filler

L5050 Ankle, Symes, molded socket, SACH foot

L5060 Ankle, Symes, metal frame, molded leather socket, articulated ankle/foot

L5100 Below knee, molded socket, shin, SACH foot

L5105 Below knee, plastic socket, joints and thigh lacer, SACH foot

L5150 Knee disarticulation (or through knee), molded socket, external knee joints, shin, SACH foot

L5160 Knee disarticulation (or through knee), molded socket, bent knee configuration, external knee joints, shin, SACH foot

L5200 Above knee, molded socket, single axis constant friction knee, shin, SACH foot

L5210 Above knee, short prosthesis, no knee joint ('stubbies'), with foot blocks, no ankle joints, each

L5220 Above knee, short prosthesis, no knee joint ('stubbies'), with articulated ankle/foot, dynamically aligned, each

L5230 Above knee, for proximal femoral focal deficiency, constant friction knee, shin, SACH foot

L5250 Hip disarticulation, Canadian type; molded socket, hip joint, single axis constant friction knee, shin, SACH foot

L5270 Hip disarticulation, tilt table type; molded socket, locking hip joint, single axis constant friction knee, shin, SACH foot

L5280 Hemipelvectomy, Canadian type; molded socket, hip joint, single axis constant friction knee, shin, SACH foot

L5301 Below knee, molded socket, shin, SACH foot, endoskeletal system

L5312 Knee disarticulation (or through knee), molded socket, single axis knee, pylon, SACH foot, endoskeletal system

L5321 Above knee, molded socket, open end, SACH foot, endoskeletal system, single axis knee

L5331 Hip disarticulation, Canadian type, molded socket, endoskeletal system, hip joint, single axis knee, SACH foot

L5341 Hemipelvectomy, Canadian type, molded socket, endoskeletal system, hip joint, single axis knee, SACH foot

Immediate Post-Surgical or Early Fitting Procedures

L5400 Immediate post-surgical or early fitting, application of initial rigid dressing, including fitting, alignment, suspension, and one cast change, below knee

L5410 Immediate post-surgical or early fitting, application of initial rigid dressing, including fitting, alignment and suspension, below knee, each additional cast change and realignment

L5420 Immediate post-surgical or early fitting, application of initial rigid dressing, including fitting, alignment and suspension and one cast change 'AK' or knee disarticulation

L5430 Immediate post-surgical or early fitting, application of initial rigid dressing, incl. fitting, alignment and suspension, 'AK' or knee disarticulation, each additional cast change and realignment

L5450 Immediate post-surgical or early fitting, application of non-weight bearing rigid dressing, below knee

L5460 Immediate post-surgical or early fitting, application of non-weight bearing rigid dressing, above knee

Initial Prosthesis

L5500 Initial, below knee 'PTB' type socket, non-alignable system, pylon, no cover, SACH foot, plaster socket, direct formed

L5505 Initial, above knee - knee disarticulation, ischial level socket, non-alignable system, pylon, no cover, SACH foot, plaster socket, direct formed

Preparatory Prosthesis

L5510 Preparatory, below knee 'PTB' type socket, non-alignable system, pylon, no cover, SACH foot, plaster socket, molded to model

L5520 Preparatory, below knee 'PTB' type socket, non-alignable system, pylon, no cover, SACH foot, thermoplastic or equal, direct formed

L5530 Preparatory, below knee 'PTB' type socket, non-alignable system, pylon, no cover, SACH foot, thermoplastic or equal, molded to model

L5535 Preparatory, below knee 'PTB' type socket, non-alignable system, no cover, SACH foot, prefabricated, adjustable open end socket

L5540 Preparatory, below knee 'PTB' type socket, non-alignable system, pylon, no cover, SACH foot, laminated socket, molded to model

L5560 Preparatory, above knee- knee disarticulation, ischial level socket, non-alignable system, pylon, no cover, SACH foot, plaster socket, molded to model

L5570 Preparatory, above knee - knee disarticulation, ischial level socket, non-alignable system, pylon, no cover, SACH foot, thermoplastic or equal, direct formed

L5580 Preparatory, above knee - knee disarticulation ischial level socket, non-alignable system, pylon, no cover, SACH foot, thermoplastic or equal, molded to model

L5585 Preparatory, above knee - knee disarticulation, ischial level socket, non-alignable system, pylon, no cover, SACH foot, prefabricated adjustable open end socket

L5590 Preparatory, above knee - knee disarticulation ischial level socket, non-alignable system, pylon no cover, SACH foot, laminated socket, molded to model

L5595 Preparatory, hip disarticulation-hemipelvectomy, pylon, no cover, SACH foot, thermoplastic or equal, molded to patient model

L5600 Preparatory, hip disarticulation-hemipelvectomy, pylon, no cover, SACH foot, laminated socket, molded to patient model

Additions To Lower Extremity

L5610 Addition to lower extremity, endoskeletal system, above knee, Hydra-Cadence system

L5611 Addition to lower extremity, endoskeletal system, above knee - knee disarticulation, 4 bar linkage, with friction swing phase control

L5613 Addition to lower extremity, endoskeletal system, above knee-knee disarticulation, 4 bar linkage, with hydraulic swing phase control

L5614 Addition to lower extremity, exoskeletal system, above knee-knee disarticulation, 4 bar linkage, with pneumatic swing phase control

● **L5615** Addition, endoskeletal knee-shin system, 4 bar linkage or multiaxial, fluid swing and stance phase control

L5616 Addition to lower extremity, endoskeletal system, above knee, universal multiplex system, friction swing phase control

L5617 Addition to lower extremity, quick change self-aligning unit, above knee or below knee, each

Additions - Test Sockets and Socket Variations

L5618 Addition to lower extremity, test socket, Symes

L5620 Addition to lower extremity, test socket, below knee

L5622 Addition to lower extremity, test socket, knee disarticulation

L5624 Addition to lower extremity, test socket, above knee

L5626 Addition to lower extremity, test socket, hip disarticulation

L5628 Addition to lower extremity, test socket, hemipelvectomy

L5629 Addition to lower extremity, below knee, acrylic socket

L5630 Addition to lower extremity, Symes type, expandable wall socket

L5631 Addition to lower extremity, above knee or knee disarticulation, acrylic socket

L5632 Addition to lower extremity, Symes type, 'PTB' brim design socket

L5634 Addition to lower extremity, Symes type, posterior opening (Canadian) socket

L5636 Addition to lower extremity, Symes type, medial opening socket

L5637 Addition to lower extremity, below knee, total contact

L5638 Addition to lower extremity, below knee, leather socket

L5639 Addition to lower extremity, below knee, wood socket

L5640 Addition to lower extremity, knee disarticulation, leather socket

L5642 Addition to lower extremity, above knee, leather socket

L5643 Addition to lower extremity, hip disarticulation, flexible inner socket, external frame

L5644 Addition to lower extremity, above knee, wood socket

L5645 Addition to lower extremity, below knee, flexible inner socket, external frame

L5646 Addition to lower extremity, below knee, air, fluid, gel or equal, cushion socket

L5647 Addition to lower extremity, below knee suction socket

L5648 Addition to lower extremity, above knee, air, fluid, gel or equal, cushion socket

L5649 Addition to lower extremity, ischial containment/narrow m-l socket

L5650 Additions to lower extremity, total contact, above knee or knee disarticulation socket

L5651 Addition to lower extremity, above knee, flexible inner socket, external frame

L5652 Addition to lower extremity, suction suspension, above knee or knee disarticulation socket

L5653 Addition to lower extremity, knee disarticulation, expandable wall socket

Additions - Socket Insert and Suspension

L5654 Addition to lower extremity, socket insert, Symes, (Kemblo, Pelite, Aliplast, Plastazote or equal)

L5655 Addition to lower extremity, socket insert, below knee (Kemblo, Pelite, Aliplast, Plastazote or equal)

L5656 Addition to lower extremity, socket insert, knee disarticulation (Kemblo, Pelite, Aliplast, Plastazote or equal)

L5658 Addition to lower extremity, socket insert, above knee (Kemblo, Pelite, Aliplast, Plastazote or equal)

L5661 Addition to lower extremity, socket insert, multi-durometer Symes

L5665 Addition to lower extremity, socket insert, multi-durometer, below knee

L5666 Addition to lower extremity, below knee, cuff suspension

L5668 Addition to lower extremity, below knee, molded distal cushion

L5670 Addition to lower extremity, below knee, molded supracondylar suspension ('pts' or similar)

L5671 Addition to lower extremity, below knee / above knee suspension locking mechanism (shuttle, lanyard or equal), excludes socket insert

L5672 Addition to lower extremity, below knee, removable medial brim suspension

L5673 Addition to lower extremity, below knee/above knee, custom fabricated from existing mold or prefabricated, socket insert, silicone gel, elastomeric or equal, for use with locking mechanism

L5676 Additions to lower extremity, below knee, knee joints, single axis, pair

L5677 Additions to lower extremity, below knee, knee joints, polycentric, pair

L5678 Additions to lower extremity, below knee, joint covers, pair

L5679 Addition to lower extremity, below knee/above knee, custom fabricated from existing mold or prefabricated, socket insert, silicone gel, elastomeric or equal, not for use with locking mechanism

L5680 Addition to lower extremity, below knee, thigh lacer, non-molded

L5681 Addition to lower extremity, below knee/above knee, custom fabricated socket insert for congenital or atypical traumatic amputee, silicone gel, elastomeric or equal, for use with or without locking mechanism, initial only (for other than initial, use code L5673 or L5679)

L5682 Addition to lower extremity, below knee, thigh lacer, gluteal/ischial, molded

L5683 Addition to lower extremity, below knee/above knee, custom fabricated socket insert for other than congenital or atypical traumatic amputee, silicone gel, elastomeric or equal, for use with or without locking mechanism, initial only (for other than initial, use code L5673 or L5679)

L5684 Addition to lower extremity, below knee, fork strap

L5685 Addition to lower extremity prosthesis, below knee, suspension/sealing sleeve, with or without valve, any material, each

L5686 Addition to lower extremity, below knee, back check (extension control)

L5688 Addition to lower extremity, below knee, waist belt, webbing

L5690 Addition to lower extremity, below knee, waist belt, padded and lined

L5692 Addition to lower extremity, above knee, pelvic control belt, light

L5694 Addition to lower extremity, above knee, pelvic control belt, padded and lined

L5695 Addition to lower extremity, above knee, pelvic control, sleeve suspension, neoprene or equal, each

L5696 Addition to lower extremity, above knee or knee disarticulation, pelvic joint

L5697 Addition to lower extremity, above knee or knee disarticulation, pelvic band

L5698 Addition to lower extremity, above knee or knee disarticulation, Silesian bandage

L5699 All lower extremity prostheses, shoulder harness

L5700 Replacement, socket, below knee, molded to patient model

L5701 Replacement, socket, above knee/knee disarticulation, including attachment plate, molded to patient model

L5702 Replacement, socket, hip disarticulation, including hip joint, molded to patient model

L5703 Ankle, Symes, molded to patient model, socket without solid ankle cushion heel (SACH) foot, replacement only

L5704 Custom shaped protective cover, below knee

L5705 Custom shaped protective cover, above knee

L5706 Custom shaped protective cover, knee disarticulation

L5707 Custom shaped protective cover, hip disarticulation

Additions - Knee-Shin System Exoskeletal

L5710 Addition, exoskeletal knee-shin system, single axis, manual lock

L5711 Additions exoskeletal knee-shin system, single axis, manual lock, ultralight material

L5712 Addition, exoskeletal knee-shin system, single axis, friction swing and stance phase control (safety knee)

L5714 Addition, exoskeletal knee-shin system, single axis, variable friction swing phase control

L5716 Addition, exoskeletal knee-shin system, polycentric, mechanical stance phase lock

L5718 Addition, exoskeletal knee-shin system, polycentric, friction swing and stance phase control

L5722 Addition, exoskeletal knee-shin system, single axis, pneumatic swing, friction stance phase control

L5724 Addition, exoskeletal knee-shin system, single axis, fluid swing phase control

L5726 Addition, exoskeletal knee-shin system, single axis, external joints fluid swing phase control

L5728 Addition, exoskeletal knee-shin system, single axis, fluid swing and stance phase control

L5780 Addition, exoskeletal knee-shin system, single axis, pneumatic/hydra pneumatic swing phase control

L5781 Addition to lower limb prosthesis, vacuum pump, residual limb volume management and moisture evacuation system

L5782 Addition to lower limb prosthesis, vacuum pump, residual limb volume management and moisture evacuation system, heavy duty

L5785 Addition, exoskeletal system, below knee, ultralight material (titanium, carbon fiber or equal)

L5790 Addition, exoskeletal system, above knee, ultralight material (titanium, carbon fiber or equal)

L5795 Addition, exoskeletal system, hip disarticulation, ultralight material (titanium, carbon fiber or equal)

Endoskeletal

L5810 Addition, endoskeletal knee-shin system, single axis, manual lock

L5811 Addition, endoskeletal knee-shin system, single axis, manual lock, ultralight material

L5812 Addition, endoskeletal knee-shin system, single axis, friction swing and stance phase control (safety knee)

L5814 Addition, endoskeletal knee-shin system, polycentric, hydraulic swing phase control, mechanical stance phase lock

L5816 Addition, endoskeletal knee-shin system, polycentric, mechanical stance phase lock

L5818 Addition, endoskeletal knee-shin system, polycentric, friction swing, and stance phase control

L5822 Addition, endoskeletal knee-shin system, single axis, pneumatic swing, friction stance phase control

L5824 Addition, endoskeletal knee-shin system, single axis, fluid swing phase control

L5826 Addition, endoskeletal knee-shin system, single axis, hydraulic swing phase control, with miniature high activity frame

L5828 Addition, endoskeletal knee-shin system, single axis, fluid swing and stance phase control

L5830 Addition, endoskeletal knee-shin system, single axis, pneumatic/ swing phase control

L5840 Addition, endoskeletal knee/shin system, 4-bar linkage or multiaxial, pneumatic swing phase control

L5845 Addition, endoskeletal, knee-shin system, stance flexion feature, adjustable

L5848 Addition to endoskeletal knee-shin system, fluid stance extension, dampening feature, with or without adjustability

L5850 Addition, endoskeletal system, above knee or hip disarticulation, knee extension assist

L5855 Addition, endoskeletal system, hip disarticulation, mechanical hip extension assist

L5856 Addition to lower extremity prosthesis, endoskeletal knee-shin system, microprocessor control feature, swing and stance phase, includes electronic sensor(s), any type

L5857 Addition to lower extremity prosthesis, endoskeletal knee-shin system, microprocessor control feature, swing phase only, includes electronic sensor(s), any type

L5858 Addition to lower extremity prosthesis, endoskeletal knee shin system, microprocessor control feature, stance phase only, includes electronic sensor(s), any type

L5859 Addition to lower extremity prosthesis, endoskeletal knee-shin system, powered and programmable flexion/extension assist control, includes any type of motor(s)

L5910 Addition, endoskeletal system, below knee, alignable system

L5920 Addition, endoskeletal system, above knee or hip disarticulation, alignable system

L5925 Addition, endoskeletal system, above knee, knee disarticulation or hip disarticulation, manual lock

● **L5926** Addition to lower extremity prosthesis, endoskeletal, knee disarticulation, above knee, hip disarticulation, positional rotation unit, any type

L5930 Addition, endoskeletal system, high activity knee control frame

L5940 Addition, endoskeletal system, below knee, ultralight material (titanium, carbon fiber or equal)

L5950 Addition, endoskeletal system, above knee, ultralight material (titanium, carbon fiber or equal)

L5960 Addition, endoskeletal system, hip disarticulation, ultralight material (titanium, carbon fiber or equal)

L5961 Addition, endoskeletal system, polycentric hip joint, pneumatic or hydraulic control, rotation control, with or without flexion and/or extension control

L5962 Addition, endoskeletal system, below knee, flexible protective outer surface covering system

L5964 Addition, endoskeletal system, above knee, flexible protective outer surface covering system

L5966 Addition, endoskeletal system, hip disarticulation, flexible protective outer surface covering system

L5968 Addition to lower limb prosthesis, multiaxial ankle with swing phase active dorsiflexion feature

L5969 Addition, endoskeletal ankle-foot or ankle system, power assist, includes any type of motor(s)

L5970 All lower extremity prostheses, foot, external keel, SACH foot

L5971 All lower extremity prosthesis, solid ankle cushion heel (SACH) foot, replacement only

L5972 All lower extremity prostheses, foot, flexible keel

L5973 Endoskeletal ankle foot system, microprocessor controlled feature, dorsiflexion and/or plantar flexion control, includes power source

L5974 All lower extremity prostheses, foot, single axis ankle/foot

L5975 All lower extremity prosthesis, combination single axis ankle and flexible keel foot

L5976 All lower extremity prostheses, energy storing foot (Seattle carbon copy ii or equal)

L5978 All lower extremity prostheses, foot, multiaxial ankle/foot

L5979 All lower extremity prosthesis, multi-axial ankle, dynamic response foot, one piece system

L5980 All lower extremity prostheses, flex foot system

L5981 All lower extremity prostheses, flex-walk system or equal

L5982 All exoskeletal lower extremity prostheses, axial rotation unit

L5984 All endoskeletal lower extremity prosthesis, axial rotation unit, with or without adjustability

L5985 All endoskeletal lower extremity prostheses, dynamic prosthetic pylon

L5986 All lower extremity prostheses, multi-axial rotation unit ('MCP' or equal)

L5987 All lower extremity prosthesis, shank foot system with vertical loading pylon

L5988 Addition to lower limb prosthesis, vertical shock reducing pylon feature

L5990 Addition to lower extremity prosthesis, user adjustable heel height

L5999 Lower extremity prosthesis, not otherwise specified

Upper Limb

NOTE: The procedures in L6000-L6599 are considered as "base" or "basic" procedures and may be modified by listing procedures from the "additions" sections. The base procedures include only standard friction wrist and control cable system unless otherwise specified.

L6000 Partial hand, thumb remaining

L6010 Partial hand, little and/or ring finger remaining

L6020 Partial hand, no finger remaining

L6026 Transcarpal/metacarpal or partial hand disarticulation prosthesis, external power, self-suspended, inner socket with removable forearm section, electrodes and cables, two batteries, charger, myoelectric control of terminal device, excludes terminal device(s)

L6050 Wrist disarticulation, molded socket, flexible elbow hinges, triceps pad

L6055 Wrist disarticulation, molded socket with expandable interface, flexible elbow hinges, triceps pad

L6100 Below elbow, molded socket, flexible elbow hinge, triceps pad

L6110 Below elbow, molded socket, (muenster or northwestern suspension types)

L6120 Below elbow, molded double wall split socket, step-up hinges, half cuff

L6130 Below elbow, molded double wall split socket, stump activated locking hinge, half cuff

L6200 Elbow disarticulation, molded socket, outside locking hinge, forearm

L6205 Elbow disarticulation, molded socket with expandable interface, outside locking hinges, forearm

L6250 Above elbow, molded double wall socket, internal locking elbow, forearm

L6300 Shoulder disarticulation, molded socket, shoulder bulkhead, humeral section, internal locking elbow, forearm

L6310 Shoulder disarticulation, passive restoration (complete prosthesis)

L6320 Shoulder disarticulation, passive restoration (shoulder cap only)

L6350 Interscapular thoracic, molded socket, shoulder bulkhead, humeral section, internal locking elbow, forearm

L6360 Interscapular thoracic, passive restoration (complete prosthesis)

L6370 Interscapular thoracic, passive restoration (shoulder cap only)

L6380 Immediate post-surgical or early fitting, application of initial rigid dressing, including fitting alignment and suspension of components, and one cast change, wrist disarticulation or below elbow

L6382 Immediate post-surgical or early fitting, application of initial rigid dressing including fitting alignment and suspension of components, and one cast change, elbow disarticulation or above elbow

L6384 Immediate post-surgical or early fitting, application of initial rigid dressing including fitting alignment and suspension of components, and one cast change, shoulder disarticulation or interscapular thoracic

L6386 Immediate post-surgical or early fitting, each additional cast change and realignment

L6388 Immediate post-surgical or early fitting, application of rigid dressing only

L6400 Below elbow, molded socket, endoskeletal system, including soft prosthetic tissue shaping

L6450 Elbow disarticulation, molded socket, endoskeletal system, including soft prosthetic tissue shaping

L6500 Above elbow, molded socket, endoskeletal system, including soft prosthetic tissue shaping

L6550 Shoulder disarticulation, molded socket, endoskeletal system, including soft prosthetic tissue shaping

L6570 Interscapular thoracic, molded socket, endoskeletal system, including soft prosthetic tissue shaping

L6580 Preparatory, wrist disarticulation or below elbow, single wall plastic socket, friction wrist, flexible elbow hinges, figure of eight harness, humeral cuff, Bowden cable control, USMC or equal pylon, no cover, molded to patient model

L6582 Preparatory, wrist disarticulation or below elbow, single wall socket, friction wrist, flexible elbow hinges, figure of eight harness, humeral cuff, Bowden cable control, USMC or equal pylon, no cover, direct formed

L6584 Preparatory, elbow disarticulation or above elbow, single wall plastic socket, friction wrist, locking elbow, figure of eight harness, fair lead cable control, USMC or equal pylon, no cover, molded to patient model

L6586 Preparatory, elbow disarticulation or above elbow, single wall socket, friction wrist, locking elbow, figure of eight harness, fair lead cable control, USMC or equal pylon, no cover, direct formed

L6588 Preparatory, shoulder disarticulation or interscapular thoracic, single wall plastic socket, shoulder joint, locking elbow, friction wrist, chest strap, fair lead cable control, USMC or equal pylon, no cover, molded to patient model

L6590 Preparatory, shoulder disarticulation or interscapular thoracic, single wall socket, shoulder joint, locking elbow, friction wrist, chest strap, fair lead cable control, USMC or equal pylon, no cover, direct formed

Additions - Upper Limb

NOTE: The following procedures, modifications and/or components may be added to other base procedures. The items in this section should reflect the additional complexity of each modification procedure, in addition to base procedure, at the time of the original order.

L6600 Upper extremity additions, polycentric hinge, pair

L6605 Upper extremity additions, single pivot hinge, pair

L6610 Upper extremity additions, flexible metal hinge, pair

L6611 Addition to upper extremity prosthesis, external powered, additional switch, any type

L6615 Upper extremity addition, disconnect locking wrist unit

L6616 Upper extremity addition, additional disconnect insert for locking wrist unit, each

L6620 Upper extremity addition, flexion/extension wrist unit, with or without friction

L6621 Upper extremity prosthesis addition, flexion/extension wrist with or without friction, for use with external powered terminal device

L6623 Upper extremity addition, spring assisted rotational wrist unit with latch release

L6624 Upper extremity addition, flexion/extension and rotation wrist unit

L6625 Upper extremity addition, rotation wrist unit with cable lock

L6628 Upper extremity addition, quick disconnect hook adapter, otto bock or equal

L6629 Upper extremity addition, quick disconnect lamination collar with coupling piece, otto bock or equal

L6630 Upper extremity addition, stainless steel, any wrist

L6632 Upper extremity addition, latex suspension sleeve, each

L6635 Upper extremity addition, lift assist for elbow

L6637 Upper extremity addition, nudge control elbow lock

L6638 Upper extremity addition to prosthesis, electric locking feature, only for use with manually powered elbow

L6640 Upper extremity additions, shoulder abduction joint, pair

L6641 Upper extremity addition, excursion amplifier, pulley type

L6642 Upper extremity addition, excursion amplifier, lever type

L6645 Upper extremity addition, shoulder flexion-abduction joint, each

L6646 Upper extremity addition, shoulder joint, multipositional locking, flexion, adjustable abduction friction control, for use with body powered or external powered system

L6647 Upper extremity addition, shoulder lock mechanism, body powered actuator

L6648 Upper extremity addition, shoulder lock mechanism, external powered actuator

L6650 Upper extremity addition, shoulder universal joint, each

L6655 Upper extremity addition, standard control cable, extra

L6660 Upper extremity addition, heavy duty control cable

L6665 Upper extremity addition, Teflon, or equal, cable lining

L6670 Upper extremity addition, hook to hand, cable adapter

L6672 Upper extremity addition, harness, chest or shoulder, saddle type

L6675 Upper extremity addition, harness, (e.g., figure of eight type), single cable design

L6676 Upper extremity addition, harness, (e.g., figure of eight type), dual cable design

L6677 Upper extremity addition, harness, triple control, simultaneous operation of terminal device and elbow

L6680 Upper extremity addition, test socket, wrist disarticulation or below elbow

L6682 Upper extremity addition, test socket, elbow disarticulation or above elbow

L6684 Upper extremity addition, test socket, shoulder disarticulation or interscapular thoracic

L6686 Upper extremity addition, suction socket

L6687 Upper extremity addition, frame type socket, below elbow or wrist disarticulation

L6688 Upper extremity addition, frame type socket, above elbow or elbow disarticulation

L6689 Upper extremity addition, frame type socket, shoulder disarticulation

L6690 Upper extremity addition, frame type socket, interscapular-thoracic

L6691 Upper extremity addition, removable insert, each

L6692 Upper extremity addition, silicone gel insert or equal, each

L6693 Upper extremity addition, locking elbow, forearm counterbalance

L6694 Addition to upper extremity prosthesis, below elbow/above elbow, custom fabricated from existing mold or prefabricated, socket insert, silicone gel, elastomeric or equal, for use with locking mechanism

L6695 Addition to upper extremity prosthesis, below elbow/above elbow, custom fabricated from existing mold or prefabricated, socket insert, silicone gel, elastomeric or equal, not for use with locking mechanism

L6696 Addition to upper extremity prosthesis, below elbow/above elbow, custom fabricated socket insert for congenital or atypical traumatic amputee, silicone gel, elastomeric or equal, for use with or without locking mechanism, initial only (for other than initial, use code L6694 or L6695)

L6697 Addition to upper extremity prosthesis, below elbow/above elbow, custom fabricated socket insert for other than congenital or atypical traumatic amputee, silicone gel, elastomeric or equal, for use with or without locking mechanism, initial only (for other than initial, use code L6694 or L6695)

L6698 Addition to upper extremity prosthesis, below elbow/above elbow, lock mechanism, excludes socket insert

Terminal Devices Hooks

L6703 Terminal device, passive hand/mitt, any material, any size

L6704 Terminal device, sport/recreational/work attachment, any material, any size

L6706 Terminal device, hook, mechanical, voluntary opening, any material, any size, lined or unlined

L6707 Terminal device, hook, mechanical, voluntary closing, any material, any size, lined or unlined

L6708 Terminal device, hand, mechanical, voluntary opening, any material, any size

L6709 Terminal device, hand, mechanical, voluntary closing, any material, any size

L6711 Terminal device, hook, mechanical, voluntary opening, any material, any size, lined or unlined, pediatric

L6712 Terminal device, hook, mechanical, voluntary closing, any material, any size, lined or unlined, pediatric

L6713 Terminal device, hand, mechanical, voluntary opening, any material, any size, pediatric

L6714 Terminal device, hand, mechanical, voluntary closing, any material, any size, pediatric

L6715 Terminal device, multiple articulating digit, includes motor(s), initial issue or replacement

L6721 Terminal device, hook or hand, heavy duty, mechanical, voluntary opening, any material, any size, lined or unlined

L6722 Terminal device, hook or hand, heavy duty, mechanical, voluntary closing, any material, any size, lined or unlined

L6805 Addition to terminal device, modifier wrist unit

L6810 Addition to terminal device, precision pinch device

Hands, Gloves and Restoration

L6880 Electric hand, switch or myoelectric controlled, independently articulating digits, any grasp pattern or combination of grasp patterns, includes motor(s)

L6881 Automatic grasp feature, addition to upper limb electric prosthetic terminal device

L6882 Microprocessor control feature, addition to upper limb prosthetic terminal device

L6883 Replacement socket, below elbow/wrist disarticulation, molded to patient model, for use with or without external power

L6884 Replacement socket, above elbow/elbow disarticulation, molded to patient model, for use with or without external power

L6885 Replacement socket, shoulder disarticulation/interscapular thoracic, molded to patient model, for use with or without external power

L6890 Addition to upper extremity prosthesis, glove for terminal device, any material, prefabricated, includes fitting and adjustment

L6895 Addition to upper extremity prosthesis, glove for terminal device, any material, custom fabricated

L6900 Hand restoration (casts, shading and measurements included), partial hand, with glove, thumb or one finger remaining

L6905 Hand restoration (casts, shading and measurements included), partial hand, with glove, multiple fingers remaining

L6910 Hand restoration (casts, shading and measurements included), partial hand, with glove, no fingers remaining

L6915 Hand restoration (shading, and measurements included), replacement glove for above

External Power Devices and Batteries

L6920 Wrist disarticulation, external power, self-suspended inner socket, removable forearm shell, otto bock or equal, switch, cables, two batteries and one charger, switch control of terminal device

L6925 Wrist disarticulation, external power, self-suspended inner socket, removable forearm shell, otto bock or equal electrodes, cables, two batteries and one charger, myoelectronic control of terminal device

L6930 Below elbow, external power, self-suspended inner socket, removable forearm shell, otto bock or equal switch, cables, two batteries and one charger, switch control of terminal device

L6935 Below elbow, external power, self-suspended inner socket, removable forearm shell, otto bock or equal electrodes, cables, two batteries and one charger, myoelectronic control of terminal device

L6940 Elbow disarticulation, external power, molded inner socket, removable humeral shell, outside locking hinges, forearm, otto bock or equal switch, cables, two batteries and one charger, switch control of terminal device

L6945 Elbow disarticulation, external power, molded inner socket, removable humeral shell, outside locking hinges, forearm, otto bock or equal electrodes, cables, two batteries and one charger, myoelectronic control of terminal device

L6950 Above elbow, external power, molded inner socket, removable humeral shell, internal locking elbow, forearm, otto bock or equal switch, cables, two batteries and one charger, switch control of terminal device

L6955 Above elbow, external power, molded inner socket, removable humeral shell, internal locking elbow, forearm, otto bock or equal electrodes, cables, two batteries and one charger, myoelectronic control of terminal device

L6960 Shoulder disarticulation, external power, molded inner socket, removable shoulder shell, shoulder bulkhead, humeral section, mechanical elbow, forearm, otto bock or equal switch, cables, two batteries and one charger, switch control of terminal device

L6965 Shoulder disarticulation, external power, molded inner socket, removable shoulder shell, shoulder bulkhead, humeral section, mechanical elbow, forearm, otto bock or equal electrodes, cables, two batteries and one charger, myoelectronic control of terminal device

L6970 Interscapular-thoracic, external power, molded inner socket, removable shoulder shell, shoulder bulkhead, humeral section, mechanical elbow, forearm, otto bock or equal switch, cables, two batteries and one charger, switch control of terminal device

L6975 Interscapular-thoracic, external power, molded inner socket, removable shoulder shell, shoulder bulkhead, humeral section, mechanical elbow, forearm, otto bock or equal electrodes, cables, two batteries and one charger, myoelectronic control of terminal device

L7007 Electric hand, switch or myoelectric controlled, adult

L7008	Electric hand, switch or myoelectric, controlled, pediatric
L7009	Electric hook, switch or myoelectric controlled, adult
L7040	Prehensile actuator, switch controlled
L7045	Electric hook, switch or myoelectric controlled, pediatric
L7170	Electronic elbow, Hosmer or equal, switch controlled
L7180	Electronic elbow, microprocessor sequential control of elbow and terminal device
L7181	Electronic elbow, microprocessor simultaneous control of elbow and terminal device
L7185	Electronic elbow, adolescent, variety village or equal, switch controlled
L7186	Electronic elbow, child, variety village or equal, switch controlled
L7190	Electronic elbow, adolescent, variety village or equal, myoelectronically controlled
L7191	Electronic elbow, child, variety village or equal, myoelectronically controlled
L7259	Electronic wrist rotator, any type
L7360	Six volt battery, each
L7362	Battery charger, six volt, each
L7364	Twelve volt battery, each
L7366	Battery charger, twelve volt, each
L7367	Lithium ion battery, rechargeable, replacement
L7368	Lithium ion battery charger, replacement only
L7400	Addition to upper extremity prosthesis, below elbow/wrist disarticulation, ultralight material (titanium, carbon fiber or equal)
L7401	Addition to upper extremity prosthesis, above elbow disarticulation, ultralight material (titanium, carbon fiber or equal)
L7402	Addition to upper extremity prosthesis, shoulder disarticulation/interscapular thoracic, ultralight material (titanium, carbon fiber or equal)
L7403	Addition to upper extremity prosthesis, below elbow/wrist disarticulation, acrylic material
L7404	Addition to upper extremity prosthesis, above elbow disarticulation, acrylic material
L7405	Addition to upper extremity prosthesis, shoulder disarticulation/interscapular thoracic, acrylic material
L7499	Upper extremity prosthesis, not otherwise specified

Repairs

L7510	Repair of prosthetic device, repair or replace minor parts
L7520	Repair prosthetic device, labor component, per 15 minutes
L7600	Prosthetic donning sleeve, any material, each
L7700	Gasket or seal, for use with prosthetic socket insert, any type, each
L7900	Male vacuum erection system
L7902	Tension ring, for vacuum erection device, any type, replacement only, each

General - Breast Prostheses

L8000	Breast prosthesis, mastectomy bra, without integrated breast prosthesis form, any size, any type
L8001	Breast prosthesis, mastectomy bra, with integrated breast prosthesis form, unilateral, any size, any type
L8002	Breast prosthesis, mastectomy bra, with integrated breast prosthesis form, bilateral, any size, any type
L8010	Breast prosthesis, mastectomy sleeve
L8015	External breast prosthesis garment, with mastectomy form, post mastectomy
L8020	Breast prosthesis, mastectomy form
L8030	Breast prosthesis, silicone or equal, without integral adhesive
L8031	Breast prosthesis, silicone or equal, with integral adhesive
L8032	Nipple prosthesis, prefabricated, reusable, any type, each
L8033	Nipple prosthesis, custom fabricated, reusable, any material, any type, each
L8035	Custom breast prosthesis, post mastectomy, molded to patient model
L8039	Breast prosthesis, not otherwise specified

General – Facial Prosthesis

L8040	Nasal prosthesis, provided by a non-physician
L8041	Midfacial prosthesis, provided by a non-physician
L8042	Orbital prosthesis, provided by a non-physician
L8043	Upper facial prosthesis, provided by a non-physician
L8044	Hemi-facial prosthesis, provided by a non-physician
L8045	Auricular prosthesis, provided by a non-physician
L8046	Partial facial prosthesis, provided by a non-physician
L8047	Nasal septal prosthesis, provided by a non-physician
L8048	Unspecified maxillofacial prosthesis, by report, provided by a non-physician
L8049	Repair or modification of maxillofacial prosthesis, labor component, 15 minute increments, provided by a non-physician

General - Trusses

L8300	Truss, single with standard pad
L8310	Truss, double with standard pads
L8320	Truss, addition to standard pad, water pad
L8330	Truss, addition to standard pad, scrotal pad

Prosthetic Socks

L8400	Prosthetic sheath, below knee, each
L8410	Prosthetic sheath, above knee, each
L8415	Prosthetic sheath, upper limb, each

L8417 Prosthetic sheath/sock, including a gel cushion layer, below knee or above knee, each

L8420 Prosthetic sock, multiple ply, below knee, each

L8430 Prosthetic sock, multiple ply, above knee, each

L8435 Prosthetic sock, multiple ply, upper limb, each

L8440 Prosthetic shrinker, below knee, each

L8460 Prosthetic shrinker, above knee, each

L8465 Prosthetic shrinker, upper limb, each

L8470 Prosthetic sock, single ply, fitting, below knee, each

L8480 Prosthetic sock, single ply, fitting, above knee, each

L8485 Prosthetic sock, single ply, fitting, upper limb, each

L8499 Unlisted procedure for miscellaneous prosthetic services

Prosthetic Implants

L8500 Artificial larynx, any type

L8501 Tracheostomy speaking valve

L8505 Artificial larynx replacement battery / accessory, any type

L8507 Tracheo-esophageal voice prosthesis, patient inserted, any type, each

L8509 Tracheo-esophageal voice prosthesis, inserted by a licensed health care provider, any type

L8510 Voice amplifier

L8511 Insert for indwelling tracheoesophageal prosthesis, with or without valve, replacement only, each

L8512 Gelatin capsules or equivalent, for use with tracheoesophageal voice prosthesis, replacement only, per 10

L8513 Cleaning device used with tracheoesophageal voice prosthesis, pipet, brush, or equal, replacement only, each

L8514 Tracheoesophageal puncture dilator, replacement only, each

L8515 Gelatin capsule, application device for use with tracheoesophageal voice prosthesis, each

Integumentary System

L8600 Implantable breast prosthesis, silicone or equal

L8603 Injectable bulking agent, collagen implant, urinary tract, 2.5 ml syringe, includes shipping and necessary supplies

L8604 Injectable bulking agent, dextranomer/hyaluronic acid copolymer implant, urinary tract, 1 ml, includes shipping and necessary supplies

L8605 Injectable bulking agent, dextranomer/hyaluronic acid copolymer implant, anal canal, 1 ml, includes shipping and necessary supplies

L8606 Injectable bulking agent, synthetic implant, urinary tract, 1 ml syringe, includes shipping and necessary supplies

L8607 Injectable bulking agent for vocal cord medialization, 0.1 ml, includes shipping and necessary supplies

L8608 Miscellaneous external component, supply or accessory for use with the argus ii retinal prosthesis system

Head (Skull, Facial Bones, and Temporomandibular Joint)

L8609 Artificial cornea

L8610 Ocular implant

L8612 Aqueous shunt

L8613 Ossicula implant

L8614 Cochlear device, includes all internal and external components

L8615 Headset/headpiece for use with cochlear implant device, replacement

L8616 Microphone for use with cochlear implant device, replacement

L8617 Transmitting coil for use with cochlear implant device, replacement

L8618 Transmitter cable for use with cochlear implant device or auditory osseointegrated device, replacement

L8619 Cochlear implant, external speech processor and controller, integrated system, replacement

L8621 Zinc air battery for use with cochlear implant device and auditory osseointegrated sound processors, replacement, each

L8622 Alkaline battery for use with cochlear implant device, any size, replacement, each

L8623 Lithium ion battery for use with cochlear implant device speech processor, other than ear level, replacement, each

L8624 Lithium ion battery for use with cochlear implant or auditory osseointegrated device speech processor, ear level, replacement, each

L8625 External recharging system for battery for use with cochlear implant or auditory osseointegrated device, replacement only, each

L8627 Cochlear implant, external speech processor, component, replacement

L8628 Cochlear implant, external controller component, replacement

L8629 Transmitting coil and cable, integrated, for use with cochlear implant device, replacement

Upper Extremity

L8630 Metacarpophalangeal joint implant

L8631 Metacarpal phalangeal joint replacement, two or more pieces, metal (e.g., stainless steel or cobalt chrome), ceramic-like material (e.g., pyrocarbon), for surgical implantation (all sizes, includes entire system)

Lower Extremity (Joint: Knee, Ankle, Toe)

L8641 Metatarsal joint implant

L8642 Hallux implant

Miscellaneous Muscular - Skeletal

L8658 Interphalangeal joint spacer, silicone or equal, each

L8659 Interphalangeal finger joint replacement, 2 or more pieces, metal (e.g., stainless steel or cobalt chrome), ceramic-like material (e.g., pyrocarbon) for surgical implantation, any size

Cardiovascular System

L8670	Vascular graft material, synthetic, implant
L8679	Implantable neurostimulator, pulse generator, any type
L8680	Implantable neurostimulator electrode, each
L8681	Patient programmer (external) for use with implantable programmable neurostimulator pulse generator, replacement only
L8682	Implantable neurostimulator radiofrequency receiver
L8683	Radiofrequency transmitter (external) for use with implantable neurostimulator radiofrequency receiver
L8684	Radiofrequency transmitter (external) for use with implantable sacral root neurostimulator receiver for bowel and bladder management, replacement
L8685	Implantable neurostimulator pulse generator, single array, rechargeable, includes extension
L8686	Implantable neurostimulator pulse generator, single array, non-rechargeable, includes extension
L8687	Implantable neurostimulator pulse generator, dual array, rechargeable, includes extension
L8688	Implantable neurostimulator pulse generator, dual array, non-rechargeable, includes extension
L8689	External recharging system for battery (internal) for use with implantable neurostimulator, replacement only
L8690	Auditory osseointegrated device, includes all internal and external components
L8691	Auditory osseointegrated device, external sound processor, excludes transducer/actuator, replacement only, each
L8692	Auditory osseointegrated device, external sound processor, used without osseointegration, body worn, includes headband or other means of external attachment
L8693	Auditory osseointegrated device abutment, any length, replacement only
L8694	Auditory osseointegrated device, transducer/actuator, replacement only, each
L8695	External recharging system for battery (external) for use with implantable neurostimulator, replacement only
L8696	Antenna (external) for use with implantable diaphragmatic/phrenic nerve stimulation device, replacement, each
L8698	Miscellaneous component, supply or accessory for use with total artificial heart system

Other

L8699	Prosthetic implant, not otherwise specified
L8701	Powered upper extremity range of motion assist device, elbow, wrist, hand with single or double upright(s), includes microprocessor, sensors, all components and accessories, custom fabricated
L8702	Powered upper extremity range of motion assist device, elbow, wrist, hand, finger, single or double upright(s), includes microprocessor, sensors, all components and accessories, custom fabricated
L9900	Orthotic and prosthetic supply, accessory, and/or service component of another HCPCS "l" code

MEDICAL SERVICES

Guidelines

In addition to the information presented in the INTRODUCTION, several other items unique to this section are defined or identified here:

1. **SUBSECTION INFORMATION:** Some of the listed subheadings or subsections have special needs or instructions unique to that section. Where these are indicated, special "notes" will be presented preceding or following the listings. Those subsections within the MEDICAL SERVICES section that have "notes" are as follows:

Subsection	Code Numbers
Office services	M0000–M0009
End-stage renal disease services	M0900–M0999

2. **SPECIAL REPORT:** A service, material or supply that is rarely provided, unusual, variable or new may require a special report in determining medical appropriateness for reimbursement purposes. Pertinent information should include an adequate definition or description of the nature, extent, and need for the service, material or supply.

3. **MODIFIERS:** Listed services may be modified under certain circumstances. When appropriate, the modifying circumstance is identified by adding a modifier to the basic procedure code. CPT and HCPCS National Level II modifiers may be used with CPT and HCPCS National Level II procedure codes. Modifiers commonly used with MEDICAL SERVICES are as follows:

   -AH Clinical psychologist

   -AJ Clinical social worker

   -CC Procedure code change (use "CC" when the procedure code submitted was changed either for administrative reasons or because an incorrect code was filed)

   -EJ Subsequent claims for a defined course of therapy (e.g., EPO, sodium hyaluronate, infliximab)

   -EM Emergency reserve supply (for ESRD benefit only)

   -EP Service provided as part of Medicaid early periodic screening diagnosis and treatment (EPSDT) program

   -FP Service provided as part of Medicaid family planning program

   -Q5 Service furnished by a substitute physician under a reciprocal billing arrangement

   -Q6 Service furnished by a locum tenens physician

   -QC Single channel monitoring

   -QD Recording and storage in solid state memory by a digital recorder

   -QT Recording and storage on tape by an analog tape recorder

   -SF Second opinion ordered by a professional review organization (PRO) per section 9401, P.L. 99-272 (100 percent reimbursement; no Medicare deductible or coinsurance)

-TC Technical component. Under certain circumstances, a charge may be made for the technical component alone. Under those circumstances, the technical component charge is identified by adding modifier -TC to the usual procedure number. Technical component charges are institutional charges and are not billed separately by physicians. However, portable x-ray suppliers bill only for the technical component and should use modifier -TC. The charge data from portable x-ray suppliers will then be used to build customary and prevailing profiles.

4. **CPT CODE CROSS-REFERENCE:** See sections for equivalent CPT code(s) for listings in this section.

Other Medical Services

M0001 Advancing cancer care MIPS value pathways

M0002 Optimal care for kidney health MIPS value pathways

M0003 Optimal care for patients with episodic neurological conditions MIPS value pathways

M0004 Supportive care for neurodegenerative conditions MIPS value pathways

▲ **M0005** Value in primary care MIPS value pathway

M0064 Brief office visit for the sole purpose of monitoring or changing drug prescriptions used in the treatment of mental psychoneurotic and personality disorders

M0075 Cellular therapy

M0076 Prolotherapy

M0100 Intragastric hypothermia using gastric freezing

▲ **M0201** Administration of pneumococcal, influenza, hepatitis b, and/or covid-19 vaccine inside a patient's home; reported only once per individual home per date of service when such vaccine administration(s) are performed at the patient's home

M0220 Injection, tixagevimab and cilgavimab, for the pre-exposure prophylaxis only, for certain adults and pediatric individuals (12 years of age and older weighing at least 40kg) with no known sars-cov-2 exposure, who either have moderate to severely compromised immune systems or for whom vaccination with any available covid-19 vaccine is not recommended due to a history of severe adverse reaction to a covid-19 vaccine(s) and/or covid-19 vaccine component(s), includes injection and post administration monitoring

M0221 Injection, tixagevimab and cilgavimab, for the pre-exposure prophylaxis only, for certain adults and pediatric individuals (12 years of age and older weighing at least 40kg) with no known sars-cov-2 exposure, who either have moderate to severely compromised immune systems or for whom vaccination with any available covid-19 vaccine is not recommended due to a history of severe adverse reaction to a covid-19 vaccine(s) and/or covid-19 vaccine component(s), includes injection and post administration monitoring in the home or residence; this includes a beneficiary's home that has been made provider-based to the hospital during the covid-19 public health emergency

M0222 Intravenous injection, bebtelovimab, includes injection and post administration monitoring

M0223 Intravenous injection, bebtelovimab, includes injection and post administration monitoring in the home or residence; this includes a beneficiary's home that has been made provider-based to the hospital during the covid-19 public health emergency

M0239 Intravenous infusion, bamlanivimab-xxxx, includes infusion and post administration monitoring

M0240 Intravenous infusion or subcutaneous injection, casirivimab and imdevimab includes infusion or injection, and post administration monitoring, subsequent repeat doses

M0241 Intravenous infusion or subcutaneous injection, casirivimab and imdevimab includes infusion or injection, and post administration monitoring in the home or residence; this includes a beneficiary's home that has been made provider-based to the hospital during the covid-19 public health emergency, subsequent repeat doses

M0243 Intravenous infusion or subcutaneous injection, casirivimab and imdevimab includes infusion or injection, and post administration monitoring

M0244 Intravenous infusion or subcutaneous injection, casirivimab and imdevimab includes infusion or injection, and post administration monitoring in the home or residence; this includes a beneficiary's home that has been made provider-based to the hospital during the covid-19 public health emergency

M0245 Intravenous infusion, bamlanivimab and etesevimab, includes infusion and post administration monitoring

M0246 Intravenous infusion, bamlanivimab and etesevimab, includes infusion and post administration monitoring in the home or residence; this includes a beneficiary's home that has been made provider based to the hospital during the covid 19 public health emergency

M0247 Intravenous infusion, sotrovimab, includes infusion and post administration monitoring

M0248 Intravenous infusion, sotrovimab, includes infusion and post administration monitoring in the home or residence; this includes a beneficiary's home that has been made provider-based to the hospital during the covid-19 public health emergency

M0249 Intravenous infusion, tocilizumab, for hospitalized adults and pediatric patients (2 years of age and older) with covid-19 who are receiving systemic corticosteroids and require supplemental oxygen, non-invasive or invasive mechanical ventilation, or extracorporeal membrane oxygenation (ECMO) only, includes infusion and post administration monitoring, first dose

M0250 Intravenous infusion, tocilizumab, for hospitalized adults and pediatric patients (2 years of age and older) with covid-19 who are receiving systemic corticosteroids and require supplemental oxygen, non-invasive or invasive mechanical ventilation, or extracorporeal membrane oxygenation (ECMO) only, includes infusion and post administration monitoring, second dose

M0300 IV chelation therapy (chemical endarterectomy)

M0301 Fabric wrapping of abdominal aneurysm

M1000 Pain screened as moderate to severe

M1001 Plan of care to address moderate to severe pain documented on or before the date of the second visit with a clinician

M1002 Plan of care for moderate to severe pain not documented on or before the date of the second visit with a clinician, reason not given

M1003 Tb screening performed and results interpreted within twelve months prior to initiation of first-time biologic and/or immune response modifier therapy

M1004 Documentation of medical reason for not screening for tb or interpreting results (i.e., patient positive for tb and documentation of past treatment; patient who has recently completed a course of anti-tb therapy)

M1005 Tb screening not performed or results not interpreted; reason not given

M1006 Disease activity not assessed; reason not given

M1007 >=50% of total number of a patient's outpatient ra encounters assessed

M1008 <50% of total number of a patient's outpatient ra encounters assessed

M1009 Discharge/discontinuation of the episode of care documented in the medical record

M1010 Discharge/discontinuation of the episode of care documented in the medical record

M1011 Discharge/discontinuation of the episode of care documented in the medical record

M1012 Discharge/discontinuation of the episode of care documented in the medical record

M1013 Discharge/discontinuation of the episode of care documented in the medical record

M1014 Discharge/discontinuation of the episode of care documented in the medical record

M1015 Discharge/discontinuation of the episode of care documented in the medical record

M1016 Female patients unable to bear children

(**M1017** Patient admitted to palliative care services
Code deleted effective 12/31/2022, no HCPCS/CPT cross-reference provided.)

M1018 Patients with an active diagnosis or history of cancer (except basal cell and squamous cell skin carcinoma), patients who are heavy tobacco smokers, lung cancer screening patients

M1019 Adolescent patients 12 to 17 years of age with major depression or dysthymia who reached remission at twelve months as demonstrated by a twelve month (+/-60 days) phq-9 or phq-9m score of less than 5

M1020 Adolescent patients 12 to 17 years of age with major depression or dysthymia who did not reach remission at twelve months as demonstrated by a twelve month (+/-60 days) phq-9 or phq-9m score of less than 5. either phq-9 or phq-9m score was not assessed or is greater than or equal to 5

M1021 Patient had only urgent care visits during the performance period

M1022 Patients who were in hospice at any time during the performance period

M1023 Adolescent patients 12 to 17 years of age with major depression or dysthymia who reached remission at six months as demonstrated by a six month (+/-60 days) phq-9 or phq-9m score of less than five

M1024 Adolescent patients 12 to 17 years of age with major depression or dysthymia who did not reach remission at six months as demonstrated by a six month (+/-60 days) phq-9 or phq-9m score of less than five. either phq-9 or phq-9m score was not assessed or is greater than or equal to five

M1025 Patients who were in hospice at any time during the performance period

M1026 Patients who were in hospice at any time during the performance period

M1027 Imaging of the head (CT or MRI) was obtained

M1028 Documentation of patients with primary headache diagnosis and imaging other than CT or MRI obtained

M1029 Imaging of the head (CT or MRI) was not obtained, reason not given

M1030 Patients with clinical indications for imaging of the head

M1031 Patients with no clinical indications for imaging of the head

M1032 Adults currently taking pharmacotherapy for oud

M1033 Pharmacotherapy for oud initiated after June 30th of performance period

M1034 Adults who have at least 180 days of continuous pharmacotherapy with a medication prescribed for oud without a gap of more than seven days

M1035 Adults who are deliberately phased out of medication assisted treatment (mat) prior to 180 days of continuous treatment

M1036 Adults who have not had at least 180 days of continuous pharmacotherapy with a medication prescribed for oud without a gap of more than seven days

M1037 Patients with a diagnosis of lumbar spine region cancer at the time of the procedure

M1038 Patients with a diagnosis of lumbar spine region fracture at the time of the procedure

M1039 Patients with a diagnosis of lumbar spine region infection at the time of the procedure

M1040 Patients with a diagnosis of lumbar idiopathic or congenital scoliosis

M1041 Patient had cancer, acute fracture or infection related to the lumbar spine or patient had neuromuscular, idiopathic or congenital lumbar scoliosis

M1042 Functional status measurement with score was obtained utilizing the Oswestry disability index (ODI version 2.1a) patient reported outcome tool within three months preoperatively and at one year (9 to 15 months) postoperatively

M1043 Functional status was not measured by the Oswestry disability index (ODI version 2.1a) at one year (9 to 15 months) postoperatively

M1044 Functional status was measured by the Oswestry disability index (ODI version 2.1a) patient reported outcome tool within three months preoperatively and at one year (9 to 15 months)

postoperatively

M1045 Functional status measured by the oxford knee score (oks) at one year (9 to 15 months) postoperatively was greater than or equal to 37 or knee injury and osteoarthritis outcome score joint replacement (koos, jr.) was greater than or equal to 71

M1046 Functional status measured by the oxford knee score (oks) at one year (9 to 15 months) postoperatively was less than 37 or the knee injury and osteoarthritis outcome score joint replacement (koos, jr.) was less than 71 postoperatively

M1047 Functional status was measured by the oxford knee score (oks) patient reported outcome tool within three months preoperatively and at one year (9 to 15 months) postoperatively

M1048 Functional status measurement with score was obtained utilizing the Oswestry disability index (ODI version 2.1a) patient reported outcome tool within three months preoperatively and at three months (6 to 20 weeks) postoperatively

M1049 Functional status was not measured by the Oswestry disability index (ODI version 2.1a) at three months (6 - 20 weeks) postoperatively

M1050 Functional status was measured by the Oswestry disability index (ODI version 2.1a) patient reported outcome tool within three months preoperatively and at three months (6 to 20 weeks) postoperatively

M1051 Patient had cancer, acute fracture or infection related to the lumbar spine or patient had neuromuscular, idiopathic or congenital lumbar scoliosis

M1052 Leg pain was not measured by the visual analog scale (vas) or numeric pain scale at one year (9 to 15 months) postoperatively

M1053 Leg pain was measured by the visual analog scale (vas) within three months preoperatively and at one year (9 to 15 months) postoperatively

M1054 Patient had only urgent care visits during the performance period

M1055 Aspirin or another antiplatelet therapy used

M1056 Prescribed anticoagulant medication during the performance period, history of GI bleeding, history of intracranial bleeding, bleeding disorder and specific provider documented reasons: allergy to aspirin or anti-platelets, use of non-steroidal anti-inflammatory agents, drug-drug interaction, uncontrolled hypertension > 180/110 mmHg or gastroesophageal reflux disease

M1057 Aspirin or another antiplatelet therapy not used, reason not given

M1058 Patient was a permanent nursing home resident at any time during the performance period

M1059 Patient was in hospice or receiving palliative care at any time during the performance period

M1060 Patient died prior to the end of the performance period

M1061 Patient pregnancy

M1062 Patient immunocompromised

M1063 Patients receiving high doses of immunosuppressive therapy

M1064 Shingrix vaccine documented as administered or previously received

M1065 Shingrix vaccine was not administered for reasons documented by clinician (e.g., patient administered vaccine other than Shingrix, patient allergy or other medical reasons, patient declined or other patient reasons, vaccine not available or other system reasons)

M1066 Shingrix vaccine not documented as administered, reason not given

M1067 Hospice services for patient provided any time during the measurement period

M1068 Adults who are not ambulatory

M1069 Patient screened for future fall risk

M1070 Patient not screened for future fall risk; reason not given

(**M1071** Patient had any additional spine procedures performed on the same date as the lumbar discectomy/laminotomy
Code deleted effective 12/31/2022, no HCPCS/CPT cross-reference provided.)

M1106 The start of an episode of care documented in the medical record

M1107 Documentation stating patient has a diagnosis of a degenerative neurological condition such as ALS, ms, or Parkinson's diagnosed at any time before or during the episode of care

M1108 Ongoing care not clinically indicated because the patient needed a home program only, referral to another provider or facility, or consultation only, as documented in the medical record

M1109 Ongoing care not medically possible because the patient was discharged early due to specific medical events, documented in the medical record, such as the patient became hospitalized or scheduled for surgery

M1110 Ongoing care not possible because the patient self-discharged early (e.g., financial or insurance reasons, transportation problems, or reason unknown)

M1111 The start of an episode of care documented in the medical record

M1112 Documentation stating patient has a diagnosis of a degenerative neurological condition such as ALS, ms, or Parkinson's diagnosed at any time before or during the episode of care

M1113 Ongoing care not clinically indicated because the patient needed a home program only, referral to another provider or facility, or consultation only, as documented in the medical record

M1114 Ongoing care not medically possible because the patient was discharged early due to specific medical events, documented in the medical record, such as the patient became hospitalized or scheduled for surgery

M1115 Ongoing care not possible because the patient self-discharged early (e.g., financial or insurance reasons, transportation problems, or reason unknown)

M1116 The start of an episode of care documented in the medical record

M1117 Documentation stating patient has a diagnosis of a degenerative neurological condition such as ALS, ms, or Parkinson's diagnosed at any time before or during the episode of care

M1118 Ongoing care not clinically indicated because the patient needed a home program only, referral to another provider or facility, or consultation only, as documented in the medical record

M1119 Ongoing care not medically possible because the patient was discharged early due to specific medical events, documented in the medical record, such as the patient became hospitalized or scheduled for surgery

M1120 Ongoing care not possible because the patient self-discharged early (e.g., financial or insurance reasons, transportation problems, or reason unknown)

M1121 The start of an episode of care documented in the medical record

M1122 Documentation stating patient has a diagnosis of a degenerative neurological condition such as ALS, ms, or Parkinson's diagnosed at any time before or during the episode of care

M1123 Ongoing care not clinically indicated because the patient needed a home program only, referral to another provider or facility, or consultation only, as documented in the medical record

M1124 Ongoing care not medically possible because the patient was discharged early due to specific medical events, documented in the medical record, such as the patient became hospitalized or scheduled for surgery

M1125 Ongoing care not possible because the patient self-discharged early (e.g., financial or insurance reasons, transportation problems, or reason unknown)

M1126 The start of an episode of care documented in the medical record

M1127 Documentation stating patient has a diagnosis of a degenerative neurological condition such as ALS, ms, or Parkinson's diagnosed at any time before or during the episode of care

M1128 Ongoing care not clinically indicated because the patient needed a home program only, referral to another provider or facility, or consultation only, as documented in the medical record

M1129 Ongoing care not medically possible because the patient was discharged early due to specific medical events, documented in the medical record, such as the patient became hospitalized or scheduled for surgery

M1130 Ongoing care not possible because the patient self-discharged early (e.g., financial or insurance reasons, transportation problems, or reason unknown)

M1131 Documentation stating patient has a diagnosis of a degenerative neurological condition such as ALS, ms, or Parkinson's diagnosed at any time before or during the episode of care

M1132 Ongoing care not clinically indicated because the patient needed a home program only, referral to another provider or facility, or consultation only, as documented in the medical record

M1133 Ongoing care not medically possible because the patient was discharged early due to specific medical events, documented in the medical record, such as the patient became hospitalized or scheduled for surgery

M1134 Ongoing care not possible because the patient self-discharged early (e.g., financial or insurance reasons, transportation problems, or reason unknown)

M1135 The start of an episode of care documented in the medical record

M1136 The start of an episode of care documented in the medical record

M1137 Documentation stating patient has a diagnosis of a degenerative neurological condition such as ALS, ms, or Parkinson's diagnosed at any time before or during the episode of care

M1138 Ongoing care not indicated, patient seen only 1-2 visits (e.g., home program only, referred to another provider or facility, consultation only)

M1139 Ongoing care not indicated, patient self-discharged early and seen only 1-2 visits (e.g., financial or insurance reasons, transportation problems, or reason unknown)

M1140 Ongoing care not indicated, patient discharged after only 1-2 visits due to specific medical events, documented in the medical record that make the treatment episode impossible such as the patient becomes hospitalized or scheduled for surgery for surgery or hospitalized

M1141 Functional status was not measured by the oxford knee score (oks), or the knee injury and osteoarthritis outcome score joint replacement (koos, jr.) at one year (9 to 15 months) postoperatively

M1142 Emergent cases

M1143 Initiated episode of rehabilitation therapy, medical, or chiropractic care for neck impairment

M1144 Ongoing care not indicated, patient seen only 1-2 visits (e.g., home program only, referred to another provider or facility, consultation only

M1145 Most favored nation (mfn) model drug add-on amount, per dose, (do not bill with line items that have the jw modifier)

M1146 Ongoing care not clinically indicated because the patient needed a home program only, referral to another provider or facility, or consultation only, as documented in the medical record

M1147 Ongoing care not medically possible because the patient was discharged early due to specific medical events, documented in the medical record, such as the patient became hospitalized or scheduled for surgery

M1148 Ongoing care not possible because the patient self-discharged early (e.g., financial or insurance reasons, transportation problems, or reason unknown)

M1149 Patient unable to complete the neck fs prom at initial evaluation and/or discharge due to blindness, illiteracy, severe mental incapacity or language incompatibility, and an adequate proxy is not available

M1150 Left ventricular ejection fraction (LVEF) less than or equal to 40% or documentation of moderately or severely depressed left ventricular systolic function

M1151 Patients with a history of heart transplant or with a left ventricular assist device (LVAD)

M1152 Patients with a history of heart transplant or with a left ventricular assist device (LVAD)

M1153 Patient with diagnosis of osteoporosis on date of encounter

M1154 Hospice services provided to patient any time during the measurement period

M1155 Patient had anaphylaxis due to the pneumococcal vaccine any time during or before the measurement period

(**M1156** Patient received active chemotherapy any time during the measurement period Code deleted effective 12/31/2023, no HCPCS/CPT cross-reference provided.)

(**M1157** Patient received bone marrow transplant any time during the measurement period Code deleted effective 12/31/2023, no HCPCS/CPT cross-reference provided.)

(**M1158** Patient had history of immunocompromising conditions prior to or during the measurement period Code deleted effective 12/31/2023, no HCPCS/CPT cross-reference provided.)

M1159 Hospice services provided to patient any time during the measurement period

M1160 Patient had anaphylaxis due to the meningococcal vaccine any time on or before the patient's 13th birthday

M1161 Patient had anaphylaxis due to the tetanus, diphtheria or pertussis vaccine any time on or before the patient's 13th birthday

M1162 Patient had encephalitis due to the tetanus, diphtheria or pertussis vaccine any time on or before the patient's 13th birthday

M1163 Patient had anaphylaxis due to the HPV vaccine any time on or before the patient's 13th birthday

M1164 Patients with dementia any time during the patient's history through the end of the measurement period

M1165 Patients who use hospice services any time during the measurement period

M1166 Pathology report for tissue specimens produced from wide local excisions or re-excisions

M1167 In hospice or using hospice services during the measurement period

M1168 Patient received an influenza vaccine on or between July 1 of the year prior to the measurement period and June 30 of the measurement period

M1169 Documentation of medical reason(s) for not administering influenza vaccine (e.g., prior anaphylaxis due to the influenza vaccine)

M1170 Patient did not receive an influenza vaccine on or between July 1 of the year prior to the measurement period and June 30 of the measurement period

M1171 Patient received at least one td vaccine or one Tdap vaccine between nine years prior to the encounter and the end of the measurement period

M1172 Documentation of medical reason(s) for not administering td or Tdap vaccine (e.g., prior anaphylaxis due to the td or Tdap vaccine or history of encephalopathy within seven days after a previous dose of a td-containing vaccine)

M1173 Patient did not receive at least one td vaccine or one Tdap vaccine between nine years prior to the encounter and the end of the measurement period

▲ **M1174** Patient received at least two doses of the herpes zoster recombinant vaccine (at least 28 days apart) anytime on or after the patient's 50th birthday before or during the measurement period

M1175 Documentation of medical reason(s) for not administering zoster vaccine (e.g., prior anaphylaxis due to the zoster vaccine)

▲ **M1176** Patient did not receive at least two doses of the herpes zoster recombinant vaccine (at least 28 days apart) anytime on or after the patient's 50th birthday before or during the measurement period

M1177 Patient received any pneumococcal conjugate or polysaccharide vaccine on or after their 60th birthday and before the end of the measurement period

M1178 Documentation of medical reason(s) for not administering pneumococcal vaccine (e.g., prior anaphylaxis due to the pneumococcal vaccine)

M1179 Patient did not receive any pneumococcal conjugate or polysaccharide vaccine, on or after their 60th birthday and before or during measurement period

M1180 Patients on immune checkpoint inhibitor therapy

M1181 Grade 2 or above diarrhea and/or grade 2 or above colitis

M1182 Patients not eligible due to pre-existing inflammatory bowel disease (IBD) (e.g., ulcerative colitis, Crohn's disease)

M1183 Documentation of immune checkpoint inhibitor therapy held and corticosteroids or immunosuppressants prescribed or administered

M1184 Documentation of medical reason(s) for not prescribing or administering corticosteroid or immunosuppressant treatment (e.g., allergy, intolerance, infectious etiology, pancreatic insufficiency, hyperthyroidism, prior bowel surgical interventions, celiac disease, receiving other medication, awaiting diagnostic workup results for alternative etiologies, other medical reasons/contraindication)

M1185 Documentation of immune checkpoint inhibitor therapy not held and/or corticosteroids or immunosuppressants prescribed or administered was not performed, reason not given

M1186 Patients who have an order for or are receiving hospice or palliative care

M1187 Patients with a diagnosis of end stage renal disease (ESRD)

M1188 Patients with a diagnosis of chronic kidney disease (CKD) stage 5

M1189 Documentation of a kidney health evaluation defined by an estimated glomerular filtration rate (EGFR) and urine albumin-creatinine ratio (uacr) performed

M1190 Documentation of a kidney health evaluation was not performed or defined by an estimated glomerular filtration rate (EGFR) and urine albumin-creatinine ratio (uacr)

M1191 Hospice services provided to patient any time during the measurement period

M1192 Patients with an existing diagnosis of squamous cell carcinoma of the esophagus

M1193 Surgical pathology reports that contain impression or conclusion of or recommendation for testing of MMR by immunohistochemistry, MSI by DNA-based testing status, or both

M1194 Documentation of medical reason(s) surgical pathology reports did not contain impression or conclusion of or recommendation for testing of MMR by immunohistochemistry, MSI by DNA-based testing status, or both tests were not included (e.g., patient will not be treated with checkpoint inhibitor therapy, no residual carcinoma is present in the sample [tissue exhausted or status post neoadjuvant treatment], insufficient tumor for testing)

M1195 Surgical pathology reports that do not contain impression or conclusion of or recommendation for testing of MMR by immunohistochemistry, MSI by DNA-based testing status, or both, reason not given

M1196 Initial (index visit) numeric rating scale (nrs), visual rating scale (VRS), or itchyquant assessment score of greater than or equal to 4

▲ **M1197** Itch severity assessment score is reduced by 3 or more points from the initial (index) assessment score to the follow-up visit score

▲ **M1198** Itch severity assessment score was not reduced by at least 3 points from initial (index) score to the follow-up visit score or assessment was not completed during the follow-up encounter

M1199 Patients receiving RRT

M1200 Ace inhibitor (ace-I) or arb therapy prescribed during the measurement period

M1201 Documentation of medical reason(s) for not prescribing ace inhibitor (ace-I) or arb therapy during

M - P CODES

the measurement period (e.g., pregnancy, history of angioedema to ace-I, other allergy to ace-I and arb, hyperkalemia or history of hyperkalemia while on ace-I or arb therapy, acute kidney injury due to ace-I or arb therapy), other medical reasons)

M1202 Documentation of patient reason(s) for not prescribing ace inhibitor or arb therapy during the measurement period, (e.g., patient declined, other patient reasons)

M1203 Ace inhibitor or arb therapy not prescribed during the measurement period; reason not given

M1204 Initial (index visit) numeric rating scale (nrs), visual rating scale (VRS), or itchyquant assessment score of greater than or equal to 4

▲ **M1205** Itch severity assessment score is reduced by 3 or more points from the initial (index) assessment score to the follow-up visit score

▲ **M1206** Itch severity assessment score was not reduced by at least 3 points from initial (index) score to the follow-up visit score or assessment was not completed during the follow-up encounter

▲ **M1207** Patient is screened for food insecurity, housing instability, transportation needs, utility difficulties, and interpersonal safety

▲ **M1208** Patient is not screened for food insecurity, housing instability, transportation needs, utility difficulties, and interpersonal safety

M1209 At least two orders for high-risk medications from the same drug class, (table 4), not ordered

M1210 At least two orders for high-risk medications from the same drug class, (table 4), not ordered

● **M1211** Most recent hemoglobin a1c level > 9.0%

● **M1212** Hemoglobin a1c level is missing, or was not performed during the measurement period (12 months)

● **M1213** No history of spirometry results with confirmed airflow obstruction (fev1/FVC < 70%) and present spirometry is >= 70%

● **M1214** Spirometry results with confirmed airflow obstruction (fev1/FVC < 70%) documented and reviewed

● **M1215** Documentation of medical reason(s) for not documenting and reviewing spirometry results (e.g., patients with dementia or tracheostomy)

● **M1216** No spirometry results with confirmed airflow obstruction (fev1/FVC < 70%) documented and/or no spirometry performed with results documented during the encounter

● **M1217** Documentation of system reason(s) for not documenting and reviewing spirometry results (e.g., spirometry equipment not available at the time of the encounter)

● **M1218** Patient has COPD symptoms (e.g., dyspnea, cough/sputum, wheezing)

● **M1219** Anaphylaxis due to the vaccine on or before the date of the encounter

● **M1220** Dilated retinal eye exam with interpretation by an ophthalmologist or optometrist or artificial intelligence (ai) interpretation documented and reviewed; with evidence of retinopathy

● **M1221** Dilated retinal eye exam with interpretation by an ophthalmologist or optometrist or artificial intelligence (ai) interpretation documented and reviewed; without evidence of retinopathy

● **M1222** Glaucoma plan of care not documented; reason not otherwise specified

● **M1223** Glaucoma plan of care documented

● **M1224** Intraocular pressure (IOP) reduced by a value less than 20% from the pre-intervention level

● **M1225** Intraocular pressure (IOP) reduced by a value of greater than or equal to 20% from the pre-intervention level

● **M1226** IOP measurement not documented, reason not otherwise specified

● **M1227** Evidence-based therapy was prescribed

- **M1228** Patient, who has a reactive HCV antibody test, and has a follow up HCV viral test that detected HCV viremia, has HCV treatment initiated within 3 months of the reactive HCV antibody test
- **M1229** Patient, who has a reactive HCV antibody test, and has a follow up HCV viral test that detected HCV viremia, is referred within 1 month of the reactive HCV antibody test to a clinician who treats HCV infection
- **M1230** Patient has a reactive HCV antibody test and does not have a follow up HCV viral test, or patient has a reactive HCV antibody test and has a follow up HCV viral test that detects HCV viremia and is not referred to a clinician who treats HCV infection within 1 month and does not have HCV treatment initiated within 3 months of the reactive HCV antibody test, reason not given
- **M1231** Patient receives HCV antibody test with nonreactive result
- **M1232** Patient receives HCV antibody test with reactive result
- **M1233** Patient does not receive HCV antibody test or patient does receive HCV antibody test but results not documented, reason not given
- **M1234** Patient has a reactive HCV antibody test, and has a follow up HCV viral test that does not detect HCV viremia
- **M1235** Documentation or patient report of HCV antibody test or HCV RNA test which occurred prior to the performance period
- **M1236** Baseline MRS > 2
- **M1237** Patient reason for not screening for food insecurity, housing instability, transportation needs, utility difficulties, and interpersonal safety (e.g., patient declined or other patient reasons)
- **M1238** Documentation that administration of second recombinant zoster vaccine could not occur during the performance period due to the recommended 2-6 month interval between doses (i.e., first dose received after October 31)
- **M1239** Patient did not respond to the question of patient felt heard and understood by this provider and team
- **M1240** Patient did not respond to the question of patient felt this provider and team put my best interests first when making recommendations about my care
- **M1241** Patient did not respond to the question of patient felt this provider and team saw me as a person, not just someone with a medical problem
- **M1242** Patient did not respond to the question of patient felt this provider and team understood what is important to me in my life
- **M1243** Patient provided a response other than "completely true" for the question of patient felt heard and understood by this provider and team
- **M1244** Patient provided a response other than "completely true" for the question of patient felt this provider and team put my best interests first when making recommendations about my care
- **M1245** Patient provided a response other than "completely true" for the question of patient felt this provider and team saw me as a person, not just someone with a medical problem
- **M1246** Patient provided a response other than "completely true" for the question of patient felt this provider and team understood what is important to me in my life
- **M1247** Patient responded "completely true" for the question of patient felt this provider and team put my best interests first when making recommendations about my care
- **M1248** Patient responded "completely true" for the question of patient felt this provider and team saw me as a person, not just someone with a medical problem
- **M1249** Patient responded "completely true" for the question of patient felt this provider and team understood what is important to me in my life
- **M1250** Patient responded as "completely true" for the question of patient felt heard and understood by this

provider and team

- ● **M1251** Patients for whom a proxy completed the entire hu survey on their behalf for any reason (no patient involvement)
- ● **M1252** Patients who did not complete at least one of the four patient experience hu survey items and return the hu survey within 60 days of the ambulatory palliative care visit
- ● **M1253** Patients who respond on the patient experience hu survey that they did not receive care by the listed ambulatory palliative care provider in the last 60 days (disavowal)
- ● **M1254** Patients who were deceased when the hu survey reached them
- ● **M1255** Patients who have another reason for visiting the clinic [not prenatal or postpartum care] and have a positive pregnancy test but have not established the clinic as an OB provider (e.g., plan to terminate the pregnancy or seek prenatal services elsewhere)
- ● **M1256** Prior history of known CVD
- ● **M1257** CVD risk assessment not performed or incomplete (e.g., CVD risk assessment was not documented), reason not otherwise specified
- ● **M1258** CVD risk assessment performed, have a documented calculated risk score
- ● **M1259** Patients listed on the kidney-pancreas transplant waitlist or who received a living donor transplant within the first year following initiation of dialysis
- ● **M1260** Patients who were not listed on the kidney-pancreas transplant waitlist or patients who did not receive a living donor transplant within the first year following initiation of dialysis
- ● **M1261** Patients that were on the kidney or kidney-pancreas waitlist prior to initiation of dialysis
- ● **M1262** Patients who had a transplant prior to initiation of dialysis
- ● **M1263** Patients in hospice on their initiation of dialysis date or during the month of evaluation
- ● **M1264** Patients aged 75 or older on their initiation of dialysis date
- ● **M1265** CMS medical evidence form 2728 for dialysis patients: initial form completed
- ● **M1266** Patients admitted to a skilled nursing facility (SNF)
- ● **M1267** Patients not on any kidney or kidney-pancreas transplant waitlist or is not in active status on any kidney or kidney-pancreas transplant waitlist as of the last day of each month during the measurement period
- ● **M1268** Patients on active status on any kidney or kidney-pancreas transplant waitlist as of the last day of each month during the measurement period
- ● **M1269** Receiving ESRD MCP dialysis services by the provider on the last day of the reporting month
- ● **M1270** Patients not on any kidney or kidney-pancreas transplant waitlist as of the last day of each month during the measurement period
- ● **M1271** Patients with dementia at any time prior to or during the month
- ● **M1272** Patients on any kidney or kidney-pancreas transplant waitlist as of the last day of each month during the measurement period
- ● **M1273** Patients who were admitted to a skilled nursing facility (SNF) within one year of dialysis initiation according to the cms-2728 form
- ● **M1274** Patients who were admitted to a skilled nursing facility (SNF) during the month of evaluation were excluded from that month
- ● **M1275** Patients determined to be in hospice were excluded from month of evaluation and the remainder of reporting period
- ● **M1276** BMI documented outside normal parameters, no follow-up plan documented, no reason given

- **M1277** Colorectal cancer screening results documented and reviewed
- **M1278** Elevated or hypertensive blood pressure reading documented, and the indicated follow-up is documented
- **M1279** Elevated or hypertensive blood pressure reading documented, indicated follow-up not documented, reason not given
- **M1280** Women who had a bilateral mastectomy or who have a history of a bilateral mastectomy or for whom there is evidence of a right and a left unilateral mastectomy
- **M1281** Blood pressure reading not documented, reason not given
- **M1282** Patient screened for tobacco use and identified as a tobacco non-user
- **M1283** Patient screened for tobacco use and identified as a tobacco user
- **M1284** Patients aged 66 or older in institutional special needs plans (SNP) or residing in long term care with pos code 32, 33, 34, 54, or 56 for more than 90 consecutive days during the measurement period
- **M1285** Screening, diagnostic, film, digital or digital breast tomosynthesis (3d) mammography results were not documented and reviewed, reason not otherwise specified
- **M1286** BMI is documented as being outside of normal parameters, follow-up plan is not completed for documented medical reason
- **M1287** BMI is documented below normal parameters, and a follow-up plan is documented
- **M1288** Documented reason for not screening or recommending a follow-up for high blood pressure
- **M1289** Patient identified as tobacco user did not receive tobacco cessation intervention during the measurement period or in the six months prior to the measurement period (counseling and/or pharmacotherapy)
- **M1290** Patient not eligible due to active diagnosis of hypertension
- **M1291** Patients 66 years of age and older with at least one claim/encounter for frailty during the measurement period and a dispensed medication for dementia during the measurement period or the year prior to the measurement period
- **M1292** Patients 66 years of age and older with at least one claim/encounter for frailty during the measurement period and either one acute inpatient encounter with a diagnosis of advanced illness or two outpatient, observation, ed or nonacute inpatient encounters on different dates of service with an advanced illness diagnosis during the measurement period or the year prior to the measurement period
- **M1293** BMI is documented above normal parameters, and a follow-up plan is documented
- **M1294** Normal blood pressure reading documented, follow-up not required
- **M1295** Patients with a diagnosis or past history of total colectomy or colorectal cancer
- **M1296** BMI is documented within normal parameters and no follow-up plan is required
- **M1297** BMI not documented due to medical reason or patient refusal of height or weight measurement
- **M1298** Documentation of patient pregnancy anytime during the measurement period prior to and including the current encounter
- **M1299** Influenza immunization administered or previously received
- **M1300** Influenza immunization was not administered for reasons documented by clinician (e.g., patient allergy or other medical reasons, patient declined or other patient reasons, vaccine not available or other system reasons)
- **M1301** Patient identified as a tobacco user received tobacco cessation intervention during the measurement period or in the six months prior to the measurement period (counseling and/or pharmacotherapy)

- • **M1302** Screening, diagnostic, film digital or digital breast tomosynthesis (3d) mammography results documented and reviewed
- • **M1303** Hospice services provided to patient any time during the measurement period
- • **M1304** Patient did not receive any pneumococcal conjugate or polysaccharide vaccine on or after their 19th birthday and before the end of the measurement period
- • **M1305** Patient received any pneumococcal conjugate or polysaccharide vaccine on or after their 19th birthday and before the end of the measurement period
- • **M1306** Patient had anaphylaxis due to the pneumococcal vaccine any time during or before the measurement period
- • **M1307** Documentation stating the patient has received or is currently receiving palliative or hospice care
- • **M1308** Influenza immunization was not administered, reason not given
- • **M1309** Palliative care services provided to patient any time during the measurement period
- • **M1310** Patient screened for tobacco use and received tobacco cessation intervention during the measurement period or in the six months prior to the measurement period (counseling, pharmacotherapy, or both), if identified as a tobacco user
- • **M1311** Anaphylaxis due to the vaccine on or before the date of the encounter
- • **M1312** Patient not screened for tobacco use
- • **M1313** Tobacco screening not performed, or tobacco cessation intervention not provided during the measurement period or in the six months prior to the measurement period
- • **M1314** BMI not documented and no reason is given
- • **M1315** Colorectal cancer screening results were not documented and reviewed; reason not otherwise specified
- • **M1316** Current tobacco non-user
- • **M1317** Patients who are counseled on connection with a CSP and explicitly opt out
- • **M1318** Patients who did not have documented contact with a CSP for at least one of their screened positive hrsns within 60 days after screening or documentation that there was no contact with a CSP
- • **M1319** Patients who had documented contact with a CSP for at least one of their screened positive hrsns within 60 days after screening
- • **M1320** Patients who screened positive for at least 1 of the 5 hrsns
- • **M1321** Patients who were not seen within 7 weeks following the date of injection for follow up or who did not have a documented IOP, or no plan of care documented if the IOP was >25 mm hg
- • **M1322** Patients seen within 7 weeks following the date of injection and are screened for elevated intraocular pressure (IOP) with tonometry with documented IOP =<25 mm hg for injected eye
- • **M1323** Patients seen within 7 weeks following the date of injection and are screened for elevated intraocular pressure (IOP) with tonometry with documented IOP >25 mm hg and a plan of care was documented
- • **M1324** Patients who had an intravitreal or periocular corticosteroid injection (e.g., triamcinolone, preservative-free triamcinolone, dexamethasone, dexamethasone intravitreal implant, or fluocinolone intravitreal implant)
- • **M1325** Patients who were not seen for reasons documented by clinician for patient or medical reasons (e.g., inadequate time for follow-up, patients who received a prior intravitreal or periocular steroid injection within the last six (6) months and had a subsequent IOP evaluation with IOP <25mm hg within seven (7) weeks of treatment)

- **M1326** Patients with a diagnosis of hypotony
- **M1327** Patients who were not appropriately evaluated during the initial exam and/or who were not re-evaluated within 8 weeks
- **M1328** Patients with a diagnosis of acute vitreous hemorrhage
- **M1329** Patients with a post-operative encounter of the eye with the acute PVD within 2 weeks before the initial encounter or 8 weeks after initial acute PVD encounter
- **M1330** Documentation of patient reason(s) for not having a follow up exam (e.g., inadequate time for follow up)
- **M1331** Patients who were appropriately evaluated during the initial exam and were re-evaluated no later than 8 weeks from initial exam
- **M1332** Patients who were not appropriately evaluated during the initial exam and/or who were not re-evaluated within 2 weeks
- **M1333** Acute vitreous hemorrhage
- **M1334** Patients with a post-operative encounter of the eye with the acute PVD within 2 weeks before the initial encounter or 2 weeks after initial acute PVD encounter
- **M1335** Documentation of patient reason(s) for not having a follow up exam (e.g., inadequate time for follow up)
- **M1336** Patients who were appropriately evaluated during the initial exam and were re-evaluated no later than 2 weeks
- **M1337** Acute PVD
- **M1338** Patients who had follow-up assessment 30 to 180 days after the index assessment who did not demonstrate positive improvement or maintenance of functioning scores during the performance period
- **M1339** Patients who had follow-up assessment 30 to 180 days after the index assessment who demonstrated positive improvement or maintenance of functioning scores during the performance period
- **M1340** Index assessment completed using the 12-item whodas 2.0 or sds during the denominator identification period
- **M1341** Patients who did not have a follow-up assessment or did not have an assessment within 30 to 180 days after the index assessment during the performance period
- **M1342** Patients who died during the performance period
- **M1343** Patients who are at pam level 4 at baseline or patients who are flagged with extreme straight line response sets on the pam
- **M1344** Patients who did not have a baseline pam score and/or a second score within 6 to 12 month of baseline pam score
- **M1345** Patients who had a baseline pam score and a second score within 6 to 12 month of baseline pam score
- **M1346** Patients who did not have a net increase in pam score of at least 6 points within a 6 to 12 month period
- **M1347** Patients who achieved a net increase in pam score of at least 3 points in a 6 to 12 month period (passing)
- **M1348** Patients who achieved a net increase in pam score of at least 6-points in a 6 to 12 month period (excellent)
- **M1349** Patients who did not have a net increase in pam score of at least 3 points within 6 to 12 month period

M - P CODES

- **M1350** Patients who had a completed suicide safety plan initiated, reviewed or updated in collaboration with their clinician (concurrent or within 24 hours) of the index clinical encounter
- **M1351** Patients who had a suicide safety plan initiated, reviewed, or updated and reviewed and updated in collaboration with the patient and their clinician concurrent or within 24 hours of clinical encounter and within 120 days after initiation
- **M1352** Suicidal ideation and/or behavior symptoms based on the c-ssrs or equivalent assessment
- **M1353** Patients who did not have a completed suicide safety plan initiated, reviewed or updated in collaboration with their clinician (concurrent or within 24 hours) of the index clinical encounter
- **M1354** Patients who did not have a suicide safety plan initiated, reviewed, or updated or reviewed and updated in collaboration with the patient and their clinician concurrent or within 24 hours of clinical encounter and within 120 days after initiation
- **M1355** Suicide risk based on their clinician's evaluation or a clinician-rated tool
- **M1356** Patients who died during the measurement period
- **M1357** Patients who had a reduction in suicidal ideation and/or behavior upon follow-up assessment within 120 days of index assessment
- **M1358** Patients who did not have a reduction in suicidal ideation and/or behavior upon follow-up assessment within 120 days of index assessment
- **M1359** Index assessment during the denominator period when the suicidal ideation and/or behavior symptoms or increased suicide risk by clinician determination occurs and a non-zero c-ssrs score is obtained
- **M1360** Suicidal ideation and/or behavior symptoms based on the c-ssrs
- **M1361** Suicide risk based on their clinician's evaluation or a clinician-rated tool
- **M1362** Patients who died during the measurement period
- **M1363** Patients who did not have a follow-up assessment within 120 days of the index assessment
- **M1364** Calculated 10-year ASCVD risk score of = 20 percent during the performance period
- **M1365** Patient encounter during the performance period with hospice and palliative care specialty code 17
- **M1366** Focusing on women's health MIPS value pathway
- **M1367** Quality care for the treatment of ear, nose, and throat disorders MIPS value pathway
- **M1368** Prevention and treatment of infectious disorders including hepatitis c and HIV MIPS value pathway
- **M1369** Quality care in mental health and substance use disorders MIPS value pathway
- **M1370** Rehabilitative support for musculoskeletal care MIPS value pathway

PATHOLOGY AND LABORATORY

Guidelines

In addition to the information presented in the INTRODUCTION, several other items unique to this section are defined or identified here:

1. **SPECIAL REPORT:** A service, material or supply that is rarely provided, unusual, variable or new may require a special report in determining medical appropriateness for reimbursement purposes. Pertinent information should include an adequate definition or description of the nature, extent, and need for the service, material or supply.

2. **MODIFIERS:** Listed services may be modified under certain circumstances. When appropriate, the modifying circumstance is identified by adding a modifier to the basic procedure code. CPT and HCPCS National Level II modifiers may be used with CPT and HCPCS National Level II procedure codes. Modifiers commonly used with PATHOLOGY AND LABORATORY SERVICES are as follows:

   -CC Procedure code change (use "CC" when the procedure code submitted was changed either for administrative reasons or because an incorrect code was filed)

   -LR Laboratory round trip

   -TC Technical component. Under certain circumstances, a charge may be made for the technical component alone. Under these circumstances, the technical component charge is identified by adding the modifier -TC to the usual procedure code. Technical component charges are institutional charges and are not billed separately by physicians. Portable x-ray suppliers bill only for the technical component however and should use modifier -TC. The charge data from portable x-ray suppliers will then be used to build customary and prevailing profiles.

3. **CPT CODE CROSS-REFERENCE:** See sections for equivalent CPT code(s) for all listings in this section.

Chemistry and Toxicology Tests

P2028 Cephalin flocculation, blood

P2029 Congo red, blood

P2031 Hair analysis (excluding arsenic)

P2033 Thymol turbidity, blood

P2038 Mucoprotein, blood (seromucoid) (medical necessity procedure)

Pathology Screening Tests

P3000 Screening Papanicolaou smear, cervical or vaginal, up to three smears, by technician under physician supervision

P3001 Screening Papanicolaou smear, cervical or vaginal, up to three smears, requiring interpretation by physician

Miscellaneous Pathology and Laboratory Tests

P7001 Culture, bacterial, urine; quantitative, sensitivity study CPT

P9010 Blood (whole), for transfusion, per unit

P9011 Blood, split unit

P9012	Cryoprecipitate, each unit
P9016	Red blood cells, leukocytes reduced, each unit
P9017	Fresh frozen plasma (single donor), frozen within 8 hours of collection, each unit
P9019	Platelets, each unit
P9020	Platelet rich plasma, each unit
P9021	Red blood cells, each unit
P9022	Red blood cells, washed, each unit
P9023	Plasma, pooled multiple donor, solvent/detergent treated, frozen, each unit
P9025	Plasma, cryoprecipitate reduced, pathogen reduced, each unit
P9026	Cryoprecipitated fibrinogen complex, pathogen reduced, each unit
P9031	Platelets, leukocytes reduced, each unit
P9032	Platelets, irradiated, each unit
P9033	Platelets, leukocytes reduced, irradiated, each unit
P9034	Platelets, pheresis, each unit
P9035	Platelets, pheresis, leukocytes reduced, each unit
P9036	Platelets, pheresis, irradiated, each unit
P9037	Platelets, pheresis, leukocytes reduced, irradiated, each unit
P9038	Red blood cells, irradiated, each unit
P9039	Red blood cells, deglycerolized, each unit
P9040	Red blood cells, leukocytes reduced, irradiated, each unit
P9041	Infusion, albumin (human), 5%, 50 ml
P9043	Infusion, plasma protein fraction (human), 5%, 50 ml
P9044	Plasma, cryoprecipitate reduced, each unit
P9045	Infusion, albumin (human), 5%, 250 ml
P9046	Infusion, albumin (human), 25%, 20 ml
P9047	Infusion, albumin (human), 25%, 50 ml
P9048	Infusion, plasma protein fraction (human), 5%, 250 ml
P9050	Granulocytes, pheresis, each unit
P9051	Whole blood or red blood cells, leukocytes reduced, CMV-negative, each unit
P9052	Platelets, HLA-matched leukocytes reduced, apheresis/pheresis, each unit
P9053	Platelets, pheresis, leukocytes reduced, CMV-negative, irradiated, each unit
P9054	Whole blood or red blood cells, leukocytes reduced, frozen, deglycerol, washed, each unit
P9055	Platelets, leukocytes reduced, CMV-negative, apheresis/pheresis, each unit
P9056	Whole blood, leukocytes reduced, irradiated, each unit
P9057	Red blood cells, frozen/deglycerolized/washed, leukocytes reduced, irradiated, each unit
P9058	Red blood cells, leukocytes reduced, CMV-negative, irradiated, each unit

P9059 Fresh frozen plasma between 8-24 hours of collection, each unit

P9060 Fresh frozen plasma, donor retested, each unit

P9070 Plasma, pooled multiple donor, pathogen reduced, frozen, each unit

P9071 Plasma (single donor), pathogen reduced, frozen, each unit

P9073 Platelets, pheresis, pathogen-reduced, each unit

P9099 Blood component or product not otherwise classified

P9100 Pathogen(s) test for platelets

P9603 Travel allowance one way in connection with medically necessary laboratory specimen collection drawn from home bound or nursing home bound patient; prorated miles actually travelled

P9604 Travel allowance one way in connection with medically necessary laboratory specimen collection drawn from home bound or nursing home bound patient; prorated trip charge.

P9612 Catheterization for collection of specimen, single patient, all places of service

P9615 Catheterization for collection of specimen(s) (multiple patients)

TEMPORARY CODES

Guidelines

In addition to the information presented in the INTRODUCTION, several other items unique to this section are defined or identified here:

1. **SUBSECTION INFORMATION:** Some of the listed subheadings or subsections have special needs or instructions unique to that section. Where these are indicated, special "notes" will be presented preceding or following the listings. Those subsections within the TEMPORARY CODES section that have "notes" are as follows:

Subsection	Code Numbers
Temporary codes	Q0000–Q9999

2. **SPECIAL REPORT:** A service, material or supply that is rarely provided, unusual, variable or new may require a special report in determining medical appropriateness for reimbursement purposes. Pertinent information should include an adequate definition or description of the nature, extent, and need for the service, material or supply.

3. **MODIFIERS:** Listed services may be modified under certain circumstances. When appropriate, the modifying circumstance is identified by adding a modifier to the basic procedure code. CPT and HCPCS National Level II modifiers may be used with CPT and HCPCS National Level II procedure codes. Modifiers commonly used with TEMPORARY CODES are as follows:

   -CC Procedure code change (use "CC" when the procedure code submitted was changed either for administrative reasons or because an incorrect code was filed)

   -LL Lease/rental (used when DME equipment rental is to be applied against the purchase price)

   -LR Laboratory round trip

   -QC Single channel monitoring

   -QD Recording and storage in solid state memory by a digital recorder

   -QE Prescribed amount of oxygen is less than 1 liter per minute (LPM)

   -QF Prescribed amount of oxygen exceeds 4 liters per minute (LPM) and portable oxygen is prescribed

   -QG Prescribed amount of oxygen is greater than 4 liters per minute (LPM)

   -QH Oxygen conserving device is being used with an oxygen delivery system

   -QT Recording and storage on tape by an analog tape recorder

   -RP Replacement and repair (may be used to indicate replacement of DME, orthotic and prosthetic devices that have been in use for some time. The claim shows the code for the part, followed by the "RP" modifier and the charge for the part.)

   -RR Rental (used when DME is to be rented)

   -TC Technical component. Under certain circumstances, a charge may be made for the technical component alone. Under these circumstances, the technical component charge is identified by adding the modifier -TC to the usual procedure code. Technical component charges are institutional charges and are not billed separately by physicians. Portable x-ray suppliers bill only for the technical component however and should use modifier -TC. The charge data from portable x-ray suppliers will then be used to build customary and prevailing profiles.

-UE Used durable medical equipment

4. **CPT CODE CROSS-REFERENCE:** See sections for equivalent CPT code(s) for all listings in this section.

Temporary Codes

NOTE: Temporary codes are national codes given by CMS on a temporary basis. The list contains current codes, as well as those which have been superseded by permanent alphanumeric codes as indicated by the cross-reference.

Q0035 Cardiokymography

Q0081 Infusion therapy, using other than chemotherapeutic drugs, per visit

Q0083 Chemotherapy administration by other than infusion technique only (e.g., subcutaneous, intramuscular, push), per visit

Q0084 Chemotherapy administration by infusion technique only, per visit

Q0085 Chemotherapy administration by both infusion technique and other technique(s) (e.g., subcutaneous, intramuscular, push), per visit

Q0091 Screening Papanicolaou smear; obtaining, preparing and conveyance of cervical or vaginal smear to laboratory

Q0092 Set-up portable x-ray equipment

Q0111 Wet mounts, including preparations of vaginal, cervical or skin specimens

Q0112 All potassium hydroxide (KOH) preparations

Q0113 Pinworm examinations

Q0114 Fern test

Q0115 Post-coital direct, qualitative examinations of vaginal or cervical mucous

Q0138 Injection, ferumoxytol, for treatment of iron deficiency anemia, 1 mg (non-ESRD use)

Q0139 Injection, ferumoxytol, for treatment of iron deficiency anemia, 1 mg (for ESRD on dialysis)

Q0144 Azithromycin dihydrate, oral, capsules/powder, 1 gram

Q0161 Chlorpromazine hydrochloride, 5 mg, oral, approved prescription anti-emetic, for use as a complete therapeutic substitute for an iv anti-emetic at the time of chemotherapy treatment, not to exceed a 48 hour dosage regimen

Q0162 Ondansetron 1 mg, oral, approved prescription anti-emetic, for use as a complete therapeutic substitute for an iv anti-emetic at the time of chemotherapy treatment, not to exceed a 48 hour dosage regimen

Q0163 Diphenhydramine hydrochloride, 50 mg, oral, approved prescription anti-emetic, for use as a complete therapeutic substitute for an iv anti-emetic at time of chemotherapy treatment not to exceed a 48 hour dosage regimen

Q0164 Prochlorperazine maleate, 5 mg, oral, approved prescription anti-emetic, for use as a complete therapeutic substitute for an iv anti-emetic at the time of chemotherapy treatment, not to exceed a 48 hour dosage regimen

Q0166 Granisetron hydrochloride, 1 mg, oral, approved prescription anti-emetic, for use as a complete therapeutic substitute for an iv anti-emetic at the time of chemotherapy treatment, not to exceed a 24 hour dosage regimen

Q0167 Dronabinol, 2.5 mg, oral, approved prescription anti-emetic, for use as a complete therapeutic substitute for an iv anti-emetic at the time of chemotherapy treatment, not to exceed a 48 hour dosage regimen

Q0169 Promethazine hydrochloride, 12.5 mg, oral, approved prescription anti-emetic, for use as a complete therapeutic substitute for an iv anti-emetic at the time of chemotherapy treatment, not to exceed a 48 hour dosage regimen

Q0173 Trimethobenzamide hydrochloride, 250 mg, oral, approved prescription anti-emetic, for use as a complete therapeutic substitute for an iv anti-emetic at the time of chemotherapy treatment, not to exceed a 48 hour dosage regimen

Q0174 Thiethylperazine maleate, 10 mg, oral, approved prescription anti-emetic, for use as a complete therapeutic substitute for an iv anti-emetic at the time of chemotherapy treatment, not to exceed a 48 hour dosage regimen

Q0175 Perphenazine, 4 mg, oral, approved prescription anti-emetic, for use as a complete therapeutic substitute for an iv anti-emetic at the time of chemotherapy treatment, not to exceed a 48 hour dosage regimen

Q0177 Hydroxyzine pamoate, 25 mg, oral, approved prescription anti-emetic, for use as a complete therapeutic substitute for an iv anti-emetic at the time of chemotherapy treatment, not to exceed a 48 hour dosage regimen

Q0180 Dolasetron mesylate, 100 mg, oral, approved prescription anti-emetic, for use as a complete therapeutic substitute for an iv anti-emetic at the time of chemotherapy treatment, not to exceed a 24 hour dosage regimen

Q0181 Unspecified oral dosage form, approved prescription anti-emetic, for use as a complete therapeutic substitute for a iv anti-emetic at the time of chemotherapy treatment, not to exceed a 48 hour dosage regimen

Q0220 Injection, tixagevimab and cilgavimab, for the pre-exposure prophylaxis only, for certain adults and pediatric individuals (12 years of age and older weighing at least 40kg) with no known sars-cov-2 exposure, who either have moderate to severely compromised immune systems or for whom vaccination with any available covid-19 vaccine is not recommended due to a history of severe adverse reaction to a covid-19 vaccine(s) and/or covid-19 vaccine component(s), 300 mg

Q0221 Injection, tixagevimab and cilgavimab, for the pre-exposure prophylaxis only, for certain adults and pediatric individuals (12 years of age and older weighing at least 40kg) with no known sars-cov-2 exposure, who either have moderate to severely compromised immune systems or for whom vaccination with any available covid-19 vaccine is not recommended due to a history of severe adverse reaction to a covid-19 vaccine(s) and/or covid-19 vaccine component(s), 600 mg

Q0222 Injection, bebtelovimab, 175 mg

Q0239 Injection, bamlanivimab-xxxx, 700 mg

Q0240 Injection, casirivimab and imdevimab, 600 mg

Q0243 Injection, casirivimab and imdevimab, 2400 mg

Q0244 Injection, casirivimab and imdevimab, 1200 mg

Q0245 Injection, bamlanivimab and etesevimab, 2100 mg

Q0247 Injection, sotrovimab, 500 mg

Q0249 Injection, tocilizumab, for hospitalized adults and pediatric patients (2 years of age and older) with covid-19 who are receiving systemic corticosteroids and require supplemental oxygen, non-invasive or invasive mechanical ventilation, or extracorporeal membrane oxygenation (ECMO) only, 1 mg

Q0247 Injection, sotrovimab, 500 mg

Q - R - S CODES

Not payable by Medicare | Non-covered by Medicare | Special coverage instructions | Carrier judgement

Q0477 Power module patient cable for use with electric or electric/pneumatic ventricular assist device, replacement only

Q0479 Power module for use with electric or electric/pneumatic ventricular assist device, replacement only

Q0480 Driver for use with pneumatic ventricular assist device, replacement only

Q0481 Microprocessor control unit for use with electric ventricular assist device, replacement only

Q0482 Microprocessor control unit for use with electric/pneumatic combination ventricular assist device, replacement only

Q0483 Monitor/display module for use with electric ventricular assist device, replacement only

Q0484 Monitor/display module for use with electric or electric/pneumatic ventricular assist device, replacement only

Q0485 Monitor control cable for use with electric ventricular assist device, replacement only

Q0486 Monitor control cable for use with electric/pneumatic ventricular assist device, replacement only

Q0487 Leads (pneumatic/electrical) for use with any type of electric/pneumatic ventricular assist device, replacement only

Q0488 Power pack base for use with electric ventricular assist device, replacement only

Q0489 Power pack base for use with electric/pneumatic ventricular assist device, replacement only

Q0490 Emergency power source for use with electric ventricular assist device, replacement only

Q0491 Emergency power source for use with electric/pneumatic ventricular assist device, replacement only

Q0492 Emergency power supply cable for use with electric ventricular assist device, replacement only

Q0493 Emergency power supply cable for use with electric/pneumatic ventricular assist device, replacement only

Q0494 Emergency hand pump for use with electric or electric/pneumatic ventricular assist device, replacement only

Q0495 Battery/power pack charger for use with electric or electric/pneumatic ventricular assist device, replacement only

Q0496 Battery, other than lithium-ion, for use with electric or electric/pneumatic ventricular assist device, replacement only

Q0497 Battery clips for use with electric or electric/pneumatic ventricular assist device, replacement only

Q0498 Holster for use with electric or electric/pneumatic ventricular assist device, replacement only

Q0499 Belt/vest/bag for use to carry external peripheral components of any type of ventricular assist device, replacement only

Q0500 Filters for use with electric or electric/pneumatic ventricular assist device, replacement only

Q0501 Shower cover for use with electric or electric/pneumatic ventricular assist device, replacement only

Q0502 Mobility cart for pneumatic ventricular assist device, replacement only

Q0503 Battery for pneumatic ventricular assist device, replacement only, each

Q0504 Power adapter for pneumatic ventricular assist device, replacement only, vehicle type

Q0506 Battery, lithium-ion, for use with electric or electric/pneumatic ventricular assist device, replacement only

Q0507 Miscellaneous supply or accessory for use with an external ventricular assist device

Q0508 Miscellaneous supply or accessory for use with an implanted ventricular assist device

Q0509 Miscellaneous supply or accessory for use with any implanted ventricular assist device for which payment was not made under Medicare part a

Q0510 Pharmacy supply fee for initial immunosuppressive drug(s), first month following transplant

Q0511 Pharmacy supply fee for oral anti-cancer, oral anti-emetic or immunosuppressive drug(s); for the first prescription in a 30-day period

Q0512 Pharmacy supply fee for oral anti-cancer, oral anti-emetic or immunosuppressive drug(s); for a subsequent prescription in a 30-day period

Q0513 Pharmacy dispensing fee for inhalation drug(s); per 30 days

Q0514 Pharmacy dispensing fee for inhalation drug(s); per 90 days

Q0515 Injection, sermorelin acetate, 1 microgram

• **Q0516** Pharmacy supplying fee for HIV pre-exposure prophylaxis FDA approved prescription drug, per 30-days

• **Q0517** Pharmacy supplying fee for HIV pre-exposure prophylaxis FDA approved prescription drug, per 60-days

• **Q0518** Pharmacy supplying fee for HIV pre-exposure prophylaxis FDA approved prescription drug, per 90-days

Q1004 New technology intraocular lens category 4 as defined in federal register notice

Q1005 New technology intraocular lens category 5 as defined in federal register notice

Q2004 Irrigation solution for treatment of bladder calculi, for example Renacidin, per 500 ml

Q2009 Injection, fosphenytoin, 50 mg phenytoin equivalent

Q2017 Injection, teniposide, 50 mg

Q2026 Injection, Radiesse, 0.1 ml

Q2028 Injection, Sculptra, 0.5 mg

Q2034 Influenza virus vaccine, split virus, for intramuscular use (Agriflu)

Q2035 Influenza virus vaccine, split virus, when administered to individuals 3 years of age and older, for intramuscular use (Afluria)

Q2036 Influenza virus vaccine, split virus, when administered to individuals 3 years of age and older, for intramuscular use (FluLaval)

Q2037 Influenza virus vaccine, split virus, when administered to individuals 3 years of age and older, for intramuscular use (Fluvirin)

Q2038 Influenza virus vaccine, split virus, when administered to individuals 3 years of age and older, for intramuscular use (Fluzone)

Q2039 Influenza virus vaccine, not otherwise specified

Q2040 Tisagenlecleucel, up to 250 million car-positive viable t cells, including leukapheresis and dose preparation procedures, per infusion

Q2041 Axicabtagene ciloleucel, up to 200 million autologous anti-cd19 car positive viable t cells, including leukapheresis and dose preparation procedures, per therapeutic dose

Q2042 Tisagenlecleucel, up to 600 million car-positive viable t cells, including leukapheresis and dose preparation procedures, per therapeutic dose

Q2043 Sipuleucel-t, minimum of 50 million autologous cd54+ cells activated with pap-gm-csf, including leukapheresis and all other preparatory procedures, per infusion

Q2049 Injection, doxorubicin hydrochloride, liposomal, imported Lipidox, 10 mg

Q2050 Injection, doxorubicin hydrochloride, liposomal, not otherwise specified, 10 mg

Q - R - S CODES

Q2052	Services, supplies and accessories used in the home under the Medicare intravenous immune globulin (IVIG) demonstration
Q2053	Brexucabtagene autoleucel, up to 200 million autologous anti-cd19 car positive viable t cells, including leukapheresis and dose preparation procedures, per therapeutic dose
Q2054	Lisocabtagene maraleucel, up to 110 million autologous anti-cd19 car-positive viable t cells, including leukapheresis and dose preparation procedures, per therapeutic dose
Q2055	Idecabtagene vicleucel, up to 460 million autologous b-cell maturation antigen (BCMA) directed car-positive t cells, including leukapheresis and dose preparation procedures, per therapeutic dose
Q2056	Ciltacabtagene autoleucel, up to 100 million autologous b-cell maturation antigen (bcma) directed car-positive t cells, including leukapheresis and dose preparation procedures, per therapeutic dose
Q3001	Radioelements for brachytherapy, any type, each
Q3014	Telehealth originating site facility fee
Q3027	Injection, interferon beta-1a, 1 mcg for intramuscular use
Q3028	Injection, interferon beta-1a, 1 mcg for subcutaneous use
Q3031	Collagen skin test
Q4001	Casting supplies, body cast adult, with or without head, plaster
Q4002	Cast supplies, body cast adult, with or without head, fiberglass
Q4003	Cast supplies, shoulder cast, adult (11 years +), plaster
Q4004	Cast supplies, shoulder cast, adult (11 years +), fiberglass
Q4005	Cast supplies, long arm cast, adult (11 years +), plaster
Q4006	Cast supplies, long arm cast, adult (11 years +), fiberglass
Q4007	Cast supplies, long arm cast, pediatric (0-10 years), plaster
Q4008	Cast supplies, long arm cast, pediatric (0-10 years), fiberglass
Q4009	Cast supplies, short arm cast, adult (11 years +), plaster
Q4010	Cast supplies, short arm cast, adult (11 years +), fiberglass
Q4011	Cast supplies, short arm cast, pediatric (0-10 years), plaster
Q4012	Cast supplies, short arm cast, pediatric (0-10 years), fiberglass
Q4013	Cast supplies, gauntlet cast (includes lower forearm and hand), adult (11 years +), plaster
Q4014	Cast supplies, gauntlet cast (includes lower forearm and hand), adult (11 years +), fiberglass
Q4015	Cast supplies, gauntlet cast (includes lower forearm and hand), pediatric (0-10 years), plaster
Q4016	Cast supplies, gauntlet cast (includes lower forearm and hand), pediatric (0-10 years), fiberglass
Q4017	Cast supplies, long arm splint, adult (11 years +), plaster
Q4018	Cast supplies, long arm splint, adult (11 years +), fiberglass
Q4019	Cast supplies, long arm splint, pediatric (0-10 years), plaster
Q4020	Cast supplies, long arm splint, pediatric (0-10 years), fiberglass
Q4021	Cast supplies, short arm splint, adult (11 years +), plaster
Q4022	Cast supplies, short arm splint, adult (11 years +), fiberglass
Q4023	Cast supplies, short arm splint, pediatric (0-10 years), plaster

Q4024 Cast supplies, short arm splint, pediatric (0-10 years), fiberglass

Q4025 Cast supplies, hip spica (one or both legs), adult (11 years +), plaster

Q4026 Cast supplies, hip spica (one or both legs), adult (11 years +), fiberglass

Q4027 Cast supplies, hip spica (one or both legs), pediatric (0-10 years), plaster

Q4028 Cast supplies, hip spica (one or both legs), pediatric (0-10 years), fiberglass

Q4029 Cast supplies, long leg cast, adult (11 years +), plaster

Q4030 Cast supplies, long leg cast, adult (11 years +), fiberglass

Q4031 Cast supplies, long leg cast, pediatric (0-10 years), plaster

Q4032 Cast supplies, long leg cast, pediatric (0-10 years), fiberglass

Q4033 Cast supplies, long leg cylinder cast, adult (11 years +), plaster

Q4034 Cast supplies, long leg cylinder cast, adult (11 years +), fiberglass

Q4035 Cast supplies, long leg cylinder cast, pediatric (0-10 years), plaster

Q4036 Cast supplies, long leg cylinder cast, pediatric (0-10 years), fiberglass

Q4037 Cast supplies, short leg cast, adult (11 years +), plaster

Q4038 Cast supplies, short leg cast, adult (11 years +), fiberglass

Q4039 Cast supplies, short leg cast, pediatric (0-10 years), plaster

Q4040 Cast supplies, short leg cast, pediatric (0-10 years), fiberglass

Q4041 Cast supplies, long leg splint, adult (11 years +), plaster

Q4042 Cast supplies, long leg splint, adult (11 years +), fiberglass

Q4043 Cast supplies, long leg splint, pediatric (0-10 years), plaster

Q4044 Cast supplies, long leg splint, pediatric (0-10 years), fiberglass

Q4045 Cast supplies, short leg splint, adult (11 years +), plaster

Q4046 Cast supplies, short leg splint, adult (11 years +), fiberglass

Q4047 Cast supplies, short leg splint, pediatric (0-10 years), plaster

Q4048 Cast supplies, short leg splint, pediatric (0-10 years), fiberglass

Q4049 Finger splint, static

Q4050 Cast supplies, for unlisted types and materials of casts

Q4051 Splint supplies, miscellaneous (includes thermoplastics, strapping, fasteners, padding and other supplies)

Q4074 Iloprost, inhalation solution,-approved final product, non-compounded, administered through DME, unit dose form, up to 20 micrograms

Injection Codes for EPO

Q4081 Injection, epoetin alfa, 100 units (for ESRD on dialysis)

Q4082 Drug or biological, not otherwise classified, part b drug competitive acquisition program (cap)

Q4100 Skin substitute, not otherwise specified

Q4101 Apligraf, per square centimeter

Q4102 Oasis wound matrix, per square centimeter

Q - R - S CODES

Q4103	Oasis burn matrix, per square centimeter
Q4104	Integra bilayer matrix wound dressing (BMWD), per square centimeter
Q4105	Integra dermal regeneration template (DRT) or Integra Omnigraft dermal regeneration matrix, per square centimeter
Q4106	Dermagraft, per square centimeter
Q4107	Graftjacket, per square centimeter
Q4108	Integra matrix, per square centimeter
Q4110	Primatrix, per square centimeter
Q4111	Gammagraft, per square centimeter
Q4112	Cymetra, injectable, 1 cc
Q4113	Graftjacket xpress, injectable, 1 cc
Q4114	Integra flowable wound matrix, injectable, 1 cc
Q4115	Alloskin, per square centimeter
Q4116	AlloDerm, per square centimeter
Q4117	Hyalomatrix, per square centimeter
Q4118	Matristem micromatrix, 1 mg
Q4121	TheraSkin, per square centimeter
Q4122	Dermacell, Dermacell awm or Dermacell awm porous, per square centimeter
Q4123	Alloskin rt, per square centimeter
Q4124	Oasis ultra tri-layer wound matrix, per square centimeter
Q4125	Arthroflex, per square centimeter
Q4126	Memoderm, dermaspan, TranZgraft or integuply, per square centimeter
Q4127	Talymed, per square centimeter
Q4128	Flex hd, Allopatch hd, or matrix hd, per square centimeter
Q4131	Epifix or EpiCord, per square centimeter
Q4132	Grafix core and grafixpl core, per square centimeter
Q4133	Grafix prime, grafixpl prime, stravix and stravixpl, per square centimeter
Q4134	Hmatrix, per square centimeter
Q4135	Mediskin, per square centimeter
Q4136	EZ-derm, per square centimeter
Q4137	Amnioexcel, Amnioexcel plus or biodexcel, per square centimeter
Q4138	Biodefense dryflex, per square centimeter
Q4139	Amniomatrix or Biomatrix, injectable, 1 cc
Q4140	Biodefense, per square centimeter
Q4141	Alloskin ac, per square centimeter
Q4142	Xcm biologic tissue matrix, per square centimeter
Q4143	Repriza, per square centimeter

Q4145	Epifix, injectable, 1 mg
Q4146	Tensix, per square centimeter
Q4147	Architect, architect px, or architect fx, extracellular matrix, per square centimeter
Q4148	Neox cord 1k, Neox cord rt, or clarix cord 1k, per square centimeter
Q4149	Excellagen, 0.1 cc
Q4150	Allowrap DS or dry, per square centimeter
Q4151	Amnioband or guardian, per square centimeter
Q4152	Dermapure, per square centimeter
Q4153	Dermavest and Plurivest, per square centimeter
Q4154	Biovance, per square centimeter
Q4155	Neoxflo or Clarixflo, 1 mg
Q4156	Neox 100 or clarix 100, per square centimeter
Q4157	Revitalon, per square centimeter
Q4158	Kerecis omega3, per square centimeter
Q4159	Affinity, per square centimeter
Q4160	Nushield, per square centimeter
Q4161	Bio-connekt wound matrix, per square centimeter
Q4162	Woundex flow, BioSkin flow, 0.5 cc
Q4163	Woundex, BioSkin, per square centimeter
Q4164	Helicoll, per square centimeter
Q4165	Keramatrix or Kerasorb, per square centimeter
Q4166	Cytal, per square centimeter
Q4167	Truskin, per square centimeter
Q4168	Amnioband, 1 mg
Q4169	Artacent wound, per square centimeter
Q4170	Cygnus, per square centimeter
Q4171	Interfyl, 1 mg
Q4173	Palingen or Palingen xplus, per square centimeter
Q4174	Palingen or Promatrx, 0.36 mg per 0.25 cc
Q4175	Miroderm, per square centimeter
Q4176	Neopatch, per square centimeter
Q4177	Floweramnioflo, 0.1 cc
Q4178	Floweramniopatch, per square centimeter
Q4179	Flowerderm, per square centimeter
Q4180	Revita, per square centimeter
Q4181	Amnio wound, per square centimeter

Q4182	TransCyte, per square centimeter
Q4183	Surgigraft, per square centimeter
Q4184	Cellesta or Cellesta duo, per square centimeter
Q4185	Cellesta flowable amnion (25 mg per cc); per 0.5 cc
Q4186	Epifix, per square centimeter
Q4187	Epicord, per square centimeter
Q4188	Amnioarmor, per square centimeter
Q4189	Artacent ac, 1 mg
Q4190	Artacent ac, per square centimeter
Q4191	Restorigin, per square centimeter
Q4192	Restorigin, 1 cc
Q4193	Coll-e-derm, per square centimeter
Q4194	Novachor, per square centimeter
Q4195	PuraPly, per square centimeter
Q4196	PuraPly am, per square centimeter
Q4197	PuraPly xt, per square centimeter
Q4198	Genesis amniotic membrane, per square centimeter
Q4199	Cygnus matrix, per square centimeter
Q4200	Skin te, per square centimeter
Q4201	Matrion, per square centimeter
Q4202	Keroxx (2.5g/cc), 1cc
Q4203	Derma-gide, per square centimeter
Q4204	Xwrap, per square centimeter
Q4205	Membrane graft or membrane wrap, per square centimeter
Q4206	Fluid flow or fluid gf, 1 cc
Q4208	Novafix, per square centimeter
Q4209	Surgraft, per square centimeter
Q4210	Axolotl graft or axolotl dualgraft, per square centimeter
Q4211	Amnion bio or axobiomembrane, per square centimeter
Q4212	Allogen, per cc
Q4213	Ascent, 0.5 mg
Q4214	Cellesta cord, per square centimeter
Q4215	Axolotl ambient or axolotl cryo, 0.1 mg
Q4216	Artacent cord, per square centimeter
Q4217	Woundfix, Biosound, Woundfix plus, biowound plus, Woundfix xplus or biowound xplus, per square centimeter
Q4218	Surgicord, per square centimeter
Q4219	Surgigraft-dual, per square centimeter
Q4220	Bellacell hd or SureDerm, per square centimeter

Q4221 Amniowrap2, per square centimeter

Q4222 Progenamatrix, per square centimeter

▲ Q4225 Amniobind or dermabind tl, per square centimeter

Q4226 Myown skin, includes harvesting and preparation procedures, per square centimeter

Q4236 Carepatch, per square centimeter

Q4237 Cryo-cord, per square centimeter

Q4238 Derm-maxx, per square centimeter

Q4239 Amnio-maxx or amnio-maxx lite, per square centimeter

Q4240 Corecyte, for topical use only, per 0.5 cc

Q4241 Polycyte, for topical use only, per 0.5 cc

Q4242 Amniocyte plus, per 0.5 cc

Q4244 Procenta, per 200 mg

Q4245 Amniotext, per cc

Q4246 Coretext or protext, per cc

Q4247 Amniotext patch, per square centimeter

Q4248 Dermacyte amniotic membrane allograft, per square centimeter

Q4249 Amniply, for topical use only, per square centimeter

Q4250 Amnioamp-mp, per square centimeter

Q4251 Vim, per square centimeter

Q4252 Vendaje, per square centimeter

Q4253 Zenith amniotic membrane, per square centimeter

Q4254 Novafix dl, per square centimeter

Q4255 Reguard, for topical use only, per square centimeter

Q4256 Mlg-complete, per square centimeter

Q4257 Relese, per square centimeter

Q4258 Enverse, per square centimeter

Q4259 Celera dual layer or celera dual membrane, per square centimeter

Q4260 Signature apatch, per square centimeter

Q4261 Tag, per square centimeter

Q4262 Dual layer impax membrane, per square centimeter

Q4263 Surgraft tl, per square centimeter

Q4264 Cocoon membrane, per square centimeter

● Q4279 Vendaje ac, per square centimeter

● Q4287 Dermabind dl, per square centimeter

● Q4288 Dermabind ch, per square centimeter

● Q4289 Revoshield + amniotic barrier, per square centimeter

● Q4290 Membrane wrap-hydro, per square centimeter

- • **Q4291** Lamellas xt, per square centimeter
- • **Q4292** Lamellas, per square centimeter
- • **Q4293** Acesso dl, per square centimeter
- • **Q4294** Amnio quad-core, per square centimeter
- • **Q4295** Amnio tri-core amniotic, per square centimeter
- • **Q4296** Rebound matrix, per square centimeter
- • **Q4297** Emerge matrix, per square centimeter
- • **Q4298** Amnicore pro, per square centimeter
- • **Q4299** Amnicore pro+, per square centimeter
- • **Q4300** Acesso tl, per square centimeter
- • **Q4301** Activate matrix, per square centimeter
- • **Q4302** Complete aca, per square centimeter
- • **Q4303** Complete aa, per square centimeter
- • **Q4304** Grafix plus, per square centimeter

Hospice or Home Health Care

Q5001 Hospice or home health care provided in patient's home/residence

Q5002 Hospice or home health care provided in assisted living facility

Q5003 Hospice care provided in nursing long term care facility (LTC) or non-skilled nursing facility (NF)

Q5004 Hospice care provided in skilled nursing facility (SNF)

Q5005 Hospice care provided in inpatient hospital

Q5006 Hospice care provided in inpatient hospice facility

Q5007 Hospice care provided in long term care facility

Q5008 Hospice care provided in inpatient psychiatric facility

Q5009 Hospice or home health care provided in place not otherwise specified (nos)

Q5010 Hospice home care provided in a hospice facility

Miscellaneous and Osmolar Contrast Material

Q5101 Injection, filgrastim-sndz, biosimilar, (zarxio), 1 microgram

Q5103 Injection, infliximab-dyyb, biosimilar, (inflectra), 10 mg

Q5104 Injection, infliximab-abda, biosimilar, (renflexis), 10 mg

Q5105 Injection, epoetin alfa-epbx, biosimilar, (retacrit) (for ESRD on dialysis), 100 units

Q5106 Injection, epoetin alfa-epbx, biosimilar, (retacrit) (for non-ESRD use), 1000 units

Q5107 Injection, bevacizumab-awwb, biosimilar, (mvasi), 10 mg

Q5108 Injection, pegfilgrastim-jmdb, biosimilar, (fulphila), 0.5 mg

Q5109 Injection, infliximab-qbtx, biosimilar, (ixifi), 10 mg

Q5110 Injection, filgrastim-aafi, biosimilar, (nivestym), 1 microgram

Q5112 Injection, trastuzumab-dttb, biosimilar, (ontruzant), 10 mg

Q5113 Injection, trastuzumab-pkrb, biosimilar, (Herzuma), 10 mg

Q5115 Injection, rituximab-abbs, biosimilar, (truxima), 10 mg

Q5116 Injection, trastuzumab-qyyp, biosimilar, (trazimera), 10 mg

Q5117 Injection, trastuzumab-anns, biosimilar, (kanjinti), 10 mg

Q5118 Injection, bevacizumab-bvzr, biosimilar, (zirabev), 10 mg

Q5122 Injection, pegfilgrastim-apgf, biosimilar, (nyvepria), 0.5 mg

Q5126 Injection, bevacizumab-maly, biosimilar, (alymsys), 10 mg

• Q5132 Injection, adalimumab-afzb (abrilada), biosimilar, 10 mg

Q9001 Assessment by chaplain services

Q9002 Counseling, individual, by chaplain services

Q9003 Counseling, group, by chaplain services

Q9004 Department of veterans affairs whole health partner services

Q9950 Injection, sulfur hexafluoride lipid microspheres, per ml

Q9951 Low osmolar contrast material, 400 or greater mg/ml iodine concentration, per ml

Q9953 Injection, iron-based magnetic resonance contrast agent, per ml

Q9954 Oral magnetic resonance contrast agent, per 100 ml

Q9955 Injection, perflexane lipid microspheres, per ml

Q9956 Injection, octafluoropropane microspheres, per ml

Q9957 Injection, perflutren lipid microspheres, per ml

Q9958 High osmolar contrast material, up to 149 mg/ml iodine concentration, per ml

Q9959 High osmolar contrast material, 150-199 mg/ml iodine concentration, per ml

Q9960 High osmolar contrast material, 200-249 mg/ml iodine concentration, per ml

Q9961 High osmolar contrast material, 250-299 mg/ml iodine concentration, per ml

Q9962 High osmolar contrast material, 300-349 mg/ml iodine concentration, per ml

Q9963 High osmolar contrast material, 350-399 mg/ml iodine concentration, per ml

Q9964 High osmolar contrast material, 400 or greater mg/ml iodine concentration, per ml

Q9965 Low osmolar contrast material, 100-199 mg/ml iodine concentration, per ml

Q9966 Low osmolar contrast material, 200-299 mg/ml iodine concentration, per ml

Q9967 Low osmolar contrast material, 300-399 mg/ml iodine concentration, per ml

Q9968 Injection, non-radioactive, non-contrast, visualization adjunct (e.g., methylene blue, isosulfan blue), 1 mg

Q9969 Tc-99m from non-highly enriched uranium source, full cost recovery add-on, per study dose

Q9970 Injection, ferric carboxymaltose, 1mg

Q9972 Injection, epoetin beta, 1 microgram, (for ESRD on dialysis)

Q9973 Injection, epoetin beta, 1 microgram, (non-ESRD use)

Q9974 Injection, morphine sulfate, preservative-free for epidural or intrathecal use, 10 mg

Q9975 Injection, factor viii fc fusion protein (recombinant), per iu

Q9976	Injection, ferric pyrophosphate citrate solution, 0.1 mg of iron
Q9977	Compounded drug, not otherwise classified
Q9978	Netupitant 300 mg and palonosetron 0.5 mg
Q9979	Injection, alemtuzumab, 1 mg
Q9980	Hyaluronan or derivative, genvisc 850, for intra-articular injection, 1 mg
Q9981	Rolapitant, oral, 1 mg
Q9982	Flutemetamol f18, diagnostic, per study dose, up to 5 millicuries
Q9983	Florbetaben f18, diagnostic, per study dose, up to 8.1 millicuries
Q9984	Levonorgestrel-releasing intrauterine contraceptive system (kyleena), 19.5 mg
Q9985	Injection, hydroxyprogesterone caproate, not otherwise specified, 10 mg
Q9986	Injection, hydroxyprogesterone caproate, (Makena), 10 mg
Q9987	Pathogen(s) test for platelets
Q9988	Platelets, pheresis, pathogen-reduced, each unit
Q9989	Ustekinumab, for intravenous injection, 1 mg
Q9991	Injection, buprenorphine extended-release (sublocade), less than or equal to 100 mg
Q9992	Injection, buprenorphine extended-release (sublocade), greater than 100 mg
Q9993	Injection, triamcinolone acetonide, preservative-free, extended-release, microsphere formulation, 1 mg
Q9994	In-line cartridge containing digestive enzyme(s) for enteral feeding, each
Q9995	Injection, emicizumab-kxwh, 0.5 mg

DIAGNOSTIC RADIOLOGY SERVICES

Guidelines

In addition to the information presented in the INTRODUCTION, several other items unique to this section are defined or identified here:

1. **SPECIAL REPORT:** A service, material or supply that is rarely provided, unusual, variable or new may require a special report in determining medical appropriateness for reimbursement purposes. Pertinent information should include an adequate definition or description of the nature, extent, and need for the service, material or supply.

2. **MODIFIERS:** Listed services may be modified under certain circumstances. When appropriate, the modifying circumstance is identified by adding a modifier to the basic procedure code. CPT and HCPCS National Level II modifiers may be used with CPT and HCPCS National Level II procedure codes. Modifiers commonly used with DIAGNOSTIC RADIOLOGY SERVICES are as follows:

   -CC Procedure code change (use "CC" when the procedure code submitted was changed either for administrative reasons or because an incorrect code was filed)

   -LT Left side (used to identify procedures performed on the left side of the body)

   -RT Right side (used to identify procedures performed on the right side of the body)

   -TC Technical component. Under certain circumstances, a charge may be made for the technical component alone. Under those circumstances, the technical component charge is identified by adding modifier -TC to the usual procedure number. Technical component charges are institutional charges and are not billed separately by physicians. However, portable x-ray suppliers bill only for the technical component and should use modifier -TC. The charge data from portable x-ray suppliers will then be used to build customary and prevailing profiles.

3. **CPT CODE CROSS-REFERENCE:** There are no equivalent CPT codes for procedures listed in this section.

Diagnostic Radiology Services

R0070 Transportation of portable x-ray equipment and personnel to home or nursing home, per trip to facility or location, one patient seen

R0075 Transportation of portable x-ray equipment and personnel to home or nursing home, per trip to facility or location, more than one patient seen

R0076 Transportation of portable EKG to facility or location, per patient

PRIVATE PAYER CODES

Guidelines

HCPCS "S" codes are temporary national codes established by the private payers for private payer use. Prior to using "S" codes on insurance claims to private payers, you should consult with the payer to confirm that the "S" codes are acceptable. "S" codes are not valid for Medicare use.

In addition to the information presented in the INTRODUCTION, several other items unique to this section are defined or identified here.

1. **SPECIAL REPORT:** A service, material or supply that is rarely provided, unusual, variable or new may require a special report in determining medical appropriateness for reimbursement purposes. Pertinent information should include an adequate definition or description of the nature, extent, and need for the service, material or supply.

2. **MODIFIERS:** Listed services may be modified under certain circumstances. When appropriate, the modifying circumstance is identified by adding a modifier to the basic procedure code. CPT and HCPCS National Level II modifiers may be used with CPT and HCPCS National Level II procedure codes.

Private Payer Codes

S0012 Butorphanol tartrate, nasal spray, 25 mg

S0013 Esketamine, nasal spray, 1 mg

S0014 Tacrine hydrochloride, 10 mg

S0017 Injection, aminocaproic acid, 5 grams

S0020 Injection, Bupivicaine hydrochloride, 30 ml

S0021 Injection, cefoperazone sodium, 1 gram

S0023 Injection, cimetidine hydrochloride, 300 mg

S0028 Injection, famotidine, 20 mg

S0030 Injection, metronidazole, 500 mg

S0032 Injection, nafcillin sodium, 2 grams

S0034 Injection, ofloxacin, 400 mg

S0039 Injection, sulfamethoxazole and trimethoprim, 10 ml

S0040 Injection, ticarcillin disodium and clavulanate potassium, 3.1 grams

S0073 Injection, aztreonam, 500 mg

S0074 Injection, cefotetan disodium, 500 mg

S0077 Injection, clindamycin phosphate, 300 mg

S0078 Injection, fosphenytoin sodium, 750 mg

S0080 Injection, pentamidine isethionate, 300 mg

S0081 Injection, piperacillin sodium, 500 mg

S0088 Imatinib, 100 mg

S0090 Sildenafil citrate, 25 mg

S0091 Granisetron hydrochloride, 1 mg (for circumstances falling under the Medicare statute, use Q0166)

S0092 Injection, hydromorphone hydrochloride, 250 mg (loading dose for infusion pump)

S0093 Injection, morphine sulfate, 500 mg (loading dose for infusion pump)

S0104 Zidovudine, oral, 100 mg

S0106 Bupropion HCL sustained release tablet, 150 mg, per bottle of 60 tablets

S0108 Mercaptopurine, oral, 50 mg

S0109 Methadone, oral, 5 mg

S0117 Tretinoin, topical, 5 grams

S0119 Ondansetron, oral, 4 mg (for circumstances falling under the Medicare statute, use HCPCS q code)

S0122 Injection, menotropins, 75 iu

S0126 Injection, follitropin alfa, 75 iu

S0128 Injection, follitropin beta, 75 iu

S0132 Injection, ganirelix acetate, 250 mcg

S0136 Clozapine, 25 mg

S0137 Didanosine (DDI), 25 mg

S0138 Finasteride, 5 mg

S0139 Minoxidil, 10 mg

S0140 Saquinavir, 200 mg

S0142 Colistimethate sodium, inhalation solution administered through DME, concentrated form, per mg

S0145 Injection, pegylated interferon alfa-2a, 180 mcg per ml

S0148 Injection, pegylated interferon alfa-2b, 10 mcg

S0155 Sterile dilutant for epoprostenol, 50 ml

S0156 Exemestane, 25 mg

S0157 Becaplermin gel 0.01%, 0.5 gm

S0160 Dextroamphetamine sulfate, 5 mg

S0164 Injection, pantoprazole sodium, 40 mg

(S0166 Injection, olanzapine, 2.5 mg

Code deleted effective 12/31/2023, no HCPCS/CPT cross-reference provided.)

S0169 Calcitrol, 0.25 microgram

S0170 Anastrozole, oral, 1 mg

(S0171 Injection, bumetanide, 0.5 mg

Code deleted effective 12/31/2023, no HCPCS/CPT cross-reference provided.)

S0172 Chlorambucil, oral, 2 mg

S0174 Dolasetron mesylate, oral 50 mg (for circumstances falling under the Medicare statute, use Q0180)

S0175 Flutamide, oral, 125 mg

S0176 Hydroxyurea, oral, 500 mg

S0177	Levamisole hydrochloride, oral, 50 mg
S0178	Lomustine, oral, 10 mg
S0179	Megestrol acetate, oral, 20 mg
S0182	Procarbazine hydrochloride, oral, 50 mg
S0183	Prochlorperazine maleate, oral, 5 mg (for circumstances falling under the Medicare statute, use Q0164)
S0187	Tamoxifen citrate, oral, 10 mg
S0189	Testosterone pellet, 75 mg
S0190	Mifepristone, oral, 200 mg
S0191	Misoprostol, oral, 200 mcg
S0194	Dialysis/stress vitamin supplement, oral, 100 capsules
S0197	Prenatal vitamins, 30-day supply
S0199	Medically induced abortion by oral ingestion of medication including all associated services and supplies (e.g., patient counseling, office visits, confirmation of pregnancy by hCG, ultrasound to confirm duration of pregnancy, ultrasound to confirm completion of abortion) except drugs
S0201	Partial hospitalization services, less than 24 hours, per diem
S0207	Paramedic intercept, non-hospital-based ALS service (non-voluntary), non-transport
S0208	Paramedic intercept, hospital-based ALS service (non-voluntary), non-transport
S0209	Wheelchair van, mileage, per mile
S0215	Non-emergency transportation; mileage, per mile
S0220	Medical conference by a physician with interdisciplinary team of health professionals or representatives of community agencies to coordinate activities of patient care (patient is present); approximately 30 minutes
S0221	Medical conference by a physician with interdisciplinary team of health professionals or representatives of community agencies to coordinate activities of patient care (patient is present); approximately 60 minutes
S0250	Comprehensive geriatric assessment and treatment planning performed by assessment team
S0255	Hospice referral visit (advising patient and family of care options) performed by nurse, social worker, or other designated staff
S0257	Counseling and discussion regarding advance directives or end of life care planning and decisions, with patient and/or surrogate (list separately in addition to code for appropriate evaluation and management service)
S0260	History and physical (outpatient or office) related to surgical procedure (list separately in addition to code for appropriate evaluation and management service)
S0265	Genetic counseling, under physician supervision, each 15 minutes
S0270	Physician management of patient home care, standard monthly case rate (per 30 days)
S0271	Physician management of patient home care, hospice monthly case rate (per 30 days)
S0272	Physician management of patient home care, episodic care monthly case rate (per 30 days)
S0274	Nurse practitioner visit at member's home, outside of a capitation arrangement
S0280	Medical home program, comprehensive care coordination and planning, initial plan
S0281	Medical home program, comprehensive care coordination and planning, maintenance of plan

Q - R - S CODES

S0302	Completed early periodic screening diagnosis and treatment (EPSDT) service (list in addition to code for appropriate evaluation and management service)
S0310	Hospitalist services (list separately in addition to code for appropriate evaluation and management service)
S0311	Comprehensive management and care coordination for advanced illness, per calendar month
S0315	Disease management program; initial assessment and initiation of the program
S0316	Disease management program, follow-up/reassessment
S0317	Disease management program; per diem
S0320	Telephone calls by a registered nurse to a disease management program member for monitoring purposes; per month
S0340	Lifestyle modification program for management of coronary artery disease, including all supportive services; first quarter / stage
S0341	Lifestyle modification program for management of coronary artery disease, including all supportive services; second or third quarter / stage
S0342	Lifestyle modification program for management of coronary artery disease, including all supportive services; fourth quarter / stage
S0353	Treatment planning and care coordination management for cancer, initial treatment
S0354	Treatment planning and care coordination management for cancer, established patient with a change of regimen
S0390	Routine foot care; removal and/or trimming of corns, calluses and/or nails and preventive maintenance in specific medical conditions (e.g., diabetes), per visit
S0395	Impression casting of a foot performed by a practitioner other than the manufacturer of the orthotic
S0400	Global fee for extracorporeal shock wave lithotripsy treatment of kidney stone(s)
S0500	Disposable contact lens, per lens
S0504	Single vision prescription lens (safety, athletic, or sunglass), per lens
S0506	Bifocal vision prescription lens (safety, athletic, or sunglass), per lens
S0508	Trifocal vision prescription lens (safety, athletic, or sunglass), per lens
S0510	Non-prescription lens (safety, athletic, or sunglass), per lens
S0512	Daily wear specialty contact lens, per lens
S0514	Color contact lens, per lens
S0515	Scleral lens, liquid bandage device, per lens
S0516	Safety eyeglass frames
S0518	Sunglasses frames
S0580	Polycarbonate lens (list this code in addition to the basic code for the lens)
S0581	Nonstandard lens (list this code in addition to the basic code for the lens)
S0590	Integral lens service, miscellaneous services reported separately
S0592	Comprehensive contact lens evaluation
S0595	Dispensing new spectacle lenses for patient supplied frame
S0596	Phakic intraocular lens for correction of refractive error

S0601	Screening proctoscopy
S0610	Annual gynecological examination, new patient
S0612	Annual gynecological examination, established patient
S0613	Annual gynecological examination; clinical breast examination without pelvic evaluation
S0618	Audiometry for hearing aid evaluation to determine the level and degree of hearing loss
S0620	Routine ophthalmological examination including refraction; new patient
S0621	Routine ophthalmological examination including refraction; established patient
S0622	Physical exam for college, new or established patient (list separately in addition to appropriate evaluation and management code)
S0630	Removal of sutures; by a physician other than the physician who originally closed the wound
S0800	Laser in situ keratomileusis (LASIK)
S0810	Photorefractive keratectomy (PRK)
S0812	Phototherapeutic keratectomy (PTK)
S1001	Deluxe item, patient aware (list in addition to code for basic item)
S1002	Customized item (list in addition to code for basic item)
S1015	IV tubing extension set
S1016	Non-PVC (polyvinyl chloride) intravenous administration set, for use with drugs that are not stable in PVC e.g., paclitaxel
S1030	Continuous noninvasive glucose monitoring device, purchase (for physician interpretation of data, use CPT code)
S1031	Continuous noninvasive glucose monitoring device, rental, including sensor, sensor replacement, and download to monitor (for physician interpretation of data, use CPT code)
S1034	Artificial pancreas device system (e.g., low glucose suspend (LGS) feature) including continuous glucose monitor, blood glucose device, insulin pump and computer algorithm that communicates with all of the devices
S1035	Sensor; invasive (e.g., subcutaneous), disposable, for use with artificial pancreas device system
S1036	Transmitter; external, for use with artificial pancreas device system
S1037	Receiver (monitor); external, for use with artificial pancreas device system
S1040	Cranial remolding orthosis, pediatric, rigid, with soft interface material, custom fabricated, includes fitting and adjustment(s)
S2053	Transplantation of small intestine and liver allografts
S2054	Transplantation of multivisceral organs
S2055	Harvesting of donor multivisceral organs, with preparation and maintenance of allografts; from cadaver donor
S2060	Lobar lung transplantation
S2061	Donor lobectomy (lung) for transplantation, living donor
S2065	Simultaneous pancreas kidney transplantation
S2066	Breast reconstruction with gluteal artery perforator (gap) flap, including harvesting of the flap, microvascular transfer, closure of donor site and shaping the flap into a breast, unilateral
S2067	Breast reconstruction of a single breast with "stacked" deep inferior epigastric perforator (DIEP) flap(s)

Q - R - S CODES

and/or gluteal artery perforator (gap) flap(s), including harvesting of the flap(s), microvascular transfer, closure of donor site(s) and shaping the flap into a breast, unilateral

S2068 Breast reconstruction with deep inferior epigastric perforator (DIEP) flap or superficial inferior epigastric artery (siea) flap, including harvesting of the flap, microvascular transfer, closure of donor site and shaping the flap into a breast, unilateral

S2070 Cystourethroscopy, with ureteroscopy and/or pyeloscopy; with endoscopic laser treatment of ureteral calculi (includes ureteral catheterization)

S2079 Laparoscopic esophagomyotomy (Heller type)

S2080 Laser-assisted uvulopalatoplasty (LAUP)

S2083 Adjustment of gastric band diameter via subcutaneous port by injection or aspiration of saline

S2095 Transcatheter occlusion or embolization for tumor destruction, percutaneous, any method, using yttrium-90 microspheres

S2102 Islet cell tissue transplant from pancreas; allogeneic

S2103 Adrenal tissue transplant to brain

S2107 Adoptive immunotherapy i.e., development of specific anti-tumor reactivity (e.g., tumor-infiltrating lymphocyte therapy) per course of treatment

S2112 Arthroscopy, knee, surgical for harvesting of cartilage (chondrocyte cells)

S2115 Osteotomy, periacetabular, with internal fixation

S2117 Arthroereisis, subtalar

S2118 Metal-on-metal total hip resurfacing, including acetabular and femoral components

S2120 Low density lipoprotein (LDL) apheresis using heparin-induced extracorporeal LDL precipitation

S2140 Cord blood harvesting for transplantation, allogeneic

S2142 Cord blood-derived stem-cell transplantation, allogeneic

S2150 Bone marrow or blood-derived stem cells (peripheral or umbilical), allogeneic or autologous, harvesting, transplantation, and related complications; including: pheresis and cell preparation/storage; marrow ablative therapy; drugs, supplies, hospitalization with outpatient follow-up; medical/surgical, diagnostic, emergency, and rehabilitative services; and the number of days of pre-and post-transplant care in the global definition

S2152 Solid organ(s), complete or segmental, single organ or combination of organs; deceased or living donor(s), procurement, transplantation, and related complications; including drugs; supplies; hospitalization with outpatient follow-up; medical/surgical, diagnostic, emergency, and rehabilitative services, and the number of days of pre- and post-transplant care in the global definition

S2202 Echosclerotherapy

S2205 Minimally invasive direct coronary artery bypass surgery involving mini-thoracotomy or mini-sternotomy surgery, performed under direct vision; using arterial graft(s), single coronary arterial graft

S2206 Minimally invasive direct coronary artery bypass surgery involving mini-thoracotomy or mini-sternotomy surgery, performed under direct vision; using arterial graft(s), two coronary arterial grafts

S2207 Minimally invasive direct coronary artery bypass surgery involving mini-thoracotomy or mini-sternotomy surgery, performed under direct vision; using venous graft only, single coronary venous graft

S2208 Minimally invasive direct coronary artery bypass surgery involving mini-thoracotomy or mini-sternotomy surgery, performed under direct vision; using single arterial and venous graft(s), single venous graft

S2209 Minimally invasive direct coronary artery bypass surgery involving mini-thoracotomy or mini-sternotomy surgery, performed under direct vision; using two arterial grafts and single venous graft

S2225 Myringotomy, laser-assisted

S2230 Implantation of magnetic component of semi-implantable hearing device on ossicles in middle ear

S2235 Implantation of auditory brain stem implant

S2260 Induced abortion, 17 to 24 weeks

S2265 Induced abortion, 25 to 28 weeks

S2266 Induced abortion, 29 to 31 weeks

S2267 Induced abortion, 32 weeks or greater

S2300 Arthroscopy, shoulder, surgical; with thermally-induced capsulorrhaphy

S2325 Hip core decompression

S2340 Chemodenervation of abductor muscle(s) of vocal cord

S2341 Chemodenervation of adductor muscle(s) of vocal cord

S2342 Nasal endoscopy for post-operative debridement following functional endoscopic sinus surgery, nasal and/or sinus cavity(s), unilateral or bilateral

S2348 Decompression procedure, percutaneous, of nucleus pulposus of intervertebral disc, using radiofrequency energy, single or multiple levels, lumbar

S2350 Diskectomy, anterior, with decompression of spinal cord and/or nerve root(s), including osteophytectomy; lumbar, single interspace

S2351 Diskectomy, anterior, with decompression of spinal cord and/or nerve root(s), including osteophytectomy; lumbar, each additional interspace (list separately in addition to code for primary procedure)

S2400 Repair, congenital diaphragmatic hernia in the fetus using temporary tracheal occlusion, procedure performed in utero

S2401 Repair, urinary tract obstruction in the fetus, procedure performed in utero

S2402 Repair, congenital cystic adenomatoid malformation in the fetus, procedure performed in utero

S2403 Repair, extralobar pulmonary sequestration in the fetus, procedure performed in utero

S2404 Repair, myelomeningocele in the fetus, procedure performed in utero

S2405 Repair of sacrococcygeal teratoma in the fetus, procedure performed in utero

S2409 Repair, congenital malformation of fetus, procedure performed in utero, not otherwise classified

S2411 Fetoscopic laser therapy for treatment of twin-to-twin transfusion syndrome

S2900 Surgical techniques requiring use of robotic surgical system (list separately in addition to code for primary procedure)

S3000 Diabetic indicator; retinal eye exam, dilated, bilateral

S3005 Performance measurement, evaluation of patient self-assessment, depression

S3600 Stat laboratory request (situations other than S3601)

S3601 Emergency stat laboratory charge for patient who is homebound or residing in a nursing facility

S3620 Newborn metabolic screening panel, includes test kit, postage and the laboratory tests specified by the

Q - R - S CODES

state for inclusion in this panel (e.g., galactose; hemoglobin, electrophoresis; hydroxyprogesterone, 17-d; phenylalanine (PKU); and thyroxine, total)

S3630 Eosinophil count, blood, direct

S3645 HIV-1 antibody testing of oral mucosal transudate

S3650 Saliva test, hormone level; during menopause

S3652 Saliva test, hormone level; to assess preterm labor risk

S3655 Antisperm antibodies test (immunobead)

S3708 Gastrointestinal fat absorption study

S3722 Dose optimization by area under the curve (AUC) analysis, for infusional 5-fluorouracil

S3800 Genetic testing for amyotrophic lateral sclerosis (ALS)

S3840 DNA analysis for germline mutations of the ret proto-oncogene for susceptibility to multiple endocrine neoplasia type 2

S3841 Genetic testing for retinoblastoma

S3842 Genetic testing for von Hippel-Lindau disease

S3844 DNA analysis of the connexin 26 gene (gjb2) for susceptibility to congenital, profound deafness

S3845 Genetic testing for alpha-thalassemia

S3846 Genetic testing for hemoglobin e beta-thalassemia

S3849 Genetic testing for Niemann-pick disease

S3850 Genetic testing for sickle cell anemia

S3852 DNA analysis for apoe epsilon 4 allele for susceptibility to Alzheimer's disease

S3853 Genetic testing for myotonic muscular dystrophy

S3854 Gene expression profiling panel for use in the management of breast cancer treatment

S3861 Genetic testing, sodium channel, voltage-gated, type v, alpha subunit (scn5a) and variants for suspected Brugada syndrome

S3865 Comprehensive gene sequence analysis for hypertrophic cardiomyopathy

S3866 Genetic analysis for a specific gene mutation for hypertrophic cardiomyopathy (HCM) in an individual with a known HCM mutation in the family

S3870 Comparative genomic hybridization (CGH) microarray testing for developmental delay, autism spectrum disorder and/or intellectual disability

S3900 Surface electromyography (EMG)

S3902 Ballistocardiogram

S3904 Masters two step

S4005 Interim labor facility global (labor occurring but not resulting in delivery)

S4011 In vitro fertilization; including but not limited to identification and incubation of mature oocytes, fertilization with sperm, incubation of embryo(s), and subsequent visualization for determination of development

S4013 Complete cycle, gamete intrafallopian transfer (gift), case rate

S4014 Complete cycle, zygote intrafallopian transfer (zift), case rate

S4015 Complete in vitro fertilization cycle, not otherwise specified, case rate

S4016	Frozen in vitro fertilization cycle, case rate
S4017	Incomplete cycle, treatment cancelled prior to stimulation, case rate
S4018	Frozen embryo transfer procedure cancelled before transfer, case rate
S4020	In vitro fertilization procedure cancelled before aspiration, case rate
S4021	In vitro fertilization procedure cancelled after aspiration, case rate
S4022	Assisted oocyte fertilization, case rate
S4023	Donor egg cycle, incomplete, case rate
S4025	Donor services for in vitro fertilization (sperm or embryo), case rate
S4026	Procurement of donor sperm from sperm bank
S4027	Storage of previously frozen embryos
S4028	Microsurgical epididymal sperm aspiration (mesa)
S4030	Sperm procurement and cryopreservation services; initial visit
S4031	Sperm procurement and cryopreservation services; subsequent visit
S4035	Stimulated intrauterine insemination (IUI), case rate
S4037	Cryopreserved embryo transfer, case rate
S4040	Monitoring and storage of cryopreserved embryos, per 30 days
S4042	Management of ovulation induction (interpretation of diagnostic tests and studies, non-face-to-face medical management of the patient), per cycle
S4981	Insertion of levonorgestrel-releasing intrauterine system
S4989	Contraceptive intrauterine device (e.g., Progestasert IUD), including implants and supplies
S4990	Nicotine patches, legend
S4991	Nicotine patches, non-legend
S4993	Contraceptive pills for birth control
S4995	Smoking cessation gum
S5000	Prescription drug, generic
S5001	Prescription drug, brand name
S5010	5% dextrose and 0.45% normal saline, 1000 ml
S5012	5% dextrose with potassium chloride, 1000 ml
S5013	5% dextrose/0.45% normal saline with potassium chloride and magnesium sulfate, 1000 ml
S5014	5% dextrose/0.45% normal saline with potassium chloride and magnesium sulfate, 1500 ml
S5035	Home infusion therapy, routine service of infusion device (e.g., pump maintenance)
S5036	Home infusion therapy, repair of infusion device (e.g., pump repair)
S5100	Day care services, adult; per 15 minutes
S5101	Day care services, adult; per half day
S5102	Day care services, adult; per diem
S5105	Day care services, center-based; services not included in program fee, per diem
S5108	Home care training to home care client, per 15 minutes

S5109 Home care training to home care client, per session

S5110 Home care training, family; per 15 minutes

S5111 Home care training, family; per session

S5115 Home care training, non-family; per 15 minutes

S5116 Home care training, non-family; per session

S5120 Chore services; per 15 minutes

S5121 Chore services; per diem

S5125 Attendant care services; per 15 minutes

S5126 Attendant care services; per diem

S5130 Homemaker service, nos; per 15 minutes

S5131 Homemaker service, nos; per diem

S5135 Companion care, adult (e.g., IADL/ADL); per 15 minutes

S5136 Companion care, adult (e.g., IADL/ADL); per diem

S5140 Foster care, adult; per diem

S5141 Foster care, adult; per month

S5145 Foster care, therapeutic, child; per diem

S5146 Foster care, therapeutic, child; per month

S5150 Unskilled respite care, not hospice; per 15 minutes

S5151 Unskilled respite care, not hospice; per diem

S5160 Emergency response system; installation and testing

S5161 Emergency response system; service fee, per month (excludes installation and testing)

S5162 Emergency response system; purchase only

S5165 Home modifications; per service

S5170 Home delivered meals, including preparation; per meal

S5175 Laundry service, external, professional; per order

S5180 Home health respiratory therapy, initial evaluation

S5181 Home health respiratory therapy, nos, per diem

S5185 Medication reminder service, non-face-to-face; per month

S5190 Wellness assessment, performed by non-physician

S5199 Personal care item, nos, each

S5497 Home infusion therapy, catheter care / maintenance, not otherwise classified; includes administrative services, professional pharmacy services, care coordination, and all necessary supplies and equipment (drugs and nursing visits coded separately), per diem

S5498 Home infusion therapy, catheter care / maintenance, simple (single lumen), includes administrative services, professional pharmacy services, care coordination and all necessary supplies and equipment, (drugs and nursing visits coded separately), per diem

S5501 Home infusion therapy, catheter care / maintenance, complex (more than one lumen), includes administrative services, professional pharmacy services, care coordination, and all necessary supplies and equipment (drugs and nursing visits coded separately), per diem

S5502 Home infusion therapy, catheter care / maintenance, implanted access device, includes administrative services, professional pharmacy services, care coordination and all necessary supplies and equipment, (drugs and nursing visits coded separately), per diem (use this code for interim maintenance of vascular access not currently in use)

S5517 Home infusion therapy, all supplies necessary for restoration of catheter patency or declotting

S5518 Home infusion therapy, all supplies necessary for catheter repair

S5520 Home infusion therapy, all supplies (including catheter) necessary for a peripherally inserted central venous catheter (PICC) line insertion

S5521 Home infusion therapy, all supplies (including catheter) necessary for a midline catheter insertion

S5522 Home infusion therapy, insertion of peripherally inserted central venous catheter (PICC), nursing services only (no supplies or catheter included)

S5523 Home infusion therapy, insertion of midline venous catheter, nursing services only (no supplies or catheter included)

S5550 Insulin, rapid onset, 5 units

S5551 Insulin, most rapid onset (lispro or aspart); 5 units

S5552 Insulin, intermediate acting (NPH or lente); 5 units

S5553 Insulin, long acting; 5 units

S5560 Insulin delivery device, reusable pen; 1.5 ml size

S5561 Insulin delivery device, reusable pen; 3 ml size

S5565 Insulin cartridge for use in insulin delivery device other than pump; 150 units

S5566 Insulin cartridge for use in insulin delivery device other than pump; 300 units

S5570 Insulin delivery device, disposable pen (including insulin); 1.5 ml size

S5571 Insulin delivery device, disposable pen (including insulin); 3 ml size

S8030 Scleral application of tantalum ring(s) for localization of lesions for proton beam therapy

S8035 Magnetic source imaging

S8037 Magnetic resonance cholangiopancreatography (MRCP)

S8040 Topographic brain mapping

S8042 Magnetic resonance imaging (MRI), low-field

S8055 Ultrasound guidance for multifetal pregnancy reduction(s), technical component (only to be used when the physician doing the reduction procedure does not perform the ultrasound, guidance is included in the CPT code for multifetal pregnancy reduction - 59866)

S8080 Scintimammography (radioimmunoscintigraphy of the breast), unilateral, including supply of radiopharmaceutical

S8085 Fluorine-18 fluorodeoxyglucose (f-18 FDG) imaging using dual-head coincidence detection system (non-dedicated pet scan)

S8092 Electron beam computed tomography (ALSo known as ultrafast CT, cine CT)

S8096 Portable peak flow meter

S8097 Asthma kit (including but not limited to portable peak expiratory flow meter, instructional video, brochure, and/or spacer)

S8100 Holding chamber or spacer for use with an inhaler or nebulizer; without mask

S8101	Holding chamber or spacer for use with an inhaler or nebulizer; with mask
S8110	Peak expiratory flow rate (physician services)
S8120	Oxygen contents, gaseous, 1 unit equals 1 cubic foot
S8121	Oxygen contents, liquid, 1 unit equals 1 pound
S8130	Interferential current stimulator, 2 channel
S8131	Interferential current stimulator, 4 channel
S8185	Flutter device
S8186	Swivel adapter
S8189	Tracheostomy supply, not otherwise classified
S8210	Mucus trap
S8265	Haberman feeder for cleft lip/palate
S8270	Enuresis alarm, using auditory buzzer and/or vibration device
S8301	Infection control supplies, not otherwise specified
S8415	Supplies for home delivery of infant
S8420	Gradient pressure aid (sleeve and glove combination), custom made
S8421	Gradient pressure aid (sleeve and glove combination), ready made
S8422	Gradient pressure aid (sleeve), custom made, medium weight
S8423	Gradient pressure aid (sleeve), custom made, heavy weight
S8424	Gradient pressure aid (sleeve), ready made
S8425	Gradient pressure aid (glove), custom made, medium weight
S8426	Gradient pressure aid (glove), custom made, heavy weight
S8427	Gradient pressure aid (glove), ready made
S8428	Gradient pressure aid (gauntlet), ready made
S8429	Gradient pressure exterior wrap
S8430	Padding for compression bandage, roll
S8431	Compression bandage, roll
S8450	Splint, prefabricated, digit (specify digit by use of modifier)
S8451	Splint, prefabricated, wrist or ankle
S8452	Splint, prefabricated, elbow
S8460	Camisole, post-mastectomy
S8490	Insulin syringes (100 syringes, any size)
S8930	Electrical stimulation of auricular acupuncture points; each 15 minutes of personal one-on-one contact with the patient
S8940	Equestrian/hippotherapy, per session
S8948	Application of a modality (requiring constant provider attendance) to one or more areas; low-level laser; each 15 minutes
S8950	Complex lymphedema therapy, each 15 minutes
S8990	Physical or manipulative therapy performed for maintenance rather than restoration

S8999 Resuscitation bag (for use by patient on artificial respiration during power failure or other catastrophic event)

S9001 Home uterine monitor with or without associated nursing services

S9007 Ultrafiltration monitor

S9024 Paranasal sinus ultrasound

S9025 Omnicardiogram/cardiointegram

S9034 Extracorporeal shockwave lithotripsy for gall stones (if performed with ERCP, use 43265)

S9055 Procuren or other growth factor preparation to promote wound healing

S9056 Coma stimulation per diem

S9061 Home administration of aerosolized drug therapy (e.g., pentamidine); administrative services, professional pharmacy services, care coordination, all necessary supplies and equipment (drugs and nursing visits coded separately), per diem

S9083 Global fee urgent care centers

S9088 Services provided in an urgent care center (list in addition to code for service)

S9090 Vertebral axial decompression, per session

S9097 Home visit for wound care

S9098 Home visit, phototherapy services (e.g., bili-lite), including equipment rental, nursing services, blood draw, supplies, and other services, per diem

S9110 Telemonitoring of patient in their home, including all necessary equipment; computer system, connections, and software; maintenance; patient education and support; per month

S9117 Back school, per visit

S9122 Home health aide or certified nurse assistant, providing care in the home; per hour

S9123 Nursing care, in the home; by registered nurse, per hour (use for general nursing care only, not to be used when CPT codes 99500-99602 can be used)

S9124 Nursing care, in the home; by licensed practical nurse, per hour

S9125 Respite care, in the home, per diem

S9126 Hospice care, in the home, per diem

S9127 Social work visit, in the home, per diem

S9128 Speech therapy, in the home, per diem

S9129 Occupational therapy, in the home, per diem

S9131 Physical therapy; in the home, per diem

S9140 Diabetic management program, follow-up visit to non-md provider

S9141 Diabetic management program, follow-up visit to md provider

S9145 Insulin pump initiation, instruction in initial use of pump (pump not included)

S9150 Evaluation by ocularist

S9152 Speech therapy, re-evaluation

S9208 Home management of preterm labor, including administrative services, professional pharmacy services, care coordination, and all necessary supplies or equipment (drugs and nursing visits coded separately), per diem (do not use this code with any home infusion per diem code)

S9209 Home management of preterm premature rupture of membranes (PPROM), including administrative services, professional pharmacy services, care coordination, and all necessary supplies or equipment (drugs and nursing visits coded separately), per diem (do not use this code with any home infusion per diem code)

S9211 Home management of gestational hypertension, includes administrative services, professional pharmacy services, care coordination and all necessary supplies and equipment (drugs and nursing visits coded separately); per diem (do not use this code with any home infusion per diem code)

S9212 Home management of postpartum hypertension, includes administrative services, professional pharmacy services, care coordination, and all necessary supplies and equipment (drugs and nursing visits coded separately), per diem (do not use this code with any home infusion per diem code)

S9213 Home management of preeclampsia, includes administrative services, professional pharmacy services, care coordination, and all necessary supplies and equipment (drugs and nursing services coded separately); per diem (do not use this code with any home infusion per diem code)

S9214 Home management of gestational diabetes, includes administrative services, professional pharmacy services, care coordination, and all necessary supplies and equipment (drugs and nursing visits coded separately); per diem (do not use this code with any home infusion per diem code)

S9325 Home infusion therapy, pain management infusion; administrative services, professional pharmacy services, care coordination, and all necessary supplies and equipment, (drugs and nursing visits coded separately), per diem (do not use this code with S9326, S9327 or S9328)

S9326 Home infusion therapy, continuous (twenty-four hours or more) pain management infusion; administrative services, professional pharmacy services, care coordination and all necessary supplies and equipment (drugs and nursing visits coded separately), per diem

S9327 Home infusion therapy, intermittent (less than twenty-four hours) pain management infusion; administrative services, professional pharmacy services, care coordination, and all necessary supplies and equipment (drugs and nursing visits coded separately), per diem

S9328 Home infusion therapy, implanted pump pain management infusion; administrative services, professional pharmacy services, care coordination, and all necessary supplies and equipment (drugs and nursing visits coded separately), per diem

S9329 Home infusion therapy, chemotherapy infusion; administrative services, professional pharmacy services, care coordination, and all necessary supplies and equipment (drugs and nursing visits coded separately), per diem (do not use this code with S9330 or S9331)

S9330 Home infusion therapy, continuous (twenty-four hours or more) chemotherapy infusion; administrative services, professional pharmacy services, care coordination, and all necessary supplies and equipment (drugs and nursing visits coded separately), per diem

S9331 Home infusion therapy, intermittent (less than twenty-four hours) chemotherapy infusion; administrative services, professional pharmacy services, care coordination, and all necessary supplies and equipment (drugs and nursing visits coded separately), per diem

S9335 Home therapy, hemodialysis; administrative services, professional pharmacy services, care coordination, and all necessary supplies and equipment (drugs and nursing services coded separately), per diem

S9336 Home infusion therapy, continuous anticoagulant infusion therapy (e.g., heparin), administrative services, professional pharmacy services, care coordination and all necessary supplies and equipment (drugs and nursing visits coded separately), per diem

S9338 Home infusion therapy, immunotherapy, administrative services, professional pharmacy services, care coordination, and all necessary supplies and equipment (drugs and nursing visits coded separately), per diem

S9339 Home therapy; peritoneal dialysis, administrative services, professional pharmacy services, care coordination and all necessary supplies and equipment (drugs and nursing visits coded separately), per diem

S9340 Home therapy; enteral nutrition; administrative services, professional pharmacy services, care coordination, and all necessary supplies and equipment (enteral formula and nursing visits coded separately), per diem

S9341 Home therapy; enteral nutrition via gravity; administrative services, professional pharmacy services, care coordination, and all necessary supplies and equipment (enteral formula and nursing visits coded separately), per diem

S9342 Home therapy; enteral nutrition via pump; administrative services, professional pharmacy services, care coordination, and all necessary supplies and equipment (enteral formula and nursing visits coded separately), per diem

S9343 Home therapy; enteral nutrition via bolus; administrative services, professional pharmacy services, care coordination, and all necessary supplies and equipment (enteral formula and nursing visits coded separately), per diem

S9345 Home infusion therapy, anti-hemophilic agent infusion therapy (e.g., factor viii); administrative services, professional pharmacy services, care coordination, and all necessary supplies and equipment (drugs and nursing visits coded separately), per diem

S9346 Home infusion therapy, alpha-1-proteinase inhibitor (e.g., Prolastin); administrative services, professional pharmacy services, care coordination, and all necessary supplies and equipment (drugs and nursing visits coded separately), per diem

S9347 Home infusion therapy, uninterrupted, long-term, controlled rate intravenous or subcutaneous infusion therapy (e.g., epoprostenol); administrative services, professional pharmacy services, care coordination, and all necessary supplies and equipment (drugs and nursing visits coded separately), per diem

S9348 Home infusion therapy, sympathomimetic/inotropic agent infusion therapy (e.g., dobutamine); administrative services, professional pharmacy services, care coordination, all necessary supplies and equipment (drugs and nursing visits coded separately), per diem

S9349 Home infusion therapy, tocolytic infusion therapy; administrative services, professional pharmacy services, care coordination, and all necessary supplies and equipment (drugs and nursing visits coded separately), per diem

S9351 Home infusion therapy, continuous or intermittent anti-emetic infusion therapy; administrative services, professional pharmacy services, care coordination, and all necessary supplies and equipment (drugs and visits coded separately), per diem

S9353 Home infusion therapy, continuous insulin infusion therapy; administrative services, professional pharmacy services, care coordination, and all necessary supplies and equipment (drugs and nursing visits coded separately), per diem

S9355 Home infusion therapy, chelation therapy; administrative services, professional pharmacy services, care coordination, and all necessary

S9357 Home infusion therapy, enzyme replacement intravenous therapy; (e.g., imiglucerase); administrative services, professional pharmacy services, care coordination, and all necessary supplies and equipment (drugs and nursing visits coded separately), per diem

S9359 Home infusion therapy, anti-tumor necrosis factor intravenous therapy; (e.g., infliximab); administrative services, professional pharmacy services, care coordination, and all necessary supplies and equipment (drugs and nursing visits coded separately), per diem

S9361 Home infusion therapy, diuretic intravenous therapy; administrative services, professional pharmacy services, care coordination, and all necessary supplies and equipment (drugs and nursing visits coded separately), per diem

S9363 Home infusion therapy, anti-spasmotic therapy; administrative services, professional pharmacy services, care coordination, and all necessary supplies and equipment (drugs and nursing visits coded separately), per diem

S9364 Home infusion therapy, total parenteral nutrition (TPN); administrative services, professional pharmacy services, care coordination, and all necessary supplies and equipment including standard TPN formula (lipids, specialty amino acid formulas, drugs other than in standard formula and nursing visits coded separately), per diem (do not use with home infusion codes S9365-S9368 using daily volume scales)

S9365 Home infusion therapy, total parenteral nutrition (TPN); one liter per day, administrative services, professional pharmacy services, care coordination, and all necessary supplies and equipment including standard TPN formula (lipids, specialty amino acid formulas, drugs other than in standard formula and nursing visits coded separately), per diem

S9366 Home infusion therapy, total parenteral nutrition (TPN); more than one liter but no more than two liters per day, administrative services, professional pharmacy services, care coordination, and all necessary supplies and equipment including standard TPN formula (lipids, specialty amino acid formulas, drugs other than in standard formula and nursing visits coded separately), per diem

S9367 Home infusion therapy, total parenteral nutrition (TPN); more than two liters but no more than three liters per day, administrative services, professional pharmacy services, care coordination, and all necessary supplies and equipment including standard TPN formula (lipids, specialty amino acid formulas, drugs other than in standard formula and nursing visits coded separately), per diem

S9368 Home infusion therapy, total parenteral nutrition (TPN); more than three liters per day, administrative services, professional pharmacy services, care coordination, and all necessary supplies and equipment including standard TPN formula (lipids, specialty amino acid formulas, drugs other than in standard formula and nursing visits coded separately), per diem

S9370 Home therapy, intermittent anti-emetic injection therapy; administrative services, professional pharmacy services, care coordination, and all necessary supplies and equipment (drugs and nursing visits coded separately), per diem

S9372 Home therapy; intermittent anticoagulant injection therapy (e.g., heparin); administrative services, professional pharmacy services, care coordination, and all necessary supplies and equipment (drugs and nursing visits coded separately), per diem (do not use this code for flushing of infusion devices with heparin to maintain patency)

S9373 Home infusion therapy, hydration therapy; administrative services, professional pharmacy services, care coordination, and all necessary supplies and equipment (drugs and nursing visits coded separately), per diem (do not use with hydration therapy codes S9374-S9377 using daily volume scales)

S9374 Home infusion therapy, hydration therapy; one liter per day, administrative services, professional pharmacy services, care coordination, and all necessary supplies and equipment (drugs and nursing visits coded separately), per diem

S9375 Home infusion therapy, hydration therapy; more than one liter but no more than two liters per day, administrative services, professional pharmacy services, care coordination, and all necessary supplies and equipment (drugs and nursing visits coded separately), per diem

S9376 Home infusion therapy, hydration therapy; more than two liters but no more than three liters per day, administrative services, professional pharmacy services, care coordination, and all necessary supplies and equipment (drugs and nursing visits coded separately), per diem

S9377 Home infusion therapy, hydration therapy; more than three liters per day, administrative services, professional pharmacy services, care coordination, and all necessary supplies (drugs and nursing visits coded separately), per diem

S9379 Home infusion therapy, infusion therapy, not otherwise classified; administrative services, professional pharmacy services, care coordination, and all necessary supplies and equipment (drugs and nursing visits coded separately), per diem

S9381 Delivery or service to high risk areas requiring escort or extra protection, per visit

S9401	Anticoagulation clinic, inclusive of all services except laboratory tests, per session
S9430	Pharmacy compounding and dispensing services
S9433	Medical food nutritionally complete, administered orally, providing 100% of nutritional intake
S9434	Modified solid food supplements for inborn errors of metabolism
S9435	Medical foods for inborn errors of metabolism
S9436	Childbirth preparation/Lamaze classes, non-physician provider, per session
S9437	Childbirth refresher classes, non-physician provider, per session
S9438	Cesarean birth classes, non-physician provider, per session
S9439	VBAC (vaginal birth after cesarean) classes, non-physician provider, per session
S9441	Asthma education, non-physician provider, per session
S9442	Birthing classes, non-physician provider, per session
S9443	Lactation classes, non-physician provider, per session
S9444	Parenting classes, non-physician provider, per session
S9445	Patient education, not otherwise classified, non-physician provider, individual, per session
S9446	Patient education, not otherwise classified, non-physician provider, group, per session
S9447	Infant safety (including CPR) classes, non-physician provider, per session
S9449	Weight management classes, non-physician provider, per session
S9451	Exercise classes, non-physician provider, per session
S9452	Nutrition classes, non-physician provider, per session
S9453	Smoking cessation classes, non-physician provider, per session
S9454	Stress management classes, non-physician provider, per session
S9455	Diabetic management program, group session
S9460	Diabetic management program, nurse visit
S9465	Diabetic management program, dietitian visit
S9470	Nutritional counseling, dietitian visit
S9472	Cardiac rehabilitation program, non-physician provider, per diem
S9473	Pulmonary rehabilitation program, non-physician provider, per diem
S9474	Enterostomal therapy by a registered nurse certified in enterostomal therapy, per diem
S9475	Ambulatory setting substance abuse treatment or detoxification services, per diem
S9476	Vestibular rehabilitation program, non-physician provider, per diem
S9480	Intensive outpatient psychiatric services, per diem
S9482	Family stabilization services, per 15 minutes
S9484	Crisis intervention mental health services, per hour
S9485	Crisis intervention mental health services, per diem
S9490	Home infusion therapy, corticosteroid infusion; administrative services, professional pharmacy services, care coordination, and all necessary supplies and equipment (drugs and nursing visits coded separately), per diem

S9494 Home infusion therapy, antibiotic, antiviral, or antifungal therapy; administrative services, professional pharmacy services, care coordination, and all necessary supplies and equipment (drugs and nursing visits coded separately), per diem (do not use this code with home infusion codes for hourly dosing schedules S9497-S9504)

S9497 Home infusion therapy, antibiotic, antiviral, or antifungal therapy; once every 3 hours; administrative services, professional pharmacy services, care coordination, and all necessary supplies and equipment (drugs and nursing visits coded separately), per diem

S9500 Home infusion therapy, antibiotic, antiviral, or antifungal therapy; once every 24 hours; administrative services, professional pharmacy services, care coordination, and all necessary supplies and equipment (drugs and nursing visits coded separately), per diem

S9501 Home infusion therapy, antibiotic, antiviral, or antifungal therapy; once every 12 hours; administrative services, professional pharmacy services, care coordination, and all necessary supplies and equipment (drugs and nursing visits coded separately), per diem

S9502 Home infusion therapy, antibiotic, antiviral, or antifungal therapy; once every 8 hours, administrative services, professional pharmacy services, care coordination, and all necessary supplies and equipment (drugs and nursing visits coded separately), per diem

S9503 Home infusion therapy, antibiotic, antiviral, or antifungal; once every 6 hours; administrative services, professional pharmacy services, care coordination, and all necessary supplies and equipment (drugs and nursing visits coded separately), per diem

S9504 Home infusion therapy, antibiotic, antiviral, or antifungal; once every 4 hours; administrative services, professional pharmacy services, care coordination, and all necessary supplies and equipment (drugs and nursing visits coded separately), per diem

S9529 Routine venipuncture for collection of specimen(s), single home bound, nursing home, or skilled nursing facility patient

S9537 Home therapy; hematopoietic hormone injection therapy (e.g., erythropoietin, g-csf, gm-csf); administrative services, professional pharmacy services, care coordination, and all necessary supplies and equipment (drugs and nursing visits coded separately), per diem

S9538 Home transfusion of blood product(s); administrative services, professional pharmacy services, care coordination and all necessary supplies and equipment (blood products, drugs, and nursing visits coded separately), per diem

S9542 Home injectable therapy, not otherwise classified, including administrative services, professional pharmacy services, care coordination, and all necessary supplies and equipment (drugs and nursing visits coded separately), per diem

S9558 Home injectable therapy; growth hormone, including administrative services, professional pharmacy services, care coordination, and all necessary supplies and equipment (drugs and nursing visits coded separately), per diem

S9559 Home injectable therapy, interferon, including administrative services, professional pharmacy services, care coordination, and all necessary supplies and equipment (drugs and nursing visits coded separately), per diem

S9560 Home injectable therapy; hormonal therapy (e.g., leuprolide, goserelin), including administrative services, professional pharmacy services, care coordination, and all necessary supplies and equipment (drugs and nursing visits coded separately), per diem

S9562 Home injectable therapy, palivizumab, including administrative services, professional pharmacy services, care coordination, and all necessary supplies and equipment (drugs and nursing visits coded separately), per diem

S9590 Home therapy, irrigation therapy (e.g., sterile irrigation of an organ or anatomical cavity); including administrative services, professional pharmacy services, care coordination, and all necessary supplies and equipment (drugs and nursing visits coded separately), per diem

S9810 Home therapy; professional pharmacy services for provision of infusion, specialty drug administration, and/or disease state management, not otherwise classified, per hour (do not use this code with any per diem code)

S9900 Services by a journal-listed Christian science practitioner for the purpose of healing, per diem

S9901 Services by a journal-listed Christian science nurse, per hour

S9960 Ambulance service, conventional air service, nonemergency transport, one way (fixed wing)

S9961 Ambulance service, conventional air service, nonemergency transport, one way (rotary wing)

S9970 Health club membership, annual

S9975 Transplant related lodging, meals and transportation, per diem

S9976 Lodging, per diem, not otherwise classified

S9977 Meals, per diem, not otherwise specified

S9981 Medical records copying fee, administrative

S9982 Medical records copying fee, per page

S9986 Not medically necessary service (patient is aware that service not medically necessary)

S9988 Services provided as part of a phase i clinical trial

S9989 Services provided outside of the united states of America (list in addition to code(s) for service(s)

S9990 Services provided as part of a phase ii clinical trial

S9991 Services provided as part of a phase iii clinical trial

S9992 Transportation costs to and from trial location and local transportation costs (e.g., fares for taxicab or bus) for clinical trial participant and one caregiver/companion

S9994 Lodging costs (e.g., hotel charges) for clinical trial participant and one caregiver/companion

S9996 Meals for clinical trial participant and one caregiver/companion

S9999 Sales tax

STATE MEDICAID AGENCY CODES

Guidelines

"T" codes were added to HCPCS in 2002. These codes are exclusively for the use of state Medicaid agencies. Prior to using "T" codes on health insurance claims to your state Medicaid processor, you should verify that these codes are acceptable. "T" codes are not valid for Medicare use.

In addition to the information presented in the INTRODUCTION, several other items unique to this section are defined or identified here.

1. **SPECIAL REPORT:** A service, material or supply that is rarely provided, unusual, variable or new may require a special report in determining medical appropriateness for reimbursement purposes. Pertinent information should include an adequate definition or description of the nature, extent, and need for the service, material or supply.

2. **MODIFIERS:** Listed services may be modified under certain circumstances. When appropriate, the modifying circumstance is identified by adding a modifier to the basic procedure code. CPT and HCPCS National Level II modifiers may be used with CPT and HCPCS National Level II procedure codes.

State Medicaid Agency Codes

T1000 Private duty / independent nursing service(s) - licensed, up to 15 minutes

T1001 Nursing assessment / evaluation

T1002 Rn services, up to 15 minutes

T1003 LPN/LVN services, up to 15 minutes

T1004 Services of a qualified nursing aide, up to 15 minutes

T1005 Respite care services, up to 15 minutes

T1006 Alcohol and/or substance abuse services, family/couple counseling

T1007 Alcohol and/or substance abuse services, treatment plan development and/or modification

T1009 Child sitting services for children of the individual receiving alcohol and/or substance abuse services

T1010 Meals for individuals receiving alcohol and/or substance abuse services (when meals not included in the program)

T1012 Alcohol and/or substance abuse services, skills development

T1013 Sign language or oral interpretive services, per 15 minutes

T1014 Telehealth transmission, per minute, professional services bill separately

T1015 Clinic visit/encounter, all-inclusive

T1016 Case management, each 15 minutes

T1017 Targeted case management, each 15 minutes

T1018 School-based individualized education program (IEP) services, bundled

T1019 Personal care services, per 15 minutes, not for an inpatient or resident of a hospital, nursing facility, ICF/MR or IMD, part of the individualized plan of treatment (code may not be used to identify services provided by home health aide or certified nurse assistant)

T1020 Personal care services, per diem, not for an inpatient or resident of a hospital, nursing facility, ICF/MR or IMD, part of the individualized plan of treatment (code may not be used to identify services provided by home health aide or certified nurse assistant)

Not payable by Medicare | Non-covered by Medicare | Special coverage instructions | Carrier judgement

T1021 Home health aide or certified nurse assistant, per visit

T1022 Contracted home health agency services, all services provided under contract, per day

T1023 Screening to determine the appropriateness of consideration of an individual for participation in a specified program, project or treatment protocol, per encounter

T1024 Evaluation and treatment by an integrated, specialty team contracted to provide coordinated care to multiple or severely handicapped children, per encounter

T1025 Intensive, extended multidisciplinary services provided in a clinic setting to children with complex medical, physical, mental and psychosocial impairments, per diem

▲ **T1026** Intensive, extended multidisciplinary services provided in a clinic setting to children with complex medical, physical, mental and psychosocial impairments, per hour

T1027 Family training and counseling for child development, per 15 minutes

T1028 Assessment of home, physical and family environment, to determine suitability to meet patient's medical needs

T1029 Comprehensive environmental lead investigation, not including laboratory analysis, per dwelling

T1030 Nursing care, in the home, by registered nurse, per diem

T1031 Nursing care, in the home, by licensed practical nurse, per diem

T1040 Medicaid certified community behavioral health clinic services, per diem

T1041 Medicaid certified community behavioral health clinic services, per month

T1502 Administration of oral, intramuscular and/or subcutaneous medication by health care agency/professional, per visit

T1503 Administration of medication, other than oral and/or injectable, by a health care agency/professional, per visit

T1505 Electronic medication compliance management device, includes all components and accessories, not otherwise classified

T1999 Miscellaneous therapeutic items and supplies, retail purchases, not otherwise classified; identify product in "remarks"

T2001 Non-emergency transportation; patient attendant/escort

T2002 Non-emergency transportation; per diem

T2003 Non-emergency transportation; encounter/trip

T2004 Non-emergency transport; commercial carrier, multi-pass

T2005 Non-emergency transportation; stretcher van

T2007 Transportation waiting time, air ambulance and non-emergency vehicle, one-half (1/2) hour increments

T2010 Preadmission screening and resident review (pasrr) level I identification screening, per screen

T2011 Preadmission screening and resident review (pasrr) level ii evaluation, per evaluation

T2012 Habilitation, educational; waiver, per diem

T2013 Habilitation, educational, waiver; per hour

T2014 Habilitation, prevocational, waiver; per diem

T2015 Habilitation, prevocational, waiver; per hour

T2016 Habilitation, residential, waiver; per diem

T2017 Habilitation, residential, waiver; 15 minutes

T2018 Habilitation, supported employment, waiver; per diem

T2019 Habilitation, supported employment, waiver; per 15 minutes

T2020 Day habilitation, waiver; per diem

T2021 Day habilitation, waiver; per 15 minutes

T2022 Case management, per month

T2023 Targeted case management; per month

T2024 Service assessment/plan of care development, waiver

T2025 Waiver services; not otherwise specified (nos)

T2026 Specialized childcare, waiver; per diem

T2027 Specialized childcare, waiver; per 15 minutes

T2028 Specialized supply, not otherwise specified, waiver

T2029 Specialized medical equipment, not otherwise specified, waiver

T2030 Assisted living, waiver; per month

T2031 Assisted living; waiver, per diem

T2032 Residential care, not otherwise specified (nos), waiver; per month

T2033 Residential care, not otherwise specified (nos), waiver; per diem

T2034 Crisis intervention, waiver; per diem

T2035 Utility services to support medical equipment and assistive technology/devices, waiver

T2036 Therapeutic camping, overnight, waiver; each session

T2037 Therapeutic camping, day, waiver; each session

T2038 Community transition, waiver; per service

T2039 Vehicle modifications, waiver; per service

T2040 Financial management, self-directed, waiver; per 15 minutes

T2041 Supports brokerage, self-directed, waiver; per 15 minutes

T2042 Hospice routine home care; per diem

T2043 Hospice continuous home care; per hour

T2044 Hospice inpatient respite care; per diem

T2045 Hospice general inpatient care; per diem

T2046 Hospice long term care, room and board only; per diem

T2048 Behavioral health; long-term care residential (non-acute care in a residential treatment program where stay is typically longer than 30 days), with room and board, per diem

T2049 Non-emergency transportation; stretcher van, mileage; per mile

T2101 Human breast milk processing, storage and distribution only

T4521 Adult sized disposable incontinence product, brief/diaper, small, each

T4522 Adult sized disposable incontinence product, brief/diaper, medium, each

T4523 Adult sized disposable incontinence product, brief/diaper, large, each

T4524	Adult sized disposable incontinence product, brief/diaper, extra-large, each
T4525	Adult sized disposable incontinence product, protective underwear/pull-on, small size, each
T4526	Adult sized disposable incontinence product, protective underwear/pull-on, medium size, each
T4527	Adult sized disposable incontinence product, protective underwear/pull-on, large size, each
T4528	Adult sized disposable incontinence product, protective underwear/pull-on, extra-large size, each
T4529	Pediatric sized disposable incontinence product, brief/diaper, small/medium size, each
T4530	Pediatric sized disposable incontinence product, brief/diaper, large size, each
T4531	Pediatric sized disposable incontinence product, protective underwear/pull-on, small/medium size, each
T4532	Pediatric sized disposable incontinence product, protective underwear/pull-on, large size, each
T4533	Youth sized disposable incontinence product, brief/diaper, each
T4534	Youth sized disposable incontinence product, protective underwear/pull-on, each
T4535	Disposable liner/shield/guard/pad/undergarment, for incontinence, each
T4536	Incontinence product, protective underwear/pull-on, reusable, any size, each
T4537	Incontinence product, protective underpad, reusable, bed size, each
T4538	Diaper service, reusable diaper, each diaper
T4539	Incontinence product, diaper/brief, reusable, any size, each
T4540	Incontinence product, protective underpad, reusable, chair size, each
T4541	Incontinence product, disposable underpad, large, each
T4542	Incontinence product, disposable underpad, small size, each
T4543	Adult sized disposable incontinence product, protective brief/diaper, above extra-large, each
T4544	Adult sized disposable incontinence product, protective underwear/pull-on, above extra-large, each
T4545	Incontinence product, disposable, penile wrap, each
T5001	Positioning seat for persons with special orthopedic needs
T5999	Supply, not otherwise specified

CORONAVIRUS DIAGNOSTIC PANEL

CDC and Non-CDC Tests

There are new HCPCS codes for healthcare providers who need to test patients for Coronavirus. Healthcare providers using the Centers for Disease Control and Prevention (CDC) 2019 Novel Coronavirus Real Time RT-PCR Diagnostic Test Panel may bill for that test using the newly created HCPCS code U0001. A second new HCPCS code (U0002) 2019-nCoV Coronavirus, SARS-CoV-2/2019-nCoV (COVID-19), any technique, multiple types or subtypes (includes all targets), non-CDC can also be used by laboratories and healthcare facilities.

Both codes can be used to bill Medicare as well as by other health insurers that choose to utilize and accept the code. Additionally, on March 13, 2020, the American Medical Association (AMA) Current Procedural Terminology (CPT) Editorial Panel has created CPT code 87635 (Infectious agent detection by nucleic acid (DNA or RNA); severe acute respiratory syndrome coronavirus 2 (SARS-CoV-2) (Coronavirus disease [COVID-19]), amplified probe technique).

U0001 CDC 2019 novel coronavirus (2019-ncov) real-time rt-PCR diagnostic panel

U0002 2019-ncov coronavirus, sars-cov-2/2019-ncov (covid-19), any technique, multiple types or subtypes (includes all targets), non-CDC

For non-CDC nucleic acid test methodologies providers should report CPT code 87635 and utilize HCPCS code U0002 for all other testing methods

High Throughput Technologies

Cleared or Approved Clinical Diagnostic Laboratory Test (CDLT) facilities making use of high throughput technologies for the detection of SARS–CoV–2 or the diagnosis of the virus that causes COVID–19, are new and involve high throughput machines which require more intensive technician training and more time intensive processes to assure quality.

A high throughput technology uses a platform that employs automated processing of more than two hundred specimens a day. Examples of high throughput technology as of April 14, 2020 include but are not limited to technologies marketed on that date as the Roche cobas 6800 System, Roche cobas 8800 System, Abbott m2000 System, Hologic Panther Fusion System, GeneXpert Infinity System, and NeuMoDx 288 Molecular.

These tests are a type of CDLT currently paid for under 3 CMS-Ruling 2020-1-R Medicare Part B. Specifically, the following codes would identify these tests:

U0003 Infectious agent detection by nucleic acid (DNA or RNA); severe acute respiratory syndrome coronavirus 2 (sars-cov-2) (coronavirus disease [covid-19]), amplified probe technique, making use of high throughput technologies as described by CMS-2020-01-r

U0004 2019-ncov coronavirus, sars-cov-2/2019-ncov (covid-19), any technique, multiple types or subtypes (includes all targets), non-CDC, making use of high throughput technologies as described by CMS-2020-01-r

HCPCS code U0003 should identify tests that would otherwise be identified by CPT code 87635 but for being performed with these high throughput technologies. HCPCS code U0004 should identify tests that would otherwise be identified by U0002 but for being performed with these high throughput technologies. Neither U0003 nor U0004 should be used for tests that detect COVID-19 antibodies.

Add-On Payment Code

Effective January 1, 2021, CMS will change the base rate for payments for COVID-19 tests run on high throughput technology to $75. However, CMS will make an add-on payment of $25 per test ($100 per test total) to labs who complete high-throughput COVID-19 diagnostic tests within two calendar days of specimen collection and who complete the majority of their COVID-19 diagnostic tests in two days or less for all of their patients (not just Medicare patients).

Because labs may not know right away whether the majority of their high throughput tests for all patients are completed in two calendar days, there are three options for billing the add-on payment:

1. Labs can bill all tests after performing them for the lower $75 payment and wait to submit adjustment claims for the add-on HCPCS code U0005 for tests from the prior month after ensuring they were able to complete the majority of high throughput tests within the two calendar day requirement.

2. Conversely, labs may choose to wait to bill the prior month's tests at all until they can verify that they met the time requirement and then bill the test code and the HCPCS U0005 add-on code, but only labs with significant cash flow capability may be able to do this.

3. Finally, labs may bill the add-on code for every test completed in two calendar days, but then submit adjustment claims if it fails to meet the majority of tests threshold.

U0005 Infectious agent detection by nucleic acid (DNA or RNA); severe acute respiratory syndrome coronavirus 2 (sars-cov-2) (coronavirus disease [covid-19]), amplified probe technique, CDC or non-CDC, making use of high throughput technologies, completed within 2 calendar days from date of specimen collection (list separately in addition to either HCPCS code U0003 or U0004) as described by CMS-2020-01-r2

Guidelines

In addition to the information presented in the INTRODUCTION, several other items unique to this section are defined or identified here:

1. **SUBSECTION INFORMATION:** Some of the listed subheadings or subsections have special needs or instructions unique to that section. Where these are indicated, special "notes" will be presented preceding or following the listings. Those subsections within the VISION SERVICES section that have "notes" are as follows:

Subsection	Code Numbers
Spectacle lenses	V2100–V2499
Contact lenses	V2500–V2599
Low vision aids	V2600–V2615

2. **UNLISTED SERVICE OR PROCEDURE:** A service or procedure may be provided that is not listed in this edition of HCPCS. When reporting such a service, the appropriate "unlisted procedure" code may be used to indicate the service, identifying it by "special report" as defined below. HCPCS terminology is inconsistent in defining unlisted procedures. The procedure definition may include the term(s) "unlisted", "not otherwise classified", "unspecified", "unclassified", "other" and "miscellaneous". Prior to using these codes, try to determine if a Local Level III code or CPT code is available. The "unlisted procedures" and accompanying codes for VISION SERVICES are as follows:

   V2199 Not otherwise classified, single vision lens, bifocal, glass or plastic
   V2499 Variable sphericity lens, other type
   V2599 Not otherwise classified, contact lens
   V2629 Prosthetic eye, other type
   V2799 Vision service, miscellaneous

3. **SPECIAL REPORT:** A service, material or supply that is rarely provided, unusual, variable or new may require a special report in determining medical appropriateness for reimbursement purposes. Pertinent information should include an adequate definition or description of the nature, extent, and need for the service, material or supply.

4. **MODIFIERS:** Listed services may be modified under certain circumstances. When appropriate, the modifying circumstance is identified by adding a modifier to the basic procedure code. CPT and HCPCS National Level II modifiers may be used with CPT and HCPCS National Level II procedure codes. Modifiers commonly used with VISION SERVICES are as follows:

   -AP Determination of refractive state was not performed in the course of diagnostic ophthalmological examination

   -CC Procedure code change (use "CC" when the procedure code submitted was changed either for administrative reasons or because an incorrect code was filed)

   -LS FDA-monitored intraocular lens implant

   -LT Left side (used to identify procedures performed on the left side of the body)

   -PL Progressive addition lenses

   -RT Right side (used to identify procedures performed on the right side of the body)

-SF Second opinion ordered by a professional review organization (PRO) per section 9401, P.L. 99-272. (100 percent reimbursement; no Medicare deductible or coinsurance)

-TC Technical component. Under certain circumstances, a charge may be made for the technical component alone. Under those circumstances, the technical component charge is identified by adding modifier -TC to the usual procedure number. Technical component charges are institutional charges and are not billed separately by physicians. However, portable x-ray suppliers bill only for the technical component and should use modifier -TC. The charge data from portable x-ray suppliers will then be used to build customary and prevailing profiles.

-VP Aphakic patient

5. **CPT CODE CROSS-REFERENCE:** See sections for equivalent CPT code(s) for all listings in this section.

Frames

V2020 Frames, purchases

V2025 Deluxe frame

Spectacle Lenses

NOTE: If CPT code 92390 or 92395 is reported, recode with the specific lens type listed below. For aphakic temporary spectacle correction, see CPT code 92358.

V2100 Sphere, single vision, plano to plus or minus 4.00, per lens

V2101 Sphere, single vision, plus or minus 4.12 to plus or minus 7.00d, per lens

V2102 Sphere, single vision, plus or minus 7.12 to plus or minus 20.00d, per lens

V2103 Spherocylinder, single vision, plano to plus or minus 4.00d sphere, .12 to 2.00d cylinder, per lens

V2104 Spherocylinder, single vision, plano to plus or minus 4.00d sphere, 2.12 to 4.00d cylinder, per lens

V2105 Spherocylinder, single vision, plano to plus or minus 4.00d sphere, 4.25 to 6.00d cylinder, per lens

V2106 Spherocylinder, single vision, plano to plus or minus 4.00d sphere, over 6.00d cylinder, per lens

V2107 Spherocylinder, single vision, plus or minus 4.25 to plus or minus 7.00 sphere, .12 to 2.00d cylinder, per lens

V2108 Spherocylinder, single vision, plus or minus 4.25d to plus or minus 7.00d sphere, 2.12 to 4.00d cylinder, per lens

V2109 Spherocylinder, single vision, plus or minus 4.25 to plus or minus 7.00d sphere, 4.25 to 6.00d cylinder, per lens

V2110 Spherocylinder, single vision, plus or minus 4.25 to 7.00d sphere, over 6.00d cylinder, per lens

V2111 Spherocylinder, single vision, plus or minus 7.25 to plus or minus 12.00d sphere, .25 to 2.25d cylinder, per lens

V2112 Spherocylinder, single vision, plus or minus 7.25 to plus or minus 12.00d sphere, 2.25d to 4.00d cylinder, per lens

V2113 Spherocylinder, single vision, plus or minus 7.25 to plus or minus 12.00d sphere, 4.25 to 6.00d cylinder, per lens

V2114 Spherocylinder, single vision, sphere over plus or minus 12.00d, per lens

V2115 Lenticular, (myodisc), per lens, single vision

V2118 Aniseikonic lens, single vision

V2121	Lenticular lens, per lens, single
V2199	Not otherwise classified, single vision lens
V2200	Sphere, bifocal, plano to plus or minus 4.00d, per lens
V2201	Sphere, bifocal, plus or minus 4.12 to plus or minus 7.00d, per lens
V2202	Sphere, bifocal, plus or minus 7.12 to plus or minus 20.00d, per lens
V2203	Spherocylinder, bifocal, plano to plus or minus 4.00d sphere, .12 to 2.00d cylinder, per lens
V2204	Spherocylinder, bifocal, plano to plus or minus 4.00d sphere, 2.12 to 4.00d cylinder, per lens
V2205	Spherocylinder, bifocal, plano to plus or minus 4.00d sphere, 4.25 to 6.00d cylinder, per lens
V2206	Spherocylinder, bifocal, plano to plus or minus 4.00d sphere, over 6.00d cylinder, per lens
V2207	Spherocylinder, bifocal, plus or minus 4.25 to plus or minus 7.00d sphere,.12 to 2.00d cylinder, per lens
V2208	Spherocylinder, bifocal, plus or minus 4.25 to plus or minus 7.00d sphere, 2.12 to 4.00d cylinder, per lens
V2209	Spherocylinder, bifocal, plus or minus 4.25 to plus or minus 7.00d sphere, 4.25 to 6.00d cylinder, per lens
V2210	Spherocylinder, bifocal, plus or minus 4.25 to plus or minus 7.00d sphere, over 6.00d cylinder, per lens
V2211	Spherocylinder, bifocal, plus or minus 7.25 to plus or minus 12.00d sphere, .25 to 2.25d cylinder, per lens
V2212	Spherocylinder, bifocal, plus or minus 7.25 to plus or minus 12.00d sphere, 2.25 to 4.00d cylinder, per lens
V2213	Spherocylinder, bifocal, plus or minus 7.25 to plus or minus 12.00d sphere, 4.25 to 6.00d cylinder, per lens
V2214	Spherocylinder, bifocal, sphere over plus or minus 12.00d, per lens
V2215	Lenticular (myodisc), per lens, bifocal
V2218	Aniseikonic, per lens, bifocal
V2219	Bifocal seg width over 28 mm
V2220	Bifocal add over 3.25d
V2221	Lenticular lens, per lens, bifocal
V2299	Specialty bifocal (by report)
V2300	Sphere, trifocal, plano to plus or minus 4.00d, per lens
V2301	Sphere, trifocal, plus or minus 4.12 to plus or minus 7.00d, per lens
V2302	Sphere, trifocal, plus or minus 7.12 to plus or minus 20.00, per lens
V2303	Spherocylinder, trifocal, plano to plus or minus 4.00d sphere, .12-2.00d cylinder, per lens
V2304	Spherocylinder, trifocal, plano to plus or minus 4.00d sphere, 2.25-4.00d cylinder, per lens
V2305	Spherocylinder, trifocal, plano to plus or minus 4.00d sphere, 4.25 to 6.00 cylinder, per lens
V2306	Spherocylinder, trifocal, plano to plus or minus 4.00d sphere, over 6.00d cylinder, per lens
V2307	Spherocylinder, trifocal, plus or minus 4.25 to plus or minus 7.00d sphere, .12 to 2.00d cylinder, per lens

V2308 Spherocylinder, trifocal, plus or minus 4.25 to plus or minus 7.00d sphere, 2.12 to 4.00d cylinder, per lens

V2309 Spherocylinder, trifocal, plus or minus 4.25 to plus or minus 7.00d sphere, 4.25 to 6.00d cylinder, per lens

V2310 Spherocylinder, trifocal, plus or minus 4.25 to plus or minus 7.00d sphere, over 6.00d cylinder, per lens

V2311 Spherocylinder, trifocal, plus or minus 7.25 to plus or minus 12.00d sphere, .25 to 2.25d cylinder, per lens

V2312 Spherocylinder, trifocal, plus or minus 7.25 to plus or minus 12.00d sphere, 2.25 to 4.00d cylinder, per lens

V2313 Spherocylinder, trifocal, plus or minus 7.25 to plus or minus 12.00d sphere, 4.25 to 6.00d cylinder, per lens

V2314 Spherocylinder, trifocal, sphere over plus or minus 12.00d, per lens

V2315 Lenticular, (myodisc), per lens, trifocal

V2318 Aniseikonic lens, trifocal

V2319 Trifocal seg width over 28 mm

V2320 Trifocal add over 3.25d

V2321 Lenticular lens, per lens, trifocal

V2399 Specialty trifocal (by report)

V2410 Variable asphericity lens, single vision, full field, glass or plastic, per lens

V2430 Variable asphericity lens, bifocal, full field, glass or plastic, per lens

V2499 Variable sphericity lens, other type

Contact Lenses (CPT 92391 or 92396)

NOTE: If CPT code 92391 or 92396 is reported, recode with specific lens type listed below, per lens.

V2500 Contact lens, PMMA, spherical, per lens

V2501 Contact lens, PMMA, toric or prism ballast, per lens

V2502 Contact lens, PMMA, bifocal, per lens

V2503 Contact lens, PMMA, color vision deficiency, per lens

V2510 Contact lens, gas permeable, spherical, per lens

V2511 Contact lens, gas permeable, toric, prism ballast, per lens

V2512 Contact lens, gas permeable, bifocal, per lens

V2513 Contact lens, gas permeable, extended wear, per lens

V2520 Contact lens, hydrophilic, spherical, per lens

V2521 Contact lens, hydrophilic, toric, or prism ballast, per lens

V2522 Contact lens, hydrophilic, bifocal, per lens

V2523 Contact lens, hydrophilic, extended wear, per lens

V2530 Contact lens, scleral, gas impermeable, per lens (for contact lens modification, see 92325)

V2531 Contact lens, scleral, gas permeable, per lens (for contact lens modification, see 92325)

V2599 Contact lens, other type

Low Vision Aids (CPT 92392)

NOTE: If CPT code 92392 is reported, record with specific systems listed below.

V2600 Hand held low vision aids and other nonspectacle mounted aids

V2610 Single lens spectacle mounted low vision aids

V2615 Telescopic and other compound lens system, including distance vision telescopic, near vision telescopes and compound microscopic lens system

Prosthetic Eye (CPT 92330 or 92393)

V2623 Prosthetic eye, plastic, custom

V2624 Polishing/resurfacing of ocular prosthesis

V2625 Enlargement of ocular prosthesis

V2626 Reduction of ocular prosthesis

V2627 Scleral cover shell

V2628 Fabrication and fitting of ocular conformer

V2629 Prosthetic eye, other type

Intraocular Lenses

V2630 Anterior chamber intraocular lens

V2631 Iris supported intraocular lens

V2632 Posterior chamber intraocular lens

Miscellaneous

V2700 Balance lens, per lens

V2702 Deluxe lens feature

V2710 Slab off prism, glass or plastic, per lens

V2715 Prism, per lens

V2718 Press-on lens, Fresnell prism, per lens

V2730 Special base curve, glass or plastic, per lens

V2744 Tint, photochromatic, per lens

V2745 Addition to lens; tint, any color, solid, gradient or equal, excludes photochromatic, any lens material, per lens

V2750 Anti-reflective coating, per lens

V2755 U-V lens, per lens

V2756 Eye glass case

V2760 Scratch resistant coating, per lens

V2761 Mirror coating, any type, solid, gradient or equal, any lens material, per lens

V2762 Polarization, any lens material, per lens

V2770 Occluder lens, per lens

V2780 Oversize lens, per lens

V2781 Progressive lens, per lens

V2782 Lens, index 1.54 to 1.65 plastic or 1.60 to 1.79 glass, excludes polycarbonate, per lens

V2783 Lens, index greater than or equal to 1.66 plastic or greater than or equal to 1.80 glass, excludes polycarbonate, per lens

V2784 Lens, polycarbonate or equal, any index, per lens

V2785 Processing, preserving and transporting corneal tissue

V2786 Specialty occupational multifocal lens, per lens

V2787 Astigmatism correcting function of intraocular lens

V2788 Presbyopia correcting function of intraocular lens

V2790 Amniotic membrane for surgical reconstruction, per procedure

V2797 Vision supply, accessory and/or service component of another HCPCS vision code

V2799 Vision item or service, miscellaneous

Guidelines

In addition to the information presented in the INTRODUCTION, several other items unique to this section are defined or identified here:

1. **PROSTHETIC DEVICES:** Prosthetic devices that replace all or part of an internal body organ or the function of a permanently inoperative or malfunctioning internal body organ are covered when furnished on a physician's order. If the medical record and attending physician indicate the condition will be indefinite, the test of permanence is met.

2. **SPEECH PATHOLOGY:** Services necessary for diagnosing and treating speech disorders that result in communication disabilities, and swallowing disorders, regardless of the presence of a disability, are covered Medicare services if reasonable and necessary. The services must be considered to be an effective treatment for the patient's condition, and the patient's condition must be at a level of severity that requires the service of a qualified speech pathologist.

3. **UNLISTED SERVICE OR PROCEDURE:** A service or procedure may be provided that is not listed in this edition of HCPCS. When reporting such a service, the appropriate "unlisted procedure" code may be used to indicate the service, identifying it by "special report" as defined below. HCPCS terminology is inconsistent in defining unlisted procedures. The procedure definition may include the term(s) "unlisted", "not otherwise classified", "unspecified", "unclassified", "other" and "miscellaneous". Prior to using these codes, try to determine if a Local Level III code or CPT code is available. The "unlisted procedures" and accompanying codes for HEARING SERVICES are as follows:

   V5299 Hearing service, miscellaneous

4. **SPECIAL REPORT:** A service, material or supply that is rarely provided, unusual, variable or new may require a special report in determining medical appropriateness for reimbursement purposes. Pertinent information should include an adequate definition or description of the nature, extent, and need for the service, material or supply.

5. **MODIFIERS:** Listed services may be modified under certain circumstances. When appropriate, the modifying circumstance is identified by adding a modifier to the basic procedure code. CPT and HCPCS National Level II modifiers may be used with CPT and HCPCS National Level II procedure codes. Modifiers commonly used with HEARING SERVICES are as follows:

   -CC Procedure code change (use "CC" when the procedure code submitted was changed either for administrative reasons or because an incorrect code was filed)

   -LT Left side (used to identify procedures performed on the left side of the body)

   -RT Right side (used to identify procedures performed on the right side of the body)

   -SF Second opinion ordered by a professional review organization (PRO) per section 9401, P.L. 99-272 (100 percent reimbursement; no Medicare deductible or coinsurance)

   -TC Technical component. Under certain circumstances, a charge may be made for the technical component alone. Under those circumstances, the technical component charge is identified by adding modifier -TC to the usual procedure number. Technical component charges are institutional charges and are not billed separately by physicians. However, portable x-ray suppliers bill only for the technical component and should use modifier -TC. The charge data from portable x-ray suppliers will then be used to build customary and prevailing profiles.

6. **CPT CODE CROSS-REFERENCE:** See sections for equivalent CPT code(s) for all listings in this section.

Hearing Services

V5008	Hearing screening
V5010	Assessment for hearing aid
V5011	Fitting/orientation/checking of hearing aid
V5014	Repair/modification of a hearing aid
V5020	Conformity evaluation
V5030	Hearing aid, monaural, body worn, air conduction
V5040	Hearing aid, monaural, body worn, bone conduction
V5050	Hearing aid, monaural, in the ear
V5060	Hearing aid, monaural, behind the ear
V5070	Glasses, air conduction
V5080	Glasses, bone conduction
V5090	Dispensing fee, unspecified hearing aid
V5095	Semi-implantable middle ear hearing prosthesis
V5100	Hearing aid, bilateral, body worn
V5110	Dispensing fee, bilateral
V5120	Binaural, body
V5130	Binaural, in the ear
V5140	Binaural, behind the ear
V5150	Binaural, glasses
V5160	Dispensing fee, binaural
V5171	Hearing aid, contralateral routing device, monaural, in the ear (ite)
V5172	Hearing aid, contralateral routing device, monaural, in the canal (itc)
V5181	Hearing aid, contralateral routing device, monaural, behind the ear (bte)
V5190	Hearing aid, CROS, glasses
V5200	Dispensing fee, contralateral, monaural
V5211	Hearing aid, contralateral routing system, binaural, ite/ite
V5212	Hearing aid, contralateral routing system, binaural, ite/itc
V5213	Hearing aid, contralateral routing system, binaural, ite/bte
V5214	Hearing aid, contralateral routing system, binaural, itc/itc
V5215	Hearing aid, contralateral routing system, binaural, itc/bte
V5221	Hearing aid, contralateral routing system, binaural, bte/bte
V5230	Hearing aid, contralateral routing system, binaural, glasses
V5240	Dispensing fee, contralateral routing system, binaural
V5241	Dispensing fee, monaural hearing aid, any type
V5242	Hearing aid, analog, monaural, cic (completely in the ear canal)
V5243	Hearing aid, analog, monaural, itc (in the canal)
V5244	Hearing aid, digitally programmable analog, monaural, cic
V5245	Hearing aid, digitally programmable, analog, monaural, itc
V5246	Hearing aid, digitally programmable analog, monaural, ite (in the ear)

T - U - V CODES

V5247	Hearing aid, digitally programmable analog, monaural, bte (behind the ear)
V5248	Hearing aid, analog, binaural, cic
V5249	Hearing aid, analog, binaural, itc
V5250	Hearing aid, digitally programmable analog, binaural, cic
V5251	Hearing aid, digitally programmable analog, binaural, itc
V5252	Hearing aid, digitally programmable, binaural, ite
V5253	Hearing aid, digitally programmable, binaural, bte
V5254	Hearing aid, digital, monaural, cic
V5255	Hearing aid, digital, monaural, itc
V5256	Hearing aid, digital, monaural, ite
V5257	Hearing aid, digital, monaural, bte
V5258	Hearing aid, digital, binaural, cic
V5259	Hearing aid, digital, binaural, itc
V5260	Hearing aid, digital, binaural, ite
V5261	Hearing aid, digital, binaural, bte
V5262	Hearing aid, disposable, any type, monaural
V5263	Hearing aid, disposable, any type, binaural
V5264	Ear mold/insert, not disposable, any type
V5265	Ear mold/insert, disposable, any type
V5266	Battery for use in hearing device
V5267	Hearing aid or assistive listening device/supplies/accessories, not otherwise specified
V5268	Assistive listening device, telephone amplifier, any type
V5269	Assistive listening device, alerting, any type
V5270	Assistive listening device, television amplifier, any type
V5271	Assistive listening device, television caption decoder
V5272	Assistive listening device, tdd
V5273	Assistive listening device, for use with cochlear implant
V5274	Assistive listening device, not otherwise specified
V5275	Ear impression, each
V5281	Assistive listening device, personal FM/dm system, monaural, (1 receiver, transmitter, microphone), any type
V5282	Assistive listening device, personal FM/dm system, binaural, (2 receivers, transmitter, microphone), any type
V5283	Assistive listening device, personal FM/dm neck, loop induction receiver
V5284	Assistive listening device, personal FM/dm, ear level receiver
V5285	Assistive listening device, personal FM/dm, direct audio input receiver
V5286	Assistive listening device, personal blue tooth FM/dm receiver
V5287	Assistive listening device, personal FM/dm receiver, not otherwise specified
V5288	Assistive listening device, personal FM/dm transmitter assistive listening device
V5289	Assistive listening device, personal FM/dm adapter/boot coupling device for receiver, any type
V5290	Assistive listening device, transmitter microphone, any type

Not payable by Medicare | Non-covered by Medicare | Special coverage instructions | Carrier judgement

V5298	Hearing aid, not otherwise classified
V5299	Hearing service, miscellaneous
V5336	Repair/modification of augmentative communicative system or device (excludes adaptive hearing aid)
V5362	Speech screening
V5363	Language screening
V5364	Dysphagia screening

ALPHABETIC INDEX

Questions regarding coding and billing guidance should be submitted to the insurer in whose jurisdiction a claim would be filed. For private sector health insurance systems, please contact the individual private insurance entity. For Medicaid systems, please contact the Medicaid Agency in the state in which the claim is being filed. For Medicare, contact the Medicare contractor.

INDEX

INDEX

INDEX

INDEX

B

INDEX

C

INDEX

INDEX

INDEX

INDEX

D

INDEX

INDEX

E

INDEX

INDEX

F

INDEX

G

INDEX

H

INDEX

INDEX

INDEX

J

K

INDEX

L

INDEX

M

INDEX

INDEX

N

INDEX

INDEX

O

INDEX

INDEX

P

INDEX

INDEX

INDEX

INDEX

Q

INDEX

R

INDEX

S

INDEX

INDEX

INDEX

INDEX

INDEX

INDEX

U

V

INDEX

W

INDEX

INDEX

X

Y

Z

INDEX

APPENDIX A: MODIFIERS

HCPCS National Level II Modifiers

A = Action [• New modifier ▲ Revised modifier ( ) Deleted modifier]

A	MOD	DESCRIPTION
	-A1	Dressing for one wound
	-A2	Dressing for two wounds
	-A3	Dressing for three wounds
	-A4	Dressing for four wounds
	-A5	Dressing for five wounds
	-A6	Dressing for six wounds
	-A7	Dressing for seven wounds
	-A8	Dressing for eight wounds
	-A9	Dressing for nine or more wounds
	-AA	Anesthesia services performed personally by anesthesiologist
	-AB	Audiology service furnished personally by an audiologist without a physician/NPP order for non-acute hearing assessment unrelated to disequilibrium, or hearing aids, or examinations for the purpose of prescribing, fitting, or changing hearing aids; service may be performed once every 12 months, per beneficiary
	-AD	Medical supervision by a physician: more than four concurrent anesthesia procedures
	-AE	Registered dietician
	-AF	Specialty physician
	-AG	Primary physician
	-AH	Clinical psychologist
	-AI	Principal physician of record
	-AJ	Clinical social worker
	-AK	Non-participating physician
	-AM	Physician, team member service
	-AO	Alternate payment method declined by provider of service
	-AP	Determination of refractive state was not performed in the course of diagnostic ophthalmological examination
	-AQ	Physician providing a service in an unlisted health professional shortage area (HPSA)
	-AR	Physician provider services in a physician scarcity area
	-AS	Physician assistant, nurse practitioner, or clinical nurse specialist services for assistant at surgery
	-AT	Acute treatment (this modifier should be used when reporting service 98940, 98941, 98942)
	-AU	Item furnished in conjunction with a urological, ostomy, or tracheostomy supply
	-AV	Item furnished in conjunction with a prosthetic device, prosthetic or orthotic
	-AW	Item furnished in conjunction with a surgical dressing
	-AX	Item furnished in conjunction with dialysis services
	-AY	Item or service furnished to an ESRD patient that is not for the treatment of ESRD

A	MOD	DESCRIPTION
	-AZ	Physician providing a service in a dental health professional shortage area for the purpose of an electronic health record incentive payment
	-BA	Item furnished in conjunction with parenteral enteral nutrition (pen) services
	-BL	Special acquisition of blood and blood products
	-BO	Orally administered nutrition, not by feeding tube
	-BP	The beneficiary has been informed of the purchase and rental options and has elected to purchase the item
	-BR	The beneficiary has been informed of the purchase and rental options and has elected to rent the item
	-BU	The beneficiary has been informed of the purchase and rental options and after 30 days has not informed the supplier of his/her decision
	-CA	Procedure payable only in the inpatient setting when performed emergently on an outpatient who expires prior to admission
	-CB	Service ordered by a renal dialysis facility (RDF) physician as part of the ESRD beneficiary's dialysis benefit, is not part of the composite rate, and is separately reimbursable
	-CC	Procedure code change (use 'cc' when the procedure code submitted was changed either for administrative reasons or because an incorrect code was filed)
	-CD	AMCC test has been ordered by an ESRD facility or MCP physician that is part of the composite rate and is not separately billable
	-CE	AMCC test has been ordered by an ESRD facility or MCP physician that is a composite rate test but is beyond the normal frequency covered under the rate and is separately reimbursable based on medical necessity
	-CF	AMCC test has been ordered by an ESRD facility or MCP physician that is not part of the composite rate and is separately billable
	-CG	Policy criteria applied
	-CH	0 percent impaired, limited or restricted
	-CI	At least 1 percent but less than 20 percent impaired, limited or restricted
	-CJ	At least 20 percent but less than 40 percent impaired, limited or restricted
	-CK	At least 40 percent but less than 60 percent impaired, limited or restricted
	-CL	At least 60 percent but less than 80 percent impaired, limited or restricted
	-CM	At least 80 percent but less than 100 percent impaired, limited or restricted
	-CN	100 percent impaired, limited or restricted
	-CO	Outpatient occupational therapy services furnished in whole or in part by an occupational therapy assistant
	-CQ	Outpatient physical therapy services furnished in whole or in part by a physical therapist assistant
	-CR	Catastrophe/disaster related
	-CS	Item or service related, in whole or in part, to an illness, injury, or condition that was caused by or exacerbated by the effects, direct or indirect, of the 2010 oil spill in the Gulf of Mexico, including but not limited to subsequent clean-up activities
	-CT	Computed tomography services furnished using equipment that does not meet each of the attributes of the national electrical manufacturers association (nema) xr-29-2013 standard
	-DA	Oral health assessment by a licensed health professional other than a dentist
	-E1	Upper left, eyelid

A	MOD	DESCRIPTION
	-E2	Lower left, eyelid
	-E3	Upper right, eyelid
	-E4	Lower right, eyelid
	-EA	Erythropoietic stimulating agent (ESA) administered to treat anemia due to anti-cancer chemotherapy
	-EB	Erythropoietic stimulating agent (ESA) administered to treat anemia due to anti-cancer radiotherapy
	-EC	Erythropoietic stimulating agent (ESA) administered to treat anemia not due to anti-cancer radiotherapy or anti-cancer chemotherapy
	-ED	Hematocrit level has exceeded 39% (or hemoglobin level has exceeded 13.0 g/dl) for 3 or more consecutive billing cycles immediately prior to and including the current cycle
	-EE	Hematocrit level has not exceeded 39% (or hemoglobin level has not exceeded 13.0 g/dl) for 3 or more consecutive billing cycles immediately prior to and including the current cycle
	-EJ	Subsequent claims for a defined course of therapy, e.g., EPO, sodium hyaluronate, infliximab
	-EM	Emergency reserve supply (for ESRD benefit only)
	-EP	Service provided as part of Medicaid early periodic screening diagnosis and treatment (EPSDT) program
	-ER	Items and services furnished by a provider-based, off-campus emergency department
	-ET	Emergency services
	-EX	Expatriate beneficiary
	-EY	No physician or other licensed health care provider order for this item or service
	-F1	Left hand, second digit
	-F2	Left hand, third digit
	-F3	Left hand, fourth digit
	-F4	Left hand, fifth digit
	-F5	Right hand, thumb
	-F6	Right hand, second digit
	-F7	Right hand, third digit
	-F8	Right hand, fourth digit
	-F9	Right hand, fifth digit
	-FA	Left hand, thumb
	-FB	Item provided without cost to provider, supplier or practitioner, or full credit received for replaced device (examples, but not limited to, covered under warranty, replaced due to defect, free samples)
	-FC	Partial credit received for replaced device
	-FP	Service provided as part of family planning program
	-FQ	The service was furnished using audio-only communication technology
	-FR	The supervising practitioner was present through two-way, audio/video communication technology
	-FS	Split (or shared) evaluation and management visit
	-FT	Unrelated evaluation and management (e/m) visit during a postoperative period, or on the same

APPENDICES

A	MOD	DESCRIPTION
		day as a procedure or another e/m visit. (report when an e/m visit is furnished within the global period but is unrelated, or when one or more additional e/m visits furnished on the same day are unrelated
	-FX	X-ray taken using film
	-FY	X-ray taken using computed radiography technology/cassette-based imaging
	-G0	Telehealth services for diagnosis, evaluation, or treatment, of symptoms of an acute stroke
	-G1	Most recent URR reading of less than 60
	-G2	Most recent URR reading of 60 to 64.9
	-G3	Most recent URR reading of 65 to 69.9
	-G4	Most recent URR reading of 70 to 74.9
	-G5	Most recent URR reading of 75 or greater
	-G6	ESRD patient for whom less than six dialysis sessions have been provided in a month
	-G7	Pregnancy resulted from rape or incest or pregnancy certified by physician as life threatening
	-G8	Monitored anesthesia care (mac) for deep complex, complicated, or markedly invasive surgical procedure
	-G9	Monitored anesthesia care for patient who has history of severe cardio-pulmonary condition
	-GA	Waiver of liability statement issued as required by payer policy, individual case
	-GB	Claim being re-submitted for payment because it is no longer covered under a global payment demonstration
	-GC	This service has been performed in part by a resident under the direction of a teaching physician
	-GE	This service has been performed by a resident without the presence of a teaching physician under the primary care exception
	-GF	Non-physician (e.g. nurse practitioner (NP), certified registered nurse anesthetist (CRNA), certified registered nurse (CRN), clinical nurse specialist (CNS), physician assistant (pa)) services in a critical access hospital
	-GG	Performance and payment of a screening mammogram and diagnostic mammogram on the same patient, same day
	-GH	Diagnostic mammogram converted from screening mammogram on same day
	-GJ	"opt out" physician or practitioner emergency or urgent service
	-GK	Reasonable and necessary item/service associated with a -GA or -GZ modifier
	-GL	Medically unnecessary upgrade provided instead of non-upgraded item, no charge, no advance beneficiary notice (ABN)
	-GM	Multiple patients on one ambulance trip
	-GN	Services delivered under an outpatient speech language pathology plan of care
	-GO	Services delivered under an outpatient occupational therapy plan of care
	-GP	Services delivered under an outpatient physical therapy plan of care
	-GQ	Via asynchronous telecommunications system
	-GR	This service was performed in whole or in part by a resident in a Department of Veterans Affairs medical `center or clinic, supervised in accordance with VA policy
	-GS	Dosage of erythropoietin stimulating agent has been reduced and maintained in response to hematocrit or hemoglobin level

A	MOD	DESCRIPTION
	-GT	Via interactive audio and video telecommunication systems
	-GU	Waiver of liability statement issued as required by payer policy, routine notice
	-GV	Attending physician not employed or paid under arrangement by the patient's hospice provider
	-GW	Service not related to the hospice patient's terminal condition
	-GX	Notice of liability issued, voluntary under payer policy
	-GY	Item or service statutorily excluded, does not meet the definition of any Medicare benefit or, for non-Medicare insurers, is not a contract benefit
	-GZ	Item or service expected to be denied as not reasonable and necessary
	-H9	Court-ordered
	-HA	Child/adolescent program
	-HB	Adult program, non-geriatric
	-HC	Adult program, geriatric
	-HD	Pregnant/parenting women's program
	-HE	Mental health program
	-HF	Substance abuse program
	-HG	Opioid addiction treatment program
	-HH	Integrated mental health/substance abuse program
	-HI	Integrated mental health and intellectual disability/developmental disabilities program
	-HJ	Employee assistance program
	-HK	Specialized mental health programs for high-risk populations
	-HL	Intern
	-HM	Less than bachelor's degree level
	-HN	Bachelor's degree level
	-HO	Master's degree level
	-HP	Doctoral level
	-HQ	Group setting
	-HR	Family/couple with client present
	-HS	Family/couple without client present
	-HT	Multi-disciplinary team
	-HU	Funded by child welfare agency
	-HV	Funded state addictions agency
	-HW	Funded by state mental health agency
	-HX	Funded by county/local agency
	-HY	Funded by juvenile justice agency
	-HZ	Funded by criminal justice agency
	-J1	Competitive acquisition program no-pay submission for a prescription number
	-J2	Competitive acquisition program, restocking of emergency drugs after emergency administration

APPENDICES

A	MOD	DESCRIPTION
	-J3	Competitive acquisition program (cap), drug not available through cap as written, reimbursed under average sales price methodology
	-J4	DMEPOS item subject to DMEPOS competitive bidding program that is furnished by a hospital upon discharge
	-J5	Off-the-shelf orthotic subject to DMEPOS competitive bidding program that is furnished as part of a physical therapist or occupational therapist professional service
	-JA	Administered intravenously
	-JB	Administered subcutaneously
	-JC	Skin substitute used as a graft
	-JD	Skin substitute not used as a graft
	-JE	Administered via dialysate
	-JG	Drug or biological acquired with 340b drug pricing program discount, reported for informational purposes
	-JW	Drug amount discarded/not administered to any patient
	-JZ	Zero drug amount discarded/not administered to any patient
	-K0	Lower extremity prosthesis functional level 0 - does not have the ability or potential to ambulate or transfer safely with or without assistance and a prosthesis does not enhance their quality of life or mobility.
	-K1	Lower extremity prosthesis functional level 1 - has the ability or potential to use a prosthesis for transfers or ambulation on level surfaces at fixed cadence. typical of the limited and unlimited household ambulator.
	-K2	Lower extremity prosthesis functional level 2 - has the ability or potential for ambulation with the ability to traverse low level environmental barriers such as curbs, stairs or uneven surfaces. typical of the limited community ambulator.
	-K3	Lower extremity prosthesis functional level 3 - has the ability or potential for ambulation with variable cadence. typical of the community ambulator who has the ability to transverse most environmental barriers and may have vocational, therapeutic, or exercise activity that demands prosthetic utilization beyond simple locomotion.
	-K4	Lower extremity prosthesis functional level 4 - has the ability or potential for prosthetic ambulation that exceeds the basic ambulation skills, exhibiting high impact, stress, or energy levels, typical of the prosthetic demands of the child, active adult, or athlete.
	-KA	Add on option/accessory for wheelchair
	-KB	Beneficiary requested upgrade for ABN, more than 4 modifiers identified on claim
	-KC	Replacement of special power wheelchair interface
	-KD	Drug or biological infused through DME
	-KE	Bid under round one of the DMEPOS competitive bidding program for use with non-competitive bid base equipment
	-KF	Item designated by FDA as class iii device
	-KG	DMEPOS item subject to DMEPOS competitive bidding program number 1
	-KH	DMEPOS item, initial claim, purchase or first month rental
	-KI	DMEPOS item, second or third month rental
	-KJ	DMEPOS item, parenteral enteral nutrition (pen) pump or capped rental, months four to fifteen
	-KK	DMEPOS item subject to DMEPOS competitive bidding program number 2

APPENDICES

A	MOD	DESCRIPTION
	-KL	DMEPOS item delivered via mail
	-KM	Replacement of facial prosthesis including new impression/moulage
	-KN	Replacement of facial prosthesis using previous master model
	-KO	Single drug unit dose formulation
	-KP	First drug of a multiple drug unit dose formulation
	-KQ	Second or subsequent drug of a multiple drug unit dose formulation
	-KR	Rental item, billing for partial month
	-KS	Glucose monitor supply for diabetic beneficiary not treated with insulin
	-KT	Beneficiary resides in a competitive bidding area and travels outside that competitive bidding area and receives a competitive bid item
	-KU	DMEPOS item subject to DMEPOS competitive bidding program number 3
	-KV	DMEPOS item subject to DMEPOS competitive bidding program that is furnished as part of a professional service
	-KW	DMEPOS item subject to DMEPOS competitive bidding program number 4
	-KX	Requirements specified in the medical policy have been met
	-KY	DMEPOS item subject to DMEPOS competitive bidding program number 5
	-KZ	New coverage not implemented by managed care
	-LC	Left circumflex coronary artery
	-LD	Left anterior descending coronary artery
	-LL	Lease/rental (use the 'LL' modifier when DME equipment rental is to be applied against the purchase price)
	-LM	Left main coronary artery
	-LR	Laboratory round trip
	-LS	FDA-monitored intraocular lens implant
	-LT	Left side (used to identify procedures performed on the left side of the body)
	-LU	Fractionated payment of car-t therapy
	-M2	Medicare secondary payer (MSP)
	-MA	Ordering professional is not required to consult a clinical decision support mechanism due to service being rendered to a patient with a suspected or confirmed emergency medical condition
	-MB	Ordering professional is not required to consult a clinical decision support mechanism due to the significant hardship exception of insufficient internet access
	-MC	Ordering professional is not required to consult a clinical decision support mechanism due to the significant hardship exception of electronic health record or clinical decision support mechanism vendor issues
	-MD	Ordering professional is not required to consult a clinical decision support mechanism due to the significant hardship exception of extreme and uncontrollable circumstances
	-ME	The order for this service adheres to appropriate use criteria in the clinical decision support mechanism consulted by the ordering professional
	-MF	The order for this service does not adhere to the appropriate use criteria in the clinical decision support mechanism consulted by the ordering professional
	-MG	The order for this service does not have applicable appropriate use criteria in the qualified clinical

APPENDICES

A	MOD	DESCRIPTION
		decision support mechanism consulted by the ordering professional
	-MH	Unknown if ordering professional consulted a clinical decision support mechanism for this service, related information was not provided to the furnishing professional or provider
	-MS	Six-month maintenance and servicing fee for reasonable and necessary parts and labor which are not covered under any manufacturer or supplier warranty
	-NB	Nebulizer system, any type, FDA-cleared for use with specific drug
	-NR	New when rented (use the 'nr' modifier when DME which was new at the time of rental is subsequently purchased)
	-NU	New equipment
	-P1	A normal healthy patient
	-P2	A patient with mild systemic disease
	-P3	A patient with severe systemic disease
	-P4	A patient with severe systemic disease that is a constant threat to life
	-P5	A moribund patient who is not expected to survive without the operation
	-P6	A declared brain-dead patient whose organs are being removed for donor purposes
	-PA	Surgical or other invasive procedure on wrong body part
	-PB	Surgical or other invasive procedure on wrong patient
	-PC	Wrong surgery or other invasive procedure on patient
	-PD	Diagnostic or related non-diagnostic item or service provided in a wholly owned or operated entity to a patient who is admitted as an inpatient within 3 days
	-PI	Positron emission tomography (pet) or pet/computed tomography (CT) to inform the initial treatment strategy of tumors that are biopsy proven or strongly suspected of being cancerous based on other diagnostic testing
	-PL	Progressive addition lenses
	-PM	Postmortem
	-PN	Non-excepted service provided at an off-campus, outpatient, provider-based department of a hospital
	-PO	Excepted service provided at an off-campus, outpatient, provider-based department of a hospital
	-PS	Positron emission tomography (pet) or pet/computed tomography (CT) to inform the subsequent treatment strategy of cancerous tumors when the beneficiary's treating physician determines that the pet study is needed to inform subsequent anti-tumor strategy
	-PT	Colorectal cancer screening test; converted to diagnostic test or other procedure
	-Q0	Investigational clinical service provided in a clinical research study that is in an approved clinical research study
	-Q1	Routine clinical service provided in a clinical research study that is in an approved clinical research study
	-Q2	Demonstration procedure/service
	-Q3	Live kidney donor surgery and related services
	-Q4	Service for ordering/referring physician qualifies as a service exemption
	-Q5	Service furnished under a reciprocal billing arrangement by a substitute physician or by a substitute physical therapist furnishing outpatient physical therapy services in a health professional shortage area, a medically underserved area, or a rural area

A	MOD	DESCRIPTION
	-Q6	Service furnished under a fee-for-time compensation arrangement by a substitute physician or by a substitute physical therapist furnishing outpatient physical therapy services in a health professional shortage area, a medically underserved area, or a rural area
	-Q7	One class a finding
	-Q8	Two class b findings
	-Q9	One class b and two class c findings
	-QA	Prescribed amounts of stationary oxygen for daytime use while at rest and nighttime use differ and the average of the two amounts is less than 1 liter per minute (lpm)
	-QB	Prescribed amounts of stationary oxygen for daytime use while at rest and nighttime use differ and the average of the two amounts exceeds 4 liters per minute (lpm) and portable oxygen is prescribed
	-QC	Single channel monitoring
	-QD	Recording and storage in solid state memory by a digital recorder
	-QE	Prescribed amount of stationary oxygen while at rest is less than 1 liter per minute (lpm)
	-QF	Prescribed amount of stationary oxygen while at rest exceeds 4 liters per minute (lpm) and portable oxygen is prescribed
	-QG	Prescribed amount of stationary oxygen while at rest is greater than 4 liters per minute (lpm)
	-QH	Oxygen conserving device is being used with an oxygen delivery system
	-QJ	Services/items provided to a prisoner or patient in state or local custody, however the state or local government, as applicable, meets the requirements in 42 CFR 411.4 (b)
	-QK	Medical direction of two, three, or four concurrent anesthesia procedures involving qualified individuals
	-QL	Patient pronounced dead after ambulance called
	-QM	Ambulance service provided under arrangement by a provider of services
	-QN	Ambulance service furnished directly by a provider of services
	-QP	Documentation is on file showing that the laboratory test(s) was ordered individually or ordered as a CPT-recognized panel other than automated profile codes 80002-80019, G0058, G0059, and G0060.
	-QQ	Ordering professional consulted a qualified clinical decision support mechanism for this service and the related data was provided to the furnishing professional
	-QR	Prescribed amounts of stationary oxygen for daytime use while at rest and nighttime use differ and the average of the two amounts is greater than 4 liters per minute (lpm)
	-QS	Monitored anesthesia care service
	-QT	Recording and storage on tape by an analog tape recorder
	-QW	CLIA waived test
	-QX	CRNA service: with medical direction by a physician
	-QY	Medical direction of one certified registered nurse anesthetist (CRNA) by an anesthesiologist
	-QZ	CRNA service: without medical direction by a physician
	-RA	Replacement of a DME, orthotic or prosthetic item
	-RB	Replacement of a part of a DME, orthotic or prosthetic item furnished as part of a repair
	-RC	Right coronary artery
	-RD	Drug provided to beneficiary, but not administered "incident-to"

A	MOD	DESCRIPTION
	-RE	Furnished in full compliance with FDA-mandated risk evaluation and mitigation strategy (rems)
	-RI	Ramus intermedius coronary artery
	-RR	Rental (use the 'RR' modifier when DME is to be rented)
	-RT	Right side (used to identify procedures performed on the right side of the body)
	-SA	Nurse practitioner rendering service in collaboration with a physician
	-SB	Nurse midwife
	-SC	Medically necessary service or supply
	-SD	Services provided by registered nurse with specialized, highly technical home infusion training
	-SE	State and/or federally funded programs/services
	-SF	Second opinion ordered by a professional review organization (pro) per section 9401, p.l. 99-272 (100% reimbursement - no Medicare deductible or coinsurance)
	-SG	Ambulatory surgical center (ASC) facility service
	-SH	Second concurrently administered infusion therapy
	-SJ	Third or more concurrently administered infusion therapy
	-SK	Member of high-risk population (use only with codes for immunization)
	-SL	State supplied vaccine
	-SM	Second surgical opinion
	-SN	Third surgical opinion
	-SQ	Item ordered by home health
	-SS	Home infusion services provided in the infusion suite of the iv therapy provider
	-ST	Related to trauma or injury
	-SU	Procedure performed in physician's office (to denote use of facility and equipment)
	-SV	Pharmaceuticals delivered to patient's home but not utilized
	-SW	Services provided by a certified diabetic educator
	-SY	Persons who are in close contact with member of high-risk population (use only with codes for immunization)
	-T1	Left foot, second digit
	-T2	Left foot, third digit
	-T3	Left foot, fourth digit
	-T4	Left foot, fifth digit
	-T5	Right foot, great toe
	-T6	Right foot, second digit
	-T7	Right foot, third digit
	-T8	Right foot, fourth digit
	-T9	Right foot, fifth digit
	-TA	Left foot, great toe
	-TB	Drug or biological acquired with 340b drug pricing program discount, reported for informational purposes for select entities

A	MOD	DESCRIPTION
	-TC	Technical component; under certain circumstances, a charge may be made for the technical component alone; under those circumstances the technical component charge is identified by adding modifier 'TC' to the usual procedure number; technical component charges are institutional charges and not billed separately by physicians; however, portable x-ray suppliers only bill for technical component and should utilize modifier TC; the charge data from portable x-ray suppliers will then be used to build customary and prevailing profiles
	-TD	RN
	-TE	LPN/LVN
	-TF	Intermediate level of care
	-TG	Complex/high tech level of care
	-TH	Obstetrical treatment/services, prenatal or postpartum
	-TJ	Program group, child and/or adolescent
	-TK	Extra patient or passenger, non-ambulance
	-TL	Early intervention/individualized family service plan (IFSP)
	-TM	Individualized education program (IEP)
	-TN	Rural/outside providers' customary service area
	-TP	Medical transport, unloaded vehicle
	-TQ	Basic life support transport by a volunteer ambulance provider
	-TR	School-based individualized education program (IEP) services provided outside the public school district responsible for the student
	-TS	Follow-up service
	-TT	Individualized service provided to more than one patient in same setting
	-TU	Special payment rate, overtime
	-TV	Special payment rates, holidays/weekends
	-TW	Back-up equipment
	-U1	Medicaid level of care 1, as defined by each state
	-U2	Medicaid level of care 2, as defined by each state
	-U3	Medicaid level of care 3, as defined by each state
	-U4	Medicaid level of care 4, as defined by each state
	-U5	Medicaid level of care 5, as defined by each state
	-U6	Medicaid level of care 6, as defined by each state
	-U7	Medicaid level of care 7, as defined by each state
	-U8	Medicaid level of care 8, as defined by each state
	-U9	Medicaid level of care 9, as defined by each state
	-UA	Medicaid level of care 10, as defined by each state
	-UB	Medicaid level of care 11, as defined by each state
	-UC	Medicaid level of care 12, as defined by each state
	-UD	Medicaid level of care 13, as defined by each state
	-UE	Used durable medical equipment

APPENDICES

A	MOD	DESCRIPTION
	-UF	Services provided in the morning
	-UG	Services provided in the afternoon
	-UH	Services provided in the evening
	-UJ	Services provided at night
	-UK	Services provided on behalf of the client to someone other than the client (collateral relationship)
	-UN	Two patients served
	-UP	Three patients served
	-UQ	Four patients served
	-UR	Five patients served
	-US	Six or more patients served
	-V1	Demonstration modifier 1
	-V2	Demonstration modifier 2
	-V3	Demonstration modifier 3
	-V4	Demonstration modifier 4
	-V5	Vascular catheter (alone or with any other vascular access)
	-V6	Arteriovenous graft (or other vascular access not including a vascular catheter)
	-V7	Arteriovenous fistula only (in use with two needles)
	-VM	Medicare diabetes prevention program (MDPP) virtual make-up session
	-VP	Aphakic patient
	-X1	Continuous/broad services: for reporting services by clinicians, who provide the principal care for a patient, with no planned endpoint of the relationship; services in this category represent comprehensive care, dealing with the entire scope of patient problems, either directly or in a care coordination role; reporting clinician service examples include, but are not limited to: primary care, and clinicians providing comprehensive care to patients in addition to specialty care
	-X2	Continuous/focused services: for reporting services by clinicians whose expertise is needed for the ongoing management of a chronic disease or a condition that needs to be managed and followed with no planned endpoint to the relationship; reporting clinician service examples include but are not limited to: a rheumatologist taking care of the patient's rheumatoid arthritis longitudinally but not providing general primary care services
	-X3	Episodic/broad services: for reporting services by clinicians who have broad responsibility for the comprehensive needs of the patient that is limited to a defined period and circumstance such as a hospitalization; reporting clinician service examples include but are not limited to the hospitalist's services rendered providing comprehensive and general care to a patient while admitted to the hospital
	-X4	Episodic/focused services: for reporting services by clinicians who provide focused care on particular types of treatment limited to a defined period and circumstance; the patient has a problem, acute or chronic, that will be treated with surgery, radiation, or some other type of generally time-limited intervention; reporting clinician service examples include but are not limited to, the orthopedic surgeon performing a knee replacement and seeing the patient through the postoperative period
	-X5	Diagnostic services requested by another clinician: for reporting services by a clinician who furnishes care to the patient only as requested by another clinician or subsequent and related services requested by another clinician; this modifier is reported for patient relationships that may not be adequately captured by the above alternative categories; reporting clinician service

A	MOD	DESCRIPTION
		examples include but are not limited to, the radiologist's interpretation of an imaging study requested by another clinician
	-XE	Separate encounter, a service that is distinct because it occurred during a separate encounter
	-XP	Separate practitioner, a service that is distinct because it was performed by a different practitioner
	-XS	Separate structure, a service that is distinct because it was performed on a separate organ/structure
	-XU	Unusual non-overlapping service, the use of a service that is distinct because it does not overlap usual components of the main service

APPENDICES

APPENDIX B: SUMMARY OF CHANGES

Summary of Official HCPCS Additions, Changes, and Deletions

- • **A4287** Disposable collection and storage bag for breast milk, any size, any type, each
- • **A4457** Enema tube, with or without adapter, any type, replacement only, each
- • **A4468** Exsufflation belt, includes all supplies and accessories
- • **A4540** Distal transcutaneous electrical nerve stimulator, stimulates peripheral nerves of the upper arm
- • **A4541** Monthly supplies for use of device coded at e0733
- • **A4542** Supplies and accessories for external upper limb tremor stimulator of the peripheral nerves of the wrist
- • **A6520** Gradient compression garment, glove, padded, for nighttime use, each
- • **A6521** Gradient compression garment, glove, padded, for nighttime use, custom, each
- • **A6522** Gradient compression garment, arm, padded, for nighttime use, each
- • **A6523** Gradient compression garment, arm, padded, for nighttime use, custom, each
- • **A6524** Gradient compression garment, lower leg and foot, padded, for nighttime use, each
- • **A6525** Gradient compression garment, lower leg and foot, padded, for nighttime use, custom, each
- • **A6526** Gradient compression garment, full leg and foot, padded, for nighttime use, each
- • **A6527** Gradient compression garment, full leg and foot, padded, for nighttime use, custom, each
- • **A6528** Gradient compression garment, bra, for nighttime use, each
- • **A6529** Gradient compression garment, bra, for nighttime use, custom, each
- ▲ **A6531** Gradient compression stocking, below knee, 30-40 mmhg, used as a surgical dressing, each
- ▲ **A6532** Gradient compression stocking, below knee, 40-50 mmhg, used as a surgical dressing, each
- ▲ **A6535** Gradient compression stocking, thigh length, 40 mmhg or greater, each
- ▲ **A6538** Gradient compression stocking, full length/chap style, 40 mmhg or greater, each
- ▲ **A6541** Gradient compression stocking, waist length, 40 mmhg or greater, each
- ▲ **A6545** Gradient compression wrap, non-elastic, below knee, 30-50 mmhg, used as a surgical dressing, each
- ▲ **A6549** Gradient compression garment, not otherwise specified
- • **A6552** Gradient compression stocking, below knee, 30-40 mmhg, each
- • **A6553** Gradient compression stocking, below knee, 30-40 mmhg, custom, each
- • **A6554** Gradient compression stocking, below knee, 40 mmhg or greater, each
- • **A6555** Gradient compression stocking, below knee, 40 mmhg or greater, custom, each
- • **A6556** Gradient compression stocking, thigh length, 18-30 mmhg, custom, each
- • **A6557** Gradient compression stocking, thigh length, 30-40 mmhg, custom, each
- • **A6558** Gradient compression stocking, thigh length, 40 mmhg or greater, custom, each
- • **A6559** Gradient compression stocking, full length/chap style, 18-30 mmhg, custom, each
- • **A6560** Gradient compression stocking, full length/chap style, 30-40 mmhg, custom, each
- • **A6561** Gradient compression stocking, full length/chap style, 40 mmhg or greater, custom, each

• **A6562** Gradient compression stocking, waist length, 18-30 mmhg, custom, each
• **A6563** Gradient compression stocking, waist length, 30-40 mmhg, custom, each
• **A6564** Gradient compression stocking, waist length, 40 mmhg or greater, custom, each
• **A6565** Gradient compression gauntlet, custom, each
• **A6566** Gradient compression garment, neck/head, each
• **A6567** Gradient compression garment, neck/head, custom, each
• **A6568** Gradient compression garment, torso and shoulder, each
• **A6569** Gradient compression garment, torso/shoulder, custom, each
• **A6570** Gradient compression garment, genital region, each
• **A6571** Gradient compression garment, genital region, custom, each
• **A6572** Gradient compression garment, toe caps, each
• **A6573** Gradient compression garment, toe caps, custom, each
• **A6574** Gradient compression arm sleeve and glove combination, custom, each
• **A6575** Gradient compression arm sleeve and glove combination, each
• **A6576** Gradient compression arm sleeve, custom, medium weight, each
• **A6577** Gradient compression arm sleeve, custom, heavy weight, each
• **A6578** Gradient compression arm sleeve, each
• **A6579** Gradient compression glove, custom, medium weight, each
• **A6580** Gradient compression glove, custom, heavy weight, each
• **A6581** Gradient compression glove, each
• **A6582** Gradient compression gauntlet, each
• **A6583** Gradient compression wrap with adjustable straps, below knee, 30-50 mmhg, each
• **A6584** Gradient compression wrap with adjustable straps, not otherwise specified
• **A6585** Gradient pressure wrap with adjustable straps, above knee, each
• **A6586** Gradient pressure wrap with adjustable straps, full leg, each
• **A6587** Gradient pressure wrap with adjustable straps, foot, each
• **A6588** Gradient pressure wrap with adjustable straps, arm, each
• **A6589** Gradient pressure wrap with adjustable straps, bra, each
• **A6593** Accessory for gradient compression garment or wrap with adjustable straps, non-otherwise specified
• **A6594** Gradient compression bandaging supply, bandage liner, lower extremity, any size or length, each
• **A6595** Gradient compression bandaging supply, bandage liner, upper extremity, any size or length, each
• **A6596** Gradient compression bandaging supply, conforming gauze, per linear yard, any width, each
• **A6597** Gradient compression bandage roll, elastic long stretch, linear yard, any width, each
• **A6598** Gradient compression bandage roll, elastic medium stretch, per linear yard, any width, each
• **A6599** Gradient compression bandage roll, inelastic short stretch, per linear yard, any width, each
• **A6600** Gradient compression bandaging supply, high density foam sheet, per 250 square centimeters, each
• **A6601** Gradient compression bandaging supply, high density foam pad, any size or shape, each

- **A6602** Gradient compression bandaging supply, high density foam roll for bandage, per linear yard, any width, each
- **A6603** Gradient compression bandaging supply, low density channel foam sheet, per 250 square centimeters, each
- **A6604** Gradient compression bandaging supply, low density flat foam sheet, per 250 square centimeters, each
- **A6605** Gradient compression bandaging supply, padded foam, per linear yard, any width, each
- **A6606** Gradient compression bandaging supply, padded textile, per linear yard, any width, each
- **A6607** Gradient compression bandaging supply, tubular protective absorption layer, per linear yard, any width, each
- **A6608** Gradient compression bandaging supply, tubular protective absorption padded layer, per linear yard, any width, each
- **A6609** Gradient compression bandaging supply, not otherwise specified
- **A6610** Gradient compression stocking, below knee, 18-30 mmhg, custom, each
- **A7023** Mechanical allergen particle barrier/inhalation filter, cream, nasal, topical
- **A9608** Flotufolastat f 18, diagnostic, 1 millicurie
- **A9609** Fludeoxyglucose f18 up to 15 millicuries
- **C1600** Catheter, transluminal intravascular lesion preparation device, bladed, sheathed (insertable)
- **C1601** Endoscope, single-use (i.e. disposable), pulmonary, imaging/illumination device (insertable)
- **C1602** Orthopedic/device/drug matrix/absorbable bone void filler, antimicrobial-eluting (implantable)
- **C1603** Retrieval device, insertable, laser (used to retrieve intravascular inferior vena cava filter)
- **C1604** Graft, transmural transvenous arterial bypass (implantable), with all delivery system components
- **C7556** Bronchoscopy, rigid or flexible, with bronchial alveolar lavage and transendoscopic endobronchial ultrasound (ebus) during bronchoscopic diagnostic or therapeutic intervention(s) for peripheral lesion(s), including fluoroscopic guidance, when performed
- **C7557** Catheter placement in coronary artery(s) for coronary angiography, including intraprocedural injection(s) for coronary angiography, imaging supervision and interpretation with left heart catheterization including intraprocedural injection(s) for left ventriculography, when performed and intraprocedural coronary fractional flow reserve (ffr) with 3d functional mapping of color-coded ffr values for the coronary tree, derived from coronary angiogram data, for real-time review and interpretation of possible atherosclerotic stenosis(es) intervention
- **C7558** Catheter placement in coronary artery(s) for coronary angiography, including intraprocedural injection(s) for coronary angiography, imaging supervision and interpretation with right and left heart catheterization including intraprocedural injection(s) for left ventriculography, when performed, catheter placement(s) in bypass graft(s) (internal mammary, free arterial, venous grafts) with bypass graft angiography with pharmacologic agent administration (eg, inhaled nitric oxide, intravenous infusion of nitroprusside, dobutamine, milrinone, or other agent) including assessing hemodynamic measurements before, during, after and repeat pharmacologic agent administration, when performed
- **C7560** Endoscopic retrograde cholangiopancreatography (ercp) with removal of foreign body(s) or stent(s) from biliary/pancreatic duct(s) and endoscopic cannulation of papilla with direct visualization of pancreatic/common bile duct(s)
- **C7561** Debridement, bone (includes epidermis, dermis, subcutaneous tissue, muscle and/or fascia, if performed); first 20 sq cm or less with manual preparation and insertion of drug-delivery device(s), deep (e.g., subfascial)

• **C7903** Group psychotherapy service for diagnosis, evaluation, or treatment of a mental health or substance use disorder provided remotely by hospital staff who are licensed to provide mental health services under applicable state law(s), when the patient is in their home, and there is no associated professional service

(**C9152** Injection, aripiprazole, (abilify asimtufii), 1 mg **Code deleted** effective 12/31/2023, no HCPCS/CPT cross-reference provided.)

(**C9153** Injection, amisulpride, 1 mg **Code deleted** effective 12/31/2023, no HCPCS/CPT cross-reference provided.)

(**C9154** Injection, buprenorphine extended-release (brixadi), 1 mg **Code deleted** effective 12/31/2023, no HCPCS/CPT cross-reference provided.)

(**C9155** Injection, epcoritamab-bysp, 0.16 mg **Code deleted** effective 12/31/2023, no HCPCS/CPT cross-reference provided.)

(**C9156** Flotufolastat f 18, diagnostic, 1 millicurie **Code deleted** effective 12/31/2023, no HCPCS/CPT cross-reference provided.)

(**C9157** Injection, tofersen, 1 mg **Code deleted** effective 12/31/2023, no HCPCS/CPT cross-reference provided.)

(**C9158** Injection, risperidone, (uzedy), 1 mg **Code deleted** effective 12/31/2023, no HCPCS/CPT cross-reference provided.)

• **C9159** Injection, prothrombin complex concentrate (human), balfaxar, per i.u. of factor ix activity

• **C9160** Injection, daxibotulinumtoxina-lanm, 1 unit

• **C9161** Injection, aflibercept hd, 1 mg

• **C9162** Injection, avacincaptad pegol, 0.1 mg

• **C9163** Injection, talquetamab-tgvs, 0.25 mg

• **C9164** Cantharidin for topical administration, 0.7%, single unit dose applicator (3.2 mg)

• **C9165** Injection, elranatamab-bcmm, 1 mg

(**C9770** Vitrectomy, mechanical, pars plana approach, with subretinal injection of pharmacologic/biologic agent **Code deleted** effective 12/31/2023, no HCPCS/CPT cross-reference provided.)

(**C9771** Nasal/sinus endoscopy, cryoablation nasal tissue(s) and/or nerve(s), unilateral or bilateral **Code deleted** effective 12/31/2023, no HCPCS/CPT cross-reference provided.)

(**C9788** Opto-acoustic imaging, breast (including axilla when performed), unilateral, with image documentation, analysis and report, obtained with ultrasound examination **Code deleted** effective 12/31/2023, no HCPCS/CPT cross-reference provided.)

• **C9793** 3d predictive model generation for pre-planning of a cardiac procedure, using data from cardiac computed tomographic angiography with report

• **C9794** Therapeutic radiology simulation-aided field setting; complex, including acquisition of pet and ct imaging data required for radiopharmaceutical-directed radiation therapy treatment planning (i.e., modeling)

• **C9795** Stereotactic body radiation therapy, treatment delivery, per fraction to 1 or more lesions, including image guidance and real-time positron emissions-based delivery adjustments to 1 or more lesions, entire course not to exceed 5 fractions

(**C9803** Hospital outpatient clinic visit specimen collection for severe acute respiratory syndrome coronavirus 2 (sars-cov-2) (coronavirus disease [covid-19]), any specimen source **Code deleted** effective 12/31/2023, no HCPCS/CPT cross-reference provided.)

• **E0492** Power source and control electronics unit for oral device/appliance for neuromuscular electrical stimulation of the tongue muscle, controlled by phone application

- **E0493** Oral device/appliance for neuromuscular electrical stimulation of the tongue muscle, used in conjunction with the power source and control electronics unit, controlled by phone application, 90-day supply
- **E0530** Electronic positional obstructive sleep apnea treatment, with sensor, includes all components and accessories, any type
- **E0678** Non-pneumatic sequential compression garment, full leg
- **E0679** Non-pneumatic sequential compression garment, half leg
- **E0680** Non-pneumatic compression controller with sequential calibrated gradient pressure
- **E0681** Non-pneumatic compression controller without calibrated gradient pressure
- **E0682** Non-pneumatic sequential compression garment, full arm
- **E0732** Cranial electrotherapy stimulation (ces) system, any type
- **E0733** Transcutaneous electrical nerve stimulator for electrical stimulation of the trigeminal nerve
- **E0734** External upper limb tremor stimulator of the peripheral nerves of the wrist
- **E0735** Non-invasive vagus nerve stimulator
- **E1301** Whirlpool tub, walk-in, portable
- **E2001** Suction pump, home model, portable or stationary, electric, any type, for use with external urine management system
- **E3000** Speech volume modulation system, any type, including all components and accessories
- **G0011** Individual counseling for pre-exposure prophylaxis (prep) by physician or qualified health care professional (qhp)to prevent human immunodeficiency virus (hiv), includes hiv risk assessment (initial or continued assessment of risk), hiv risk reduction and medication adherence, 15-30 minutes
- **G0012** Injection of pre-exposure prophylaxis (prep) drug for hiv prevention, under skin or into muscle
- **G0013** Individual counseling for pre-exposure prophylaxis (prep) by clinical staff to prevent human immunodeficiency virus (hiv), includes: hiv risk assessment (initial or continued assessment of risk), hiv risk reduction and medication adherence
- **G0017** Psychotherapy for crisis furnished in an applicable site of service (any place of service at which the non-facility rate for psychotherapy for crisis services applies, other than the office setting); first 60 minutes
- **G0018** Psychotherapy for crisis furnished in an applicable site of service (any place of service at which the non-facility rate for psychotherapy for crisis services applies, other than the office setting); each additional 30 minutes (list separately in addition to code for primary service)
- **G0019** Community health integration services performed by certified or trained auxiliary personnel, including a community health worker, under the direction of a physician or other practitioner; 60 minutes per calendar month, in the following activities to address social determinants of health (sdoh) need(s) that are significantly limiting the ability to diagnose or treat problem(s) addressed in an initiating visit: person-centered assessment, performed to better understand the individualized context of the intersection between the sdoh need(s) and the problem(s) addressed in the initiating visit. ++ conducting a person-centered assessment to understand patient's life story, strengths, needs, goals, preferences and desired outcomes, including understanding cultural and linguistic factors and including unmet sdoh needs (that are not separately billed). ++ facilitating patient-driven goal-setting and establishing an action plan. ++ providing tailored support to the patient as needed to accomplish the practitioner's treatment plan. practitioner, home-, and community-based care coordination. ++ coordinating receipt of needed services from healthcare practitioners, providers, and facilities; and from home- and community-based service providers, social service providers, and caregiver (if applicable). ++ communication with practitioners, home- and community-based service providers, hospitals, and skilled nursing facilities (or other health care facilities) regarding the patient's psychosocial strengths and needs, functional deficits, goals, preferences, and desired outcomes, including cultural and linguistic factors. ++ coordination of

care transitions between and among health care practitioners and settings, including transitions involving referral to other clinicians; follow-up after an emergency department visit; or follow-up after discharges from hospitals, skilled nursing facilities or other health care facilities. ++ facilitating access to community-based social services (e.g., housing, utilities, transportation, food assistance) to address the sdoh need(s). health education- helping the patient contextualize health education provided by the patient's treatment team with the patient's individual needs, goals, and preferences, in the context of the sdoh need(s), and educating the patient on how to best participate in medical decision-making. building patient self-advocacy skills, so that the patient can interact with members of the health care team and related community-based services addressing the sdoh need(s), in ways that are more likely to promote personalized and effective diagnosis or treatment. health care access / health system navigation. ++ helping the patient access healthcare, including identifying appropriate practitioners or providers for clinical care and helping secure appointments with them. facilitating behavioral change as necessary for meeting diagnosis and treatment goals, including promoting patient motivation to participate in care and reach person-centered diagnosis or treatment goals. facilitating and providing social and emotional support to help the patient cope with the problem(s) addressed in the initiating visit, the sdoh need(s), and adjust daily routines to better meet diagnosis and treatment goals. leveraging lived experience when applicable to provide support, mentorship, or inspiration to meet treatment goals

• **G0022** Community health integration services, each additional 30 minutes per calendar month (list separately in addition to g0019)

• **G0023** Principal illness navigation services by certified or trained auxiliary personnel under the direction of a physician or other practitioner, including a patient navigator; 60 minutes per calendar month, in the following activities: person-centered assessment, performed to better understand the individual context of the serious, high-risk condition. ++ conducting a person-centered assessment to understand the patient's life story, strengths, needs, goals, preferences, and desired outcomes, including understanding cultural and linguistic factors and including unmet sdoh needs (that are not separately billed). ++ facilitating patient-driven goal setting and establishing an action plan. ++ providing tailored support as needed to accomplish the practitioner's treatment plan. identifying or referring patient (and caregiver or family, if applicable) to appropriate supportive services. practitioner, home, and community-based care coordination. ++ coordinating receipt of needed services from healthcare practitioners, providers, and facilities; home- and community-based service providers; and caregiver (if applicable). ++ communication with practitioners, home-, and community-based service providers, hospitals, and skilled nursing facilities (or other health care facilities) regarding the patient's psychosocial strengths and needs, functional deficits, goals, preferences, and desired outcomes, including cultural and linguistic factors. ++ coordination of care transitions between and among health care practitioners and settings, including transitions involving referral to other clinicians; follow-up after an emergency department visit; or follow-up after discharges from hospitals, skilled nursing facilities or other health care facilities. ++ facilitating access to community-based social services (e.g., housing, utilities, transportation, likely to promote personalized and effective treatment of their condition. health care access / health system navigation. ++ helping the patient access healthcare, including identifying appropriate practitioners or providers for clinical care, and helping secure appointments with them. ++ providing the patient with information/resources to consider participation in clinical trials or clinical research as applicable. facilitating behavioral change as necessary for meeting diagnosis and treatment goals, including promoting patient motivation to participate in care and reach person-centered diagnosis or treatment goals. facilitating and providing social and emotional support to help the patient cope with the condition, sdoh need(s), and adjust daily routines to better meet diagnosis and treatment goals. leverage knowledge of the serious, high-risk condition and/or lived experience when applicable to provide support, mentorship, or inspiration to meet treatment goals

• **G0024** Principal illness navigation services, additional 30 minutes per calendar month (list separately in addition to g0023)

(**G0056** Optimizing chronic disease management mips value pathways **Code deleted** effective 12/31/2023, no HCPCS/CPT cross-reference provided.)

▲ **G0129** Occupational therapy services requiring the skills of a qualified occupational therapist, furnished as a component of a partial hospitalization or intensive outpatient treatment program, per session (45 minutes or more)

APPENDICES

• **G0136** Administration of a standardized, evidence-based social determinants of health risk assessment tool, 5-15 minutes

• **G0137** Intensive outpatient services; weekly bundle, minimum of 9 services over a 7 contiguous day period, which can include individual and group therapy with physicians or psychologists (or other mental health professionals to the extent authorized under state law); occupational therapy requiring the skills of a qualified occupational therapist; services of social workers, trained psychiatric nurses, and other staff trained to work with psychiatric patients; individualized activity therapies that are not primarily recreational or diversionary; family counseling (the primary purpose of which is treatment of the individual's condition); patient training and education (to the extent that training and educational activities are closely and clearly related to individual's care and treatment); diagnostic services; and such other items and services (excluding meals and transportation) that are reasonable and necessary for the diagnosis or active treatment of the individual's condition, reasonably expected to improve or maintain the individual's condition and functional level and to prevent relapse or hospitalization, and furnished pursuant to such guidelines relating to frequency and duration of services in accordance with a physician certification and plan of treatment (provision of the services by a medicare-enrolled opioid treatment program); list separately in addition to code for primary procedure

• **G0140** Principal illness navigation - peer support by certified or trained auxiliary personnel under the direction of a physician or other practitioner, including a certified peer specialist; 60 minutes per calendar month, in the following activities: person-centered interview, performed to better understand the individual context of the serious, high-risk condition. ++ conducting a person-centered interview to understand the patient's life story, strengths, needs, goals, preferences, and desired outcomes, including understanding cultural and linguistic factors, and including unmet sdoh needs (that are not billed separately). ++ facilitating patient-driven goal setting and establishing an action plan. ++ providing tailored support as needed to accomplish the person-centered goals in the practitioner's treatment plan. identifying or referring patient (and caregiver or family, if applicable) to appropriate supportive services. practitioner, home, and community-based care communication. ++ assist the patient in communicating with their practitioners, home-, and community-based service providers, hospitals, and skilled nursing facilities (or other health care facilities) regarding the patient's psychosocial strengths and needs, goals, preferences, and desired outcomes, including cultural and linguistic factors. ++ facilitating access to community-based social services (e.g., housing, utilities, transportation, food assistance) as needed to address sdoh need(s). health education. helping the patient contextualize health education provided by the patient's treatment team with the patient's individual needs, goals, preferences, and sdoh need(s), and educating the patient (and caregiver if applicable) on how to best participate in medical decision-making. building patient self-advocacy skills, so that the patient can interact with members of the health care team and related community-based services (as needed), in ways that are more likely to promote personalized and effective treatment of their condition. developing and proposing strategies to help meet person-centered treatment goals and supporting the patient in using chosen strategies to reach person-centered treatment goals. facilitating and providing social and emotional support to help the patient cope with the condition, sdoh need(s), and adjust daily routines to better meet person-centered diagnosis and treatment goals. leverage knowledge of the serious, high-risk condition and/or lived experience when applicable to provide support, mentorship, or inspiration to meet treatment goals

• **G0146** Principal illness navigation - peer support, additional 30 minutes per calendar month (list separately in addition to g0140)

▲ **G0410** Group psychotherapy other than of a multiple-family group, in a partial hospitalization or intensive outpatient setting, approximately 45 to 50 minutes

▲ **G0411** Interactive group psychotherapy, in a partial hospitalization or intensive outpatient setting, approximately 45 to 50 minutes

(**G2066** Interrogation device evaluation(s), (remote) up to 30 days; implantable cardiovascular physiologic monitor system, implantable loop recorder system, or subcutaneous cardiac rhythm monitor system, remote data acquisition(s), receipt of transmissions and technician review, technical support and distribution of results **Code deleted** effective 12/31/2023, no HCPCS/CPT cross-reference provided.)

APPENDICES

(**G2108** Patient age 66 or older in institutional special needs plans (snp) or residing in long-term care with pos code 32, 33, 34, 54 or 56 for more than 90 consecutive days during the measurement period Code deleted effective 12/31/2023, no HCPCS/CPT cross-reference provided.)

(**G2109** Patients 66 years of age and older with at least one claim/encounter for frailty during the measurement period and a dispensed medication for dementia during the measurement period or the year prior to the measurement period Code deleted effective 12/31/2023, no HCPCS/CPT cross-reference provided.)

(**G2110** Patients 66 years of age and older with at least one claim/encounter for frailty during the measurement period and either one acute inpatient encounter with a diagnosis of advanced illness or two outpatient, observation, ed or nonacute inpatient encounters on different dates of service with an advanced illness diagnosis during the measurement period or the year prior to the measurement period Code deleted effective 12/31/2023, no HCPCS/CPT cross-reference provided.)

▲ **G2137** Back pain measured by the visual analog scale (vas) or numeric pain scale at three months (6 - 20 weeks) postoperatively was greater than 3.0 and back pain measured by the visual analog scale (vas) or numeric pain scale within three months preoperatively and at three months (6 - 20 weeks) postoperatively demonstrated improvement of less than 5.0 points

▲ **G2139** Back pain measured by the visual analog scale (vas) or numeric pain scale at one year (9 to 15 months) postoperatively was greater than 3.0 and back pain measured by the visual analog scale (vas) or numeric pain scale within three months preoperatively and at one year (9 to 15 months) postoperatively demonstrated improvement of less than 5.0 points

▲ **G2141** Leg pain measured by the visual analog scale (vas) or numeric pain scale at three months (6 - 20 weeks) postoperatively was greater than 3.0 and leg pain measured by the visual analog scale (vas) or numeric pain scale within three months preoperatively and at three months (6 - 20 weeks) postoperatively demonstrated improvement of less than 5.0 points

▲ **G2147** Leg pain measured by the visual analog scale (vas) or numeric pain scale at one year (9 to 15 months) postoperatively was greater than 3.0 and leg pain measured by the visual analog scale (vas) or numeric pain scale within three months preoperatively and at one year (9 to 15 months) postoperatively demonstrated improvement of less than 5.0 points

▲ **G2174** Uri episodes where the patient is taking antibiotics (table 1) in the 30 days prior to the episode date

▲ **G8474** Angiotensin converting enzyme (ace) inhibitor or angiotensin receptor blocker (arb) therapy not prescribed for reasons documented by the clinician (e.g., allergy, intolerance, pregnancy, renal failure due to ace inhibitor, diseases of the aortic or mitral valve, other medical reasons) or (e.g., patient declined, other patient reasons)

(**G8506** Patient receiving angiotensin converting enzyme (ace) inhibitor or angiotensin receptor blocker (arb) therapy Code deleted effective 12/31/2023, no HCPCS/CPT cross-reference provided.)

▲ **G8535** Elder maltreatment screen not documented; documentation that patient is not eligible for the elder maltreatment screen at the time of the encounter related to one of the following reasons: (1) patient refuses to participate in the screening and has reasonable decisional capacity for self-protection, or (2) patient is in an urgent or emergent situation where time is of the essence and to delay treatment to perform the screening would jeopardize the patient's health status

▲ **G8601** Iv thrombolytic therapy not initiated within 4.5 hours (<= 270 minutes) of time last known well for reasons documented by clinician (e.g. patient enrolled in clinical trial for stroke, patient admitted for elective carotid intervention)

▲ **G8807** Trans-abdominal or trans-vaginal ultrasound not performed for reasons documented by clinician (e.g., patient has a documented intrauterine pregnancy [iup])

(**G8818** Patient discharge to home no later than post-operative day #7 Code deleted effective 12/31/2023, no HCPCS/CPT cross-reference provided.)

(**G8825** Patient not discharged to home by post-operative day #7 Code deleted effective 12/31/2023, no HCPCS/CPT cross-reference provided.)

▲ **G8851** Adherence to therapy was assessed at least annually through an objective informatics system or through self-reporting (if objective reporting is not available, documented)

(**G8852** Positive airway pressure therapy was prescribed **Code deleted** effective 12/31/2023, no HCPCS/CPT cross-reference provided.)

▲ **G8854** Documentation of reason(s) for not objectively reporting adherence to evidence-based therapy (e.g., patients who have been diagnosed with a terminal or advanced disease with an expected life span of less than 6 months, patients who decline therapy, patients who do not return for follow-up at least annually, patients unable to access/afford therapy, patient's insurance will not cover therapy)

▲ **G8855** Adherence to therapy was not assessed at least annually through an objective informatics system or through self-reporting (if objective reporting is not available), reason not given

(**G8883** Biopsy results reviewed, communicated, tracked and documented **Code deleted** effective 12/31/2023, no HCPCS/CPT cross-reference provided.)

(**G8884** Clinician documented reason that patient's biopsy results were not reviewed **Code deleted** effective 12/31/2023, no HCPCS/CPT cross-reference provided.)

(**G8885** Biopsy results not reviewed, communicated, tracked or documented **Code deleted** effective 12/31/2023, no HCPCS/CPT cross-reference provided.)

▲ **G8924** Spirometry results documented (fev1/fvc < 70%)

▲ **G8936** Clinician documented that patient was not an eligible candidate for angiotensin converting enzyme (ace) inhibitor or angiotensin receptor blocker (arb) therapy (eg, allergy, intolerance, pregnancy, renal failure due to ace inhibitor, diseases of the aortic or mitral valve, other medical reasons) or (eg, patient declined, other patient reasons)

(**G8941** Elder maltreatment screen documented as positive, follow-up plan not documented, documentation the patient is not eligible for follow-up plan at the time of the encounter **Code deleted** effective 12/31/2023, no HCPCS/CPT cross-reference provided.)

▲ **G8942** Functional outcome assessment using a standardized tool is documented within the previous 30 days and a care plan, based on identified deficiencies is documented within two days of the functional outcome assessment

(**G8963** Cardiac stress imaging performed primarily for monitoring of asymptomatic patient who had pci within 2 years **Code deleted** effective 12/31/2023, no HCPCS/CPT cross-reference provided.)

(**G8964** Cardiac stress imaging test performed primarily for any other reason than monitoring of asymptomatic patient who had pci within 2 years (e.g., symptomatic patient, patient greater than 2 years since pci, initial evaluation, etc) **Code deleted** effective 12/31/2023, no HCPCS/CPT cross-reference provided.)

▲ **G8968** Documentation of medical reason(s) for not prescribing an fda-approved anticoagulant (e.g., present or planned atrial appendage occlusion or ligation or patient being currently enrolled in a clinical trial related to af/atrial flutter treatment)

(**G9192** Documentation of system reason(s) for not prescribing beta-blocker therapy (eg, other reasons attributable to the health care system) **Code deleted** effective 12/31/2023, no HCPCS/CPT cross-reference provided.)

(**G9229** Chlamydia, gonorrhea, and syphilis screening results not documented (patient refusal is the only allowed exception) **Code deleted** effective 12/31/2023, no HCPCS/CPT cross-reference provided.)

▲ **G9380** Patient offered assistance with end of life issues or existing end of life plan was reviewed or updated during the measurement period

▲ **G9382** Patient not offered assistance with end of life issues or existing end of life plan was not reviewed or updated during the measurement period

(**G9451** Patient received one-time screening for hcv infection **Code deleted** effective 12/31/2023, no HCPCS/CPT cross-reference provided.)

▲ **G9452** Documentation of medical reason(s) for not receiving hcv antibody test due to limited life expectancy

(**G9453** Documentation of patient reason(s) for not receiving one-time screening for hcv infection (e.g., patient declined, other patient reasons) Code deleted effective 12/31/2023, no HCPCS/CPT cross-reference provided.)

(**G9454** One-time screening for hcv infection not received within 12-month reporting period and no documentation of prior screening for hcv infection, reason not given Code deleted effective 12/31/2023, no HCPCS/CPT cross-reference provided.)

(**G9596** Pediatric patient had a head ct for trauma ordered by someone other than an emergency care provider or was ordered for a reason other than trauma Code deleted effective 12/31/2023, no HCPCS/CPT cross-reference provided.)

(**G9612** Photodocumentation of two or more cecal landmarks to establish a complete examination Code deleted effective 12/31/2023, no HCPCS/CPT cross-reference provided.)

(**G9613** Documentation of post-surgical anatomy (e.g., right hemicolectomy, ileocecal resection, etc.) Code deleted effective 12/31/2023, no HCPCS/CPT cross-reference provided.)

(**G9614** Photodocumentation of less than two cecal landmarks (i.e., no cecal landmarks or only one cecal landmark) to establish a complete examination Code deleted effective 12/31/2023, no HCPCS/CPT cross-reference provided.)

▲ **G9696** Documentation of medical reason(s) for not prescribing a long-acting inhaled bronchodilator (e.g., patient intolerance or history of side effects)

(**G9697** Documentation of patient reason(s) for not prescribing a long-acting inhaled bronchodilator Code deleted effective 12/31/2023, no HCPCS/CPT cross-reference provided.)

▲ **G9698** Documentation of system reason(s) for not prescribing a long-acting inhaled bronchodilator (e.g., cost of treatment or lack of insurance)

▲ **G9703** Episodes where the patient is taking antibiotics (table 1) in the 30 days prior to the episode date

(**G9715** Patients who use hospice services any time during the measurement period Code deleted effective 12/31/2023, no HCPCS/CPT cross-reference provided.)

▲ **G9717** Documentation stating the patient has had a diagnosis of bipolar disorder

(**G9725** Patients who use hospice services any time during the measurement period Code deleted effective 12/31/2023, no HCPCS/CPT cross-reference provided.)

▲ **G9771** At least 1 body temperature measurement equal to or greater than 35.5 degrees celsius (or 95.9 degrees fahrenheit) achieved within the 30 minutes immediately before or 15 minutes immediately after anesthesia end time

▲ **G9772** Documentation of medical reason(s) for not achieving at least 1 body temperature measurement equal to or greater than 35.5 degrees celsius (or 95.9 degrees fahrenheit) within the 30 minutes immediately before or 15 minutes immediately after anesthesia end time (e.g., emergency cases, intentional hypothermia, etc.)

▲ **G9773** At least 1 body temperature measurement equal to or greater than 35.5 degrees celsius (or 95.9 degrees fahrenheit) not achieved within the 30 minutes immediately before or 15 minutes immediately after anesthesia end time, reason not given

▲ **G9779** Patients who are breastfeeding at any time during the performance period

▲ **G9780** Patients who have a diagnosis of rhabdomyolysis at any time during the performance period

(**G9852** Patients who died from cancer Code deleted effective 12/31/2023, no HCPCS/CPT cross-reference provided.)

(**G9853** Patient admitted to the icu in the last 30 days of life Code deleted effective 12/31/2023, no HCPCS/CPT cross-reference provided.)

(**G9854** Patient was not admitted to the icu in the last 30 days of life Code deleted effective 12/31/2023, no HCPCS/CPT cross-reference provided.)

▲ **G9914** Patient initiated an anti-tnf agent

(**G9927** Documentation of system reason(s) for not prescribing an fda-approved anticoagulation due to patient being currently enrolled in a clinical trial related to af/atrial flutter treatment Code deleted effective 12/31/2023, no HCPCS/CPT cross-reference provided.)

▲ **G9938** Patients aged 66 or older in institutional special needs plans (snp) or residing in long-term care with pos code 32, 33, 34, 54, or 56 for more than 90 consecutive days during the six months prior to the measurement period through december 31 of the measurement period

▲ **G9990** Patient did not receive any pneumococcal conjugate or polysaccharide vaccine on or after their 19th birthday and before the end of the measurement period

▲ **G9991** Patient received any pneumococcal conjugate or polysaccharide vaccine on or after their 19th birthday and before the end of the measurement period

(**G9995** Patients who use palliative care services any time during the measurement period Code deleted effective 12/31/2023, no HCPCS/CPT cross-reference provided.)

▲ **G9998** Documentation of medical reason(s) for an interval of less than 3 years since the last colonoscopy (e.g., last colonoscopy incomplete, last colonoscopy had inadequate prep, piecemeal removal of adenomas, or sessile serrated polyps >= 20 mm in size, last colonoscopy found greater than 10 adenomas, lower gastrointestinal bleeding, or patient at high risk for colon cancer due to underlying medical history ([i.e. crohn's disease, ulcerative colitis, personal or family history of colon cancer, hereditary colorectal cancer syndromes])

• **J0184** Injection, amisulpride, 1 mg

• **J0217** Injection, velmanase alfa-tycv, 1 mg

• **J0391** Injection, artesunate, 1 mg

• **J0402** Injection, aripiprazole (abilify asimtufii), 1 mg

• **J0576** Injection, buprenorphine extended-release (brixadi), 1 mg

• **J0688** Injection, cefazolin sodium (hikma), not therapeutically equivalent to j0690, 500 mg

▲ **J0739** Injection, cabotegravir, 1mg, fda approved prescription, only for use as hiv pre-exposure prophylaxis (not for use as treatment for hiv)

• **J0750** Emtricitabine 200mg and tenofovir disoproxil fumarate 300mg, oral, fda approved prescription, only for use as hiv pre-exposure prophylaxis (not for use as treatment of hiv)

• **J0751** Emtricitabine 200mg and tenofovir alafenamide 25mg, oral, fda approved prescription, only for use as hiv pre-exposure prophylaxis (not for use as treatment of hiv)

• **J0799** Fda approved prescription drug, only for use as hiv pre-exposure prophylaxis (not for use as treatment of hiv), not otherwise classified

• **J0873** Injection, daptomycin (xellia) not therapeutically equivalent to j0878, 1 mg

• **J1105** Dexmedetomidine, oral, 1 mcg

• **J1246** Injection, dinutuximab, 0.1 mg

• **J1304** Injection, tofersen, 1 mg

• **J1412** Injection, valoctocogene roxaparvovec-rvox, per ml, containing nominal 2 x 10^13 vector genomes

• **J1413** Injection, delandistrogene moxeparvovec-rokl, per therapeutic dose

• **J1596** Injection, glycopyrrolate, 0.1 mg

• **J1939** Injection, bumetanide, 0.5 mg

APPENDICES

- **J2404** Injection, nicardipine, 0.1 mg
- **J2508** Injection, pegunigalsidase alfa-iwxj, 1 mg
- **J2679** Injection, fluphenazine hcl, 1.25 mg
- **J2799** Injection, risperidone (uzedy), 1 mg
- **J3401** Beremagene geperpavec-svdt for topical administration, containing nominal 5 x 10^9 pfu/ml vector genomes, per 0.1 ml
- **J3425** Injection, hydroxocobalamin, 10 mcg
- **J9052** Injection, carmustine (accord), not therapeutically equivalent to j9050, 100 mg
- **J9072** Injection, cyclophosphamide, (dr. reddy's), 5 mg

(**J9160** Injection, denileukin diftitox, 300 micrograms Code deleted effective 12/31/2023, no HCPCS/CPT cross-reference provided.)

- **J9172** Injection, docetaxel (ingenus) not therapeutically equivalent to j9171, 1 mg
- **J9255** Injection, methotrexate (accord) not therapeutically equivalent to j9250 and j9260, 50 mg
- **J9258** Injection, paclitaxel protein-bound particles (teva) not therapeutically equivalent to j9264, 1 mg
- **J9286** Injection, glofitamab-gxbm, 2.5 mg
- **J9321** Injection, epcoritamab-bysp, 0.16 mg
- **J9324** Injection, pemetrexed (pemrydi rtu), 10 mg
- **J9333** Injection, rozanolixizumab-noli, 1 mg
- **J9334** Injection, efgartigimod alfa, 2 mg and hyaluronidase-qvfc

(**K1001** Electronic positional obstructive sleep apnea treatment, with sensor, includes all components and accessories, any type Code deleted effective 12/31/2023, no HCPCS/CPT cross-reference provided.)

(**K1002** Cranial electrotherapy stimulation (ces) system, any type Code deleted effective 12/31/2023, no HCPCS/CPT cross-reference provided.)

(**K1003** Whirlpool tub, walk-in, portable Code deleted effective 12/31/2023, no HCPCS/CPT cross-reference provided.)

(**K1005** Disposable collection and storage bag for breast milk, any size, any type, each Code deleted effective 12/31/2023, no HCPCS/CPT cross-reference provided.)

(**K1006** Suction pump, home model, portable or stationary, electric, any type, for use with external urine management system Code deleted effective 12/31/2023, no HCPCS/CPT cross-reference provided.)

(**K1009** Speech volume modulation system, any type, including all components and accessories Code deleted effective 12/31/2023, no HCPCS/CPT cross-reference provided.)

(**K1013** Enema tube, with or without adapter, any type, replacement only, each Code deleted effective 12/31/2023, no HCPCS/CPT cross-reference provided.)

(**K1014** Addition, endoskeletal knee-shin system, 4 bar linkage or multiaxial, fluid swing and stance phase control Code deleted effective 12/31/2023, no HCPCS/CPT cross-reference provided.)

(**K1015** Foot, adductus positioning device, adjustable Code deleted effective 12/31/2023, no HCPCS/CPT cross-reference provided.)

(**K1016** Transcutaneous electrical nerve stimulator for electrical stimulation of the trigeminal nerve Code deleted effective 12/31/2023, no HCPCS/CPT cross-reference provided.)

(**K1017** Monthly supplies for use of device coded at k1016 Code deleted effective 12/31/2023, no HCPCS/CPT cross-reference provided.)

(**K1018** External upper limb tremor stimulator of the peripheral nerves of the wrist Code deleted effective 12/31/2023, no HCPCS/CPT cross-reference provided.)

(**K1019** Supplies and accessories for external upper limb tremor stimulator of the peripheral nerves of the wrist Code deleted effective 12/31/2023, no HCPCS/CPT cross-reference provided.)

(**K1020** Non-invasive vagus nerve stimulator Code deleted effective 12/31/2023, no HCPCS/CPT cross-reference provided.)

(**K1021** Exsufflation belt, includes all supplies and accessories Code deleted effective 12/31/2023, no HCPCS/CPT cross-reference provided.)

(**K1022** Addition to lower extremity prosthesis, endoskeletal, knee disarticulation, above knee, hip disarticulation, positional rotation unit, any type Code deleted effective 12/31/2023, no HCPCS/CPT cross-reference provided.)

(**K1023** Distal transcutaneous electrical nerve stimulator, stimulates peripheral nerves of the upper arm Code deleted effective 12/31/2023, no HCPCS/CPT cross-reference provided.)

(**K1024** Non-pneumatic compression controller with sequential calibrated gradient pressure Code deleted effective 12/31/2023, no HCPCS/CPT cross-reference provided.)

(**K1025** Non-pneumatic sequential compression garment, full arm Code deleted effective 12/31/2023, no HCPCS/CPT cross-reference provided.)

(**K1026** Mechanical allergen particle barrier/inhalation filter, cream, nasal, topical Code deleted effective 12/31/2023, no HCPCS/CPT cross-reference provided.)

(**K1028** Power source and control electronics unit for oral device/appliance for neuromuscular electrical stimulation of the tongue muscle, controlled by phone application Code deleted effective 12/31/2023, no HCPCS/CPT cross-reference provided.)

(**K1029** Oral device/appliance for neuromuscular electrical stimulation of the tongue muscle, used in conjunction with the power source and control electronics unit, controlled by phone application, 90-day supply Code deleted effective 12/31/2023, no HCPCS/CPT cross-reference provided.)

(**K1031** Non-pneumatic compression controller without calibrated gradient pressure Code deleted effective 12/31/2023, no HCPCS/CPT cross-reference provided.)

(**K1032** Non-pneumatic sequential compression garment, full leg Code deleted effective 12/31/2023, no HCPCS/CPT cross-reference provided.)

(**K1033** Non-pneumatic sequential compression garment, half leg Code deleted effective 12/31/2023, no HCPCS/CPT cross-reference provided.)

• **L3161** Foot, adductus positioning device, adjustable

• **L5615** Addition, endoskeletal knee-shin system, 4 bar linkage or multiaxial, fluid swing and stance phase control

• **L5926** Addition to lower extremity prosthesis, endoskeletal, knee disarticulation, above knee, hip disarticulation, positional rotation unit, any type

▲ **M0005** Value in primary care mips value pathway

▲ **M0201** Administration of pneumococcal, influenza, hepatitis b, and/or covid-19 vaccine inside a patient's home; reported only once per individual home per date of service when such vaccine administration(s) are performed at the patient's home

(**M1156** Patient received active chemotherapy any time during the measurement period Code deleted effective 12/31/2023, no HCPCS/CPT cross-reference provided.)

(**M1157** Patient received bone marrow transplant any time during the measurement period Code deleted effective 12/31/2023, no HCPCS/CPT cross-reference provided.)

(**M1158** Patient had history of immunocompromising conditions prior to or during the measurement period Code deleted effective 12/31/2023, no HCPCS/CPT cross-reference provided.)

▲ **M1174** Patient received at least two doses of the herpes zoster recombinant vaccine (at least 28 days apart) anytime on or after the patient's 50th birthday before or during the measurement period

▲ **M1176** Patient did not receive at least two doses of the herpes zoster recombinant vaccine (at least 28 days apart) anytime on or after the patient's 50th birthday before or during the measurement period

▲ **M1197** Itch severity assessment score is reduced by 3 or more points from the initial (index) assessment score to the follow-up visit score

▲ **M1198** Itch severity assessment score was not reduced by at least 3 points from initial (index) score to the follow-up visit score or assessment was not completed during the follow-up encounter

▲ **M1205** Itch severity assessment score is reduced by 3 or more points from the initial (index) assessment score to the follow-up visit score

▲ **M1206** Itch severity assessment score was not reduced by at least 3 points from initial (index) score to the follow-up visit score or assessment was not completed during the follow-up encounter

▲ **M1207** Patient is screened for food insecurity, housing instability, transportation needs, utility difficulties, and interpersonal safety

▲ **M1208** Patient is not screened for food insecurity, housing instability, transportation needs, utility difficulties, and interpersonal safety

• **M1211** Most recent hemoglobin a1c level > 9.0%

• **M1212** Hemoglobin a1c level is missing, or was not performed during the measurement period (12 months)

• **M1213** No history of spirometry results with confirmed airflow obstruction (fev1/fvc < 70%) and present spirometry is >= 70%

• **M1214** Spirometry results with confirmed airflow obstruction (fev1/fvc < 70%) documented and reviewed

• **M1215** Documentation of medical reason(s) for not documenting and reviewing spirometry results (e.g., patients with dementia or tracheostomy)

• **M1216** No spirometry results with confirmed airflow obstruction (fev1/fvc < 70%) documented and/or no spirometry performed with results documented during the encounter

• **M1217** Documentation of system reason(s) for not documenting and reviewing spirometry results (e.g., spirometry equipment not available at the time of the encounter)

• **M1218** Patient has copd symptoms (e.g., dyspnea, cough/sputum, wheezing)

• **M1219** Anaphylaxis due to the vaccine on or before the date of the encounter

• **M1220** Dilated retinal eye exam with interpretation by an ophthalmologist or optometrist or artificial intelligence (ai) interpretation documented and reviewed; with evidence of retinopathy

• **M1221** Dilated retinal eye exam with interpretation by an ophthalmologist or optometrist or artificial intelligence (ai) interpretation documented and reviewed; without evidence of retinopathy

• **M1222** Glaucoma plan of care not documented, reason not otherwise specified

• **M1223** Glaucoma plan of care documented

• **M1224** Intraocular pressure (iop) reduced by a value less than 20% from the pre-intervention level

• **M1225** Intraocular pressure (iop) reduced by a value of greater than or equal to 20% from the pre-intervention level

• **M1226** Iop measurement not documented, reason not otherwise specified

• **M1227** Evidence-based therapy was prescribed

- **M1228** Patient, who has a reactive hcv antibody test, and has a follow up hcv viral test that detected hcv viremia, has hcv treatment initiated within 3 months of the reactive hcv antibody test
- **M1229** Patient, who has a reactive hcv antibody test, and has a follow up hcv viral test that detected hcv viremia, is referred within 1 month of the reactive hcv antibody test to a clinician who treats hcv infection
- **M1230** Patient has a reactive hcv antibody test and does not have a follow up hcv viral test, or patient has a reactive hcv antibody test and has a follow up hcv viral test that detects hcv viremia and is not referred to a clinician who treats hcv infection within 1 month and does not have hcv treatment initiated within 3 months of the reactive hcv antibody test, reason not given
- **M1231** Patient receives hcv antibody test with nonreactive result
- **M1232** Patient receives hcv antibody test with reactive result
- **M1233** Patient does not receive hcv antibody test or patient does receive hcv antibody test but results not documented, reason not given
- **M1234** Patient has a reactive hcv antibody test, and has a follow up hcv viral test that does not detect hcv viremia
- **M1235** Documentation or patient report of hcv antibody test or hcv rna test which occurred prior to the performance period
- **M1236** Baseline mrs > 2
- **M1237** Patient reason for not screening for food insecurity, housing instability, transportation needs, utility difficulties, and interpersonal safety (e.g., patient declined or other patient reasons)
- **M1238** Documentation that administration of second recombinant zoster vaccine could not occur during the performance period due to the recommended 2-6 month interval between doses (i.e, first dose received after october 31)
- **M1239** Patient did not respond to the question of patient felt heard and understood by this provider and team
- **M1240** Patient did not respond to the question of patient felt this provider and team put my best interests first when making recommendations about my care
- **M1241** Patient did not respond to the question of patient felt this provider and team saw me as a person, not just someone with a medical problem
- **M1242** Patient did not respond to the question of patient felt this provider and team understood what is important to me in my life
- **M1243** Patient provided a response other than "completely true" for the question of patient felt heard and understood by this provider and team
- **M1244** Patient provided a response other than "completely true" for the question of patient felt this provider and team put my best interests first when making recommendations about my care
- **M1245** Patient provided a response other than "completely true" for the question of patient felt this provider and team saw me as a person, not just someone with a medical problem
- **M1246** Patient provided a response other than "completely true" for the question of patient felt this provider and team understood what is important to me in my life
- **M1247** Patient responded "completely true" for the question of patient felt this provider and team put my best interests first when making recommendations about my care
- **M1248** Patient responded "completely true" for the question of patient felt this provider and team saw me as a person, not just someone with a medical problem
- **M1249** Patient responded "completely true" for the question of patient felt this provider and team understood what is important to me in my life

APPENDICES

- • **M1250** Patient responded as "completely true" for the question of patient felt heard and understood by this provider and team
- • **M1251** Patients for whom a proxy completed the entire hu survey on their behalf for any reason (no patient involvement)
- • **M1252** Patients who did not complete at least one of the four patient experience hu survey items and return the hu survey within 60 days of the ambulatory palliative care visit
- • **M1253** Patients who respond on the patient experience hu survey that they did not receive care by the listed ambulatory palliative care provider in the last 60 days (disavowal)
- • **M1254** Patients who were deceased when the hu survey reached them
- • **M1255** Patients who have another reason for visiting the clinic [not prenatal or postpartum care] and have a positive pregnancy test but have not established the clinic as an ob provider (e.g., plan to terminate the pregnancy or seek prenatal services elsewhere)
- • **M1256** Prior history of known cvd
- • **M1257** Cvd risk assessment not performed or incomplete (e.g., cvd risk assessment was not documented), reason not otherwise specified
- • **M1258** Cvd risk assessment performed, have a documented calculated risk score
- • **M1259** Patients listed on the kidney-pancreas transplant waitlist or who received a living donor transplant within the first year following initiation of dialysis
- • **M1260** Patients who were not listed on the kidney-pancreas transplant waitlist or patients who did not receive a living donor transplant within the first year following initiation of dialysis
- • **M1261** Patients that were on the kidney or kidney-pancreas waitlist prior to initiation of dialysis
- • **M1262** Patients who had a transplant prior to initiation of dialysis
- • **M1263** Patients in hospice on their initiation of dialysis date or during the month of evaluation
- • **M1264** Patients age 75 or older on their initiation of dialysis date
- • **M1265** Cms medical evidence form 2728 for dialysis patients: initial form completed
- • **M1266** Patients admitted to a skilled nursing facility (snf)
- • **M1267** Patients not on any kidney or kidney-pancreas transplant waitlist or is not in active status on any kidney or kidney-pancreas transplant waitlist as of the last day of each month during the measurement period
- • **M1268** Patients on active status on any kidney or kidney-pancreas transplant waitlist as of the last day of each month during the measurement period
- • **M1269** Receiving esrd mcp dialysis services by the provider on the last day of the reporting month
- • **M1270** Patients not on any kidney or kidney-pancreas transplant waitlist as of the last day of each month during the measurement period
- • **M1271** Patients with dementia at any time prior to or during the month
- • **M1272** Patients on any kidney or kidney-pancreas transplant waitlist as of the last day of each month during the measurement period
- • **M1273** Patients who were admitted to a skilled nursing facility (snf) within one year of dialysis initiation according to the cms-2728 form
- • **M1274** Patients who were admitted to a skilled nursing facility (snf) during the month of evaluation were excluded from that month
- • **M1275** Patients determined to be in hospice were excluded from month of evaluation and the remainder of reporting period
- • **M1276** Bmi documented outside normal parameters, no follow-up plan documented, no reason given

APPENDICES

- **M1277** Colorectal cancer screening results documented and reviewed
- **M1278** Elevated or hypertensive blood pressure reading documented, and the indicated follow-up is documented
- **M1279** Elevated or hypertensive blood pressure reading documented, indicated follow-up not documented, reason not given
- **M1280** Women who had a bilateral mastectomy or who have a history of a bilateral mastectomy or for whom there is evidence of a right and a left unilateral mastectomy
- **M1281** Blood pressure reading not documented, reason not given
- **M1282** Patient screened for tobacco use and identified as a tobacco non-user
- **M1283** Patient screened for tobacco use and identified as a tobacco user
- **M1284** Patients age 66 or older in institutional special needs plans (snp) or residing in long term care with pos code 32, 33, 34, 54, or 56 for more than 90 consecutive days during the measurement period
- **M1285** Screening, diagnostic, film, digital or digital breast tomosynthesis (3d) mammography results were not documented and reviewed, reason not otherwise specified
- **M1286** Bmi is documented as being outside of normal parameters, follow-up plan is not completed for documented medical reason
- **M1287** Bmi is documented below normal parameters and a follow-up plan is documented
- **M1288** Documented reason for not screening or recommending a follow-up for high blood pressure
- **M1289** Patient identified as tobacco user did not receive tobacco cessation intervention during the measurement period or in the six months prior to the measurement period (counseling and/or pharmacotherapy)
- **M1290** Patient not eligible due to active diagnosis of hypertension
- **M1291** Patients 66 years of age and older with at least one claim/encounter for frailty during the measurement period and a dispensed medication for dementia during the measurement period or the year prior to the measurement period
- **M1292** Patients 66 years of age and older with at least one claim/encounter for frailty during the measurement period and either one acute inpatient encounter with a diagnosis of advanced illness or two outpatient, observation, ed or nonacute inpatient encounters on different dates of service with an advanced illness diagnosis during the measurement period or the year prior to the measurement period
- **M1293** Bmi is documented above normal parameters and a follow-up plan is documented
- **M1294** Normal blood pressure reading documented, follow-up not required
- **M1295** Patients with a diagnosis or past history of total colectomy or colorectal cancer
- **M1296** Bmi is documented within normal parameters and no follow-up plan is required
- **M1297** Bmi not documented due to medical reason or patient refusal of height or weight measurement
- **M1298** Documentation of patient pregnancy anytime during the measurement period prior to and including the current encounter
- **M1299** Influenza immunization administered or previously received
- **M1300** Influenza immunization was not administered for reasons documented by clinician (e.g., patient allergy or other medical reasons, patient declined or other patient reasons, vaccine not available or other system reasons)
- **M1301** Patient identified as a tobacco user received tobacco cessation intervention during the measurement period or in the six months prior to the measurement period (counseling and/or pharmacotherapy)
- **M1302** Screening, diagnostic, film digital or digital breast tomosynthesis (3d) mammography results documented and reviewed

- **M1303** Hospice services provided to patient any time during the measurement period
- **M1304** Patient did not receive any pneumococcal conjugate or polysaccharide vaccine on or after their 19th birthday and before the end of the measurement period
- **M1305** Patient received any pneumococcal conjugate or polysaccharide vaccine on or after their 19th birthday and before the end of the measurement period
- **M1306** Patient had anaphylaxis due to the pneumococcal vaccine any time during or before the measurement period
- **M1307** Documentation stating the patient has received or is currently receiving palliative or hospice care
- **M1308** Influenza immunization was not administered, reason not given
- **M1309** Palliative care services provided to patient any time during the measurement period
- **M1310** Patient screened for tobacco use and received tobacco cessation intervention during the measurement period or in the six months prior to the measurement period (counseling, pharmacotherapy, or both), if identified as a tobacco user
- **M1311** Anaphylaxis due to the vaccine on or before the date of the encounter
- **M1312** Patient not screened for tobacco use
- **M1313** Tobacco screening not performed or tobacco cessation intervention not provided during the measurement period or in the six months prior to the measurement period
- **M1314** Bmi not documented and no reason is given
- **M1315** Colorectal cancer screening results were not documented and reviewed; reason not otherwise specified
- **M1316** Current tobacco non-user
- **M1317** Patients who are counseled on connection with a csp and explicitly opt out
- **M1318** Patients who did not have documented contact with a csp for at least one of their screened positive hrsns within 60 days after screening or documentation that there was no contact with a csp
- **M1319** Patients who had documented contact with a csp for at least one of their screened positive hrsns within 60 days after screening
- **M1320** Patients who screened positive for at least 1 of the 5 hrsns
- **M1321** Patients who were not seen within 7 weeks following the date of injection for follow up or who did not have a documented iop or no plan of care documented if the iop was >25 mm hg
- **M1322** Patients seen within 7 weeks following the date of injection and are screened for elevated intraocular pressure (iop) with tonometry with documented iop =<25 mm hg for injected eye
- **M1323** Patients seen within 7 weeks following the date of injection and are screened for elevated intraocular pressure (iop) with tonometry with documented iop >25 mm hg and a plan of care was documented
- **M1324** Patients who had an intravitreal or periocular corticosteroid injection (e.g., triamcinolone, preservative-free triamcinolone, dexamethasone, dexamethasone intravitreal implant, or fluocinolone intravitreal implant)
- **M1325** Patients who were not seen for reasons documented by clinician for patient or medical reasons (e.g., inadequate time for follow-up, patients who received a prior intravitreal or periocular steroid injection within the last six (6) months and had a subsequent iop evaluation with iop <25mm hg within seven (7) weeks of treatment)
- **M1326** Patients with a diagnosis of hypotony
- **M1327** Patients who were not appropriately evaluated during the initial exam and/or who were not re-evaluated within 8 weeks
- **M1328** Patients with a diagnosis of acute vitreous hemorrhage

APPENDICES

- **M1329** Patients with a post-operative encounter of the eye with the acute pvd within 2 weeks before the initial encounter or 8 weeks after initial acute pvd encounter
- **M1330** Documentation of patient reason(s) for not having a follow up exam (e.g., inadequate time for follow up)
- **M1331** Patients who were appropriately evaluated during the initial exam and were re-evaluated no later than 8 weeks from initial exam
- **M1332** Patients who were not appropriately evaluated during the initial exam and/or who were not re-evaluated within 2 weeks
- **M1333** Acute vitreous hemorrhage
- **M1334** Patients with a post-operative encounter of the eye with the acute pvd within 2 weeks before the initial encounter or 2 weeks after initial acute pvd encounter
- **M1335** Documentation of patient reason(s) for not having a follow up exam (e.g., inadequate time for follow up)
- **M1336** Patients who were appropriately evaluated during the initial exam and were re-evaluated no later than 2 weeks
- **M1337** Acute pvd
- **M1338** Patients who had follow-up assessment 30 to 180 days after the index assessment who did not demonstrate positive improvement or maintenance of functioning scores during the performance period
- **M1339** Patients who had follow-up assessment 30 to 180 days after the index assessment who demonstrated positive improvement or maintenance of functioning scores during the performance period
- **M1340** Index assessment completed using the 12-item whodas 2.0 or sds during the denominator identification period
- **M1341** Patients who did not have a follow-up assessment or did not have an assessment within 30 to 180 days after the index assessment during the performance period
- **M1342** Patients who died during the performance period
- **M1343** Patients who are at pam level 4 at baseline or patients who are flagged with extreme straight line response sets on the pam
- **M1344** Patients who did not have a baseline pam score and/or a second score within 6 to 12 month of baseline pam score
- **M1345** Patients who had a baseline pam score and a second score within 6 to 12 month of baseline pam score
- **M1346** Patients who did not have a net increase in pam score of at least 6 points within a 6 to 12 month period
- **M1347** Patients who achieved a net increase in pam score of at least 3 points in a 6 to 12 month period (passing)
- **M1348** Patients who achieved a net increase in pam score of at least 6-points in a 6 to 12 month period (excellent)
- **M1349** Patients who did not have a net increase in pam score of at least 3 points within 6 to 12 month period
- **M1350** Patients who had a completed suicide safety plan initiated, reviewed or updated in collaboration with their clinician (concurrent or within 24 hours) of the index clinical encounter
- **M1351** Patients who had a suicide safety plan initiated, reviewed, or updated and reviewed and updated in collaboration with the patient and their clinician concurrent or within 24 hours of clinical encounter and within 120 days after initiation
- **M1352** Suicidal ideation and/or behavior symptoms based on the c-ssrs or equivalent assessment

APPENDICES

• **M1353** Patients who did not have a completed suicide safety plan initiated, reviewed or updated in collaboration with their clinician (concurrent or within 24 hours) of the index clinical encounter

• **M1354** Patients who did not have a suicide safety plan initiated, reviewed, or updated or reviewed and updated in collaboration with the patient and their clinician concurrent or within 24 hours of clinical encounter and within 120 days after initiation

• **M1355** Suicide risk based on their clinician's evaluation or a clinician-rated tool

• **M1356** Patients who died during the measurement period

• **M1357** Patients who had a reduction in suicidal ideation and/or behavior upon follow-up assessment within 120 days of index assessment

• **M1358** Patients who did not have a reduction in suicidal ideation and/or behavior upon follow-up assessment within 120 days of index assessment

• **M1359** Index assessment during the denominator period when the suicidal ideation and/or behavior symptoms or increased suicide risk by clinician determination occurs and a non-zero c-ssrs score is obtained

• **M1360** Suicidal ideation and/or behavior symptoms based on the c-ssrs

• **M1361** Suicide risk based on their clinician's evaluation or a clinician-rated tool

• **M1362** Patients who died during the measurement period

• **M1363** Patients who did not have a follow-up assessment within 120 days of the index assessment

• **M1364** Calculated 10-year ascvd risk score of = 20 percent during the performance period

• **M1365** Patient encounter during the performance period with hospice and palliative care specialty code 17

• **M1366** Focusing on women's health mips value pathway

• **M1367** Quality care for the treatment of ear, nose, and throat disorders mips value pathway

• **M1368** Prevention and treatment of infectious disorders including hepatitis c and hiv mips value pathway

• **M1369** Quality care in mental health and substance use disorders mips value pathway

• **M1370** Rehabilitative support for musculoskeletal care mips value pathway

• **Q0516** Pharmacy supplying fee for hiv pre-exposure prophylaxis fda approved prescription drug, per 30-days

• **Q0517** Pharmacy supplying fee for hiv pre-exposure prophylaxis fda approved prescription drug, per 60-days

• **Q0518** Pharmacy supplying fee for hiv pre-exposure prophylaxis fda approved prescription drug, per 90-days

▲ **Q4225** Amniobind or dermabind tl, per square centimeter

• **Q4279** Vendaje ac, per square centimeter

• **Q4287** Dermabind dl, per square centimeter

• **Q4288** Dermabind ch, per square centimeter

• **Q4289** Revoshield + amniotic barrier, per square centimeter

• **Q4290** Membrane wrap-hydro, per square centimeter

• **Q4291** Lamellas xt, per square centimeter

• **Q4292** Lamellas, per square centimeter

• **Q4293** Acesso dl, per square centimeter

• **Q4294** Amnio quad-core, per square centimeter

• **Q4295** Amnio tri-core amniotic, per square centimeter

• **Q4296** Rebound matrix, per square centimeter

- **Q4297** Emerge matrix, per square centimeter
- **Q4298** Amnicore pro, per square centimeter
- **Q4299** Amnicore pro+, per square centimeter
- **Q4300** Acesso tl, per square centimeter
- **Q4301** Activate matrix, per square centimeter
- **Q4302** Complete aca, per square centimeter
- **Q4303** Complete aa, per square centimeter
- **Q4304** Grafix plus, per square centimeter
- **Q5132** Injection, adalimumab-afzb (abrilada), biosimilar, 10 mg

(**S0166** Injection, olanzapine, 2.5 mg **Code deleted** effective 12/31/2023, no HCPCS/CPT cross-reference provided.)

(**S0171** Injection, bumetanide, 0.5 mg **Code deleted** effective 12/31/2023, no HCPCS/CPT cross-reference provided.)

▲ **T1026** Intensive, extended multidisciplinary services provided in a clinic setting to children with complex medical, physical, mental and psychosocial impairments, per hour

APPENDICES

APPENDIX C: TABLE OF DRUGS

HCPCS Table of Drugs

Directions for the Use of the Table:

1. All drugs are listed in strict alphabetical order by generic drug name.

2. HCPCS code numbers for drugs are listed only under the generic drug name. Users should first look for entries under generic names of drugs. When a drug is known only by brand name, look for the brand name and you will be directed to the generic name of the drug (see "generic name".

3. Information which is indented and appears beneath the first line for a drug is to be considered a continuation of the line preceding it. All drug entries should be checked for indented lines beneath it as a continuation of that entry.

4. When one drug has more than one entry as a result of different routes of administration or different amounts, the drug name is not repeated. All entries for the same drug are listed beneath that drug.

5. The following abbreviations are used in the "routes of administration" column:

Amp	=	ampules
DME	=	durable medical equipment
EPI	=	epidural
G	=	gram
IA	=	intra-arterial administration
IM	=	intramuscular administration
INF	=	infusion
INH	=	administration by inhaled solution
INJ	=	injection
IO	=	intraocular
IT	=	intrathecal
IU	=	international unit
IV	=	intravenous administration
mcg	=	microgram
mg	=	milligram
ml	=	milliliter
ORAL	=	administered orally
OTH	=	other routes of administration
PAR	=	parenteral
SC	=	subcutaneous administration
TABS	=	tablets
U	=	units

DRUG	DOSE	ROUTE	HCPCS
A			
Abatacept	10 mg	IV	J0129
Abbokinase, *see* Urokinase			
Abbokinase, Open Cath, *see* Urokinase			
Abciximab	10 mg	IV	J0130
Abelcet, *see* Amphotericin B Lipid Complex			
ABLC, *see* Amphotericin B			
Abobotulinumtoxin type A	5 units	IM	J0586
Acetaminophen	10 mg	IV	J0131
Acetazolamide sodium	up to 500 mg	IM, IV	J1120
Acetylcysteine, Injection	100 mg	IV	J0132
Acetylcysteine, unit dose form	per gram	INH	J7604, J7608
Achromycin, *see* Tetracycline			
Actemra, *see* Tocilizumab			
ACTH, *see* Corticotropin			
Acthar, *see* Corticotropin			
Actimmune, *see* Interferon gamma 1-B			
Activase, *see* Alteplase recombinant			
Acyclovir	5 mg		J0133
Adalimumab	20 mg	SC	J0135
Adcetris, *see* Brentuximab Vedotin			
Adenocard, *see* Adenosine			
Adenoscan, *see* Adenosine			
Adenosine	1 mg	IV	J0153
Ado-trastuzumab Emtansine	1 mg	IV	J9354
Adrenalin Chloride, *see* Adrenalin, epinephrine			
Adrenalin, epinephrine	0.1 mg	SC, IM	J0171
Adriamycin PFS, *see* Doxorubicin HCl			
Adriamycin RDF, *see* Doxorubicin HCl			
Adrucil, *see* Fluorouracil			
Afamelanotide implant	1 mg	IV	J7352
Aflibercept	1 mg	OTH	J0178
Agalsidase beta	1 mg	IV	J0180
Aggrastat, *see* Tirofiban hydrochloride			
A-hydroCort, *see* Hydrocortisone sodium phosphate			
Akineton, *see* Biperiden			
Alatrofloxacin mesylate, injection	100 mg	IV	J0200
Albuterol	0.5 mg	INH	J7620
Albuterol, concentrated form	1 mg	INH	J7610, J7611
Albuterol, unit dose form	1 mg	INH	J7609, J7613
Aldesleukin	per single use vial	IM, IV	J9015

DRUG	DOSE	ROUTE	HCPCS
Aldomet, *see* Methyldopate HCl			
Alefacept	0.5 mg	IM, IV	J0215
Alferon N, *see* Interferon alfa-n3			
Alglucerase	per 10 units	IV	J0205
Alglucosidase alfa	10 mg	IV	J0220, J0221
Alkaban-AQ, *see* Vinblastine sulfate			
Alkeran, *see* Melphalan, oral			
Alpha 1-proteinase inhibitor, human	10 mg	IV	J0256, J0257
Alphanate			J7186
Alprostadil, Injection	1.25 mcg	OTH	J0270
Alprostadil, urethral suppository		OTH	J0275
Alteplase recombinant	1 mg	IV	J2997
Alupent, *see* Metaproterenol sulfate or Metaproterenol, compounded			
Amcort, *see* Triamcinolone diacetate			
A-methaPred, *see* Methylprednisolone sodium succinate			
Amisulpride	1 mg	IM	J0184
Amgen, *see* Interferon alphacon-1			
Amifostine	500 mg	IV	J0207
Amikacin sulfate	100 mg		J0278
Aminolevulinic acid HCl unit does	354 mg	OTH	J7308
Aminolevulinic acid HCl 10% Gel	10 mg	OTH	J7345
Aminolevulinate	1 gm	OTH	J7309
Aminophylline/Aminophyllin	up to 250 mg	IV	J0280
Amiodarone HCl	30 mg	IV	J0282
Amitriptyline HCl	up to 20 mg	IM	J1320
Amobarbital	up to 125 mg	IM, IV	J0300
Amphocin, *see* Amphotericin B			
Amphotericin B	50 mg	IV	J0285
Amphotericin B, lipid complex	10 mg	IV	J0287-J0289
Ampicillin sodium	up to 500 mg	IM, IV	J0290
Ampicillin sodium/sulbactam sodium	per 1.5 gm	IM, IV	J0295
Amygdalin, *see* Laetrile, Amygdalin, vitamin B-17			
Amytal, *see* Amobarbital			
Anabolin LA 100, *see* Nandrolone decanoate			
Anidulafungin	1 mg	IV	J0348
Anascorp, *see* Centruroides Immune F(ab)			
Ancef, *see* Cefazolin sodium			
Andrest 90-4, *see* Testosterone enanthate and estradiol valerate			
Andro-Cyp, *see* Testosterone cypionate			
Andro-Cyp 200, *see* Testosterone cypionate			
Andro L.A. 200, *see* Testosterone enanthate			

DRUG	DOSE	ROUTE	HCPCS
Andro-Estro 90-4, *see* Testosterone enanthate and estradiol valerate			
Andro/Fem, *see* Testosterone cypionate and estradiol cypionate			
Androgyn L.A., *see* Testosterone enanthate and estradiol valerate			
Androlone-50, *see* Nandrolone phenpropionate			
Androlone-D 100, *see* Nandrolone decanoate			
Andronaq-50, *see* Testosterone suspension			
Andronaq-LA, *see* Testosterone cypionate			
Andronate, *see* Testosterone cypionate			
Andropository 100, *see* Testosterone enanthate			
Andryl 200, *see* Testosterone enanthate			
Anectine, *see* Succinylcholine chloride			
Anergan 25, *see* Promethazine HCl			
Anergan 50, *see* Promethazine HCl			
Anistreplase	30 units	IV	J0350
Anti-Inhibitor	per IU	IV	J7198
Antispas, *see* Dicyclomine HCl			
Antithrombin III (human)	per IU	IV	J7197
Antithrombin recombinant	50 IU	IV	J7196
Anzemet, *see* Dolasetron mesylate Injection			
A.P.L., *see* Chorionic gonadotropin			
Apomorphine Hydrochloride	1 mg	SC	J0364
Apresoline, *see* Hydralazine HCl			
Aprepitant	1 mg	IV	J0185
Aprotinin	10,000 kiu		J0365
AquaMEPHYTON, *see* Vitamin K			
Aralen, *see* Chloroquine HCl			
Aramine, *see* Metaraminol			
Aranesp, *see* Darbepoetin Alfa			
Arbutamine	1 mg	IV	J0395
Arcalyst, *see* Rilonacept			
Aredia, *see* Pamidronate disodium			
Arfonad, *see* Trimethaphan camsylate			
Arformoterol tartrate	15 mcg	INH	J7605
Argatroban (for non-ESRD use)	1 mg	IV	J0883
(for ESRD use)	1 mg	IV	J0884
Aridol, *see* Mannitol			
Aripiprazole	0.25 mg	IM	J0400
Aripiprazole, extended release	1 mg	IV	J0401
Aripiprazole lauroxil	1 mg	IV	J1942
Aripiprazole lauroxil (aristada)	1 mg	IV	J1944

DRUG	DOSE	ROUTE	HCPCS
Aripiprazole lauroxil (aristada initio)	1 mg	IV	J1943
Aristocort Forte, *see* Triamcinolone diacetate			
Aristocort Intralesional, *see* Triamcinolone diacetate			
Aristospan Intra-Articular, *see* Triamcinolone hexacetonide			
Aristospan Intralesional, *see* Triamcinolone hexacetonide			
Arrestin, *see* Trimethobenzamide HCl			
Arsenic trioxide	1 mg	IV	J9017
Artesunate	1 mg	IM	J0391
Arzerra, *see* Ofatumumab			
Asparaginase	1,000 units	IV, IM	J9019
	10,000 units	IV, IM	J9020
Astramorph PF, *see* Morphine sulfate			
Atezolizumab	10 mg	IV	J9022
Atgam, *see* Lymphocyte Immune globulin			
Ativan, *see* Lorazepam			
Atropine, concentrated form	per mg	INH	J7635
Atropine, unit dose form	per mg	INH	J7636
Atropine sulfate	0.01 mg	IV, IM, SC	J0461
Atrovent, *see* Ipratropium bromide			
Atryn, *see* Antithrombin recombinant			
Aurothioglucose	up to 50 mg	IM	J2910
Autologous cultured chondrocytes Implant		OTH	J7330
Autoplex T, *see* Hemophilia clotting factors			
Avacincaptad pegol	0.1 mg	IM	C9162
Avelumab	10 mg	IV	J9023
Avonex, *see* Interferon beta-1a			
Azacitidine	1 mg	SC	J9025
Azathioprine	50 mg	ORAL	J7500
Azathioprine, parenteral	100 mg	IV	J7501
Azithromycin, dihydrate	1 gm	ORAL	Q0144
Azithromycin, Injection	500 mg	IV	J0456
B			
Baclofen	10 mg	IT	J0475
	50 mcg	OTH	J0476
Bactocill, *see* Oxacillin sodium			
BAL in oil, *see* Dimercaprol			
Banflex, *see* Orphenadrine citrate			
Basiliximab	20 mg		J0480
BCG live intravesical instillation	1 mg	OTH	J9030
BCG (Bacillus Calmette and Guérin), live	per vial instillation	IV	J9031

DRUG	DOSE	ROUTE	HCPCS
Beclomethasone inhalation solution, unit dose form	per mg	INH	J7622
Belatacept	1 mg	IV	J0485
Belimumab	10 mg	IV	J0490
Belinostat	10 mg	IV	J9032
Bena-D, *see* Diphenhydramine HCl			
Benadryl, *see* Diphenhydramine HCl			
Benahist, *see* Diphenhydramine HCl			
Ben-Allergin-50, *see* Diphenhydramine HCl			
Bendamustine HCl (Treanda)	1 mg	IV	J9033
Bendamustine HCl (Bendeka)	1 mg	IV	J9034
Bendamustine HCl (Belrapzo/bendamustine)	1 mg	IV	J9036
BeneFIX, *see* Factor IX, recombinant			
Benlysta, *see* Belimumab			
Benoject, *see* Diphenhydramine HCl			
Benralizumab	1 mg	IV	J0517
Bentyl, *see* Dicyclomine			
Benztropine mesylate	per 1 mg	IM, IV	J0515
Beremagene geperpavec-svdt for topical administration	0.1 ml	OTH	J3401
Berinert, *see* C-1 esterase inhibitor			
Berubigen, *see* Vitamin B-12 cyanocobalamin			
Beta amyloid	per study dose	OTH	A9599
Betalin 12, *see* Vitamin B-12 cyanocobalamin			
Betameth, *see* Betamethasone sodium phosphate			
Betamethasone acetate & betamethasone sodium phosphate	per 3 mg	IM	J0702
Betamethasone inhalation solution, unit dose form	per mg	INH	J7624
Betaseron, *see* Interferon beta-1b			
Bethanechol chloride	up to 5 mg	SC	J0520
Bevacizumab	10 mg	IV	J9035
Bevacizumab-awwb	10 mg	IV	Q5107
Bevacizumab- bvzr (Zirabev)	10 mg	IV	Q5118
Bezlotoxumab	10 mg	IV	J0565
Bicillin L-A, *see* Penicillin G benzathine			
Bicillin C-R 900/300, *see* Penicillin G procaine and penicillin G benzathine			
Bicillin C-R, *see* Penicillin G benzathine and penicillin G procaine			
BiCNU, *see* Carmustine			
Biperiden lactate	per 5 mg	IM, IV	J0190
Bitolterol mesylate, concentrated form	per mg	INH	J7628
Bitolterol mesylate, unit dose form	per mg	INH	J7629
Bivalirudin	1 mg	IV	J0583

DRUG	DOSE	ROUTE	HCPCS
Blenoxane, *see* Bleomycin sulfate			
Bleomycin sulfate	15 units	IM, IV, SC	J9040
Blinatumomab	1 microgram	IV	J9039
Bortezomib	0.1 mg	IV	J9041
Bortezomib, not otherwise specified	0.1 mg		J9044
Botox, *see* OnabotulinumtoxinA			
Brentuximab Vedotin	1 mg	IV	J9042
Brethine, *see* Terbutaline sulfate or Terbutaline, compounded			
Bricanyl Subcutaneous, *see* Terbutaline sulfate			
Brolucizumab- dbll	1 mg	IV	J0179
Brompheniramine maleate	per 10 mg	IM, SC, IV	J0945
Bronkephrine, *see* Ethylnorepinephrine HCl			
Bronkosol, *see* Isoetharine HCl			
Budesonide inhalation solution, concentrated form	0.25 mg	INH	J7633, J7634
Budesonide inhalation solution, unit dose form	0.5 mg	INH	J7626, J7627
Bumetanide	0.5 mg	IM	J1939
Buprenorphine Hydrochloride	0.1 mg	IM	J0592
Buprenorphine/Naloxone	1 mg	ORAL	J0571
	< = 3 mg	ORAL	J0572
	> 3 mg but < = 6 mg	ORAL	J0573
	> 6 mg but < = 10 mg	ORAL	J0574
Buprenorphine extended release	<=100 mg	ORAL	Q9991
	>100 mg	ORAL	Q9992
Buprenorphine extended-release (brixadi)	1 mg	IM	J0576
Burosumab-twza	1 mg	IV	J0584
	> 10 mg	ORAL	J0575
Busulfan	1 mg	IV	J0594
Busulfan	2 mg	ORAL	J8510
Butorphanol tartrate	1 mg		J0595
C			
C1 Esterase Inhibitor	10 units	IV	J0596-J0599
Cabazitaxel	1 mg	IV	J9043
Cabergoline	.25 mg	ORAL	J8515
Cabotegravir FDA approved prescription	1 mg	IM	J0739
Cafcit, *see* Caffeine citrate			
Caffeine citrate	5 mg	IV	J0706
Caine, *see* Lidocaine HCl			
Calaspargase pegol – mknl	10 units	IV	J9118
Calcijex, *see* Calcitriol			
Calcimar, *see* Calcitonin-salmon			

DRUG	DOSE	ROUTE	HCPCS
Calcitonin-salmon	up to 400 units	SC, IM	J0630
Calcitriol	0.1 mcg	IM	J0636
Calcium Disodium Versenate, *see* Edetate calcium disodium			
Calcium gluconate	per 10 ml	IV	J0610
Calcium glycerophosphate & calcium lactate	per 10 ml	IM, SC	J0620
Caldolor, *see* Ibuprofen			
Calphosan, *see* Calcium glycerophosphate and calcium lactate			
Camptosar, *see* Irinotecan			
Canakinumab	1 mg	SC	J0638
Cantharidin for topical administration, single unit dose	3.2 mg	OTH	C9164
Capecitabine	150 mg	ORAL	J8520
	500 mg	ORAL	J8521
Capsaicin patch	per sq cm	OTH	J7336
Carbidopa 5 mg/levodopa	20 mg enteral suspension	IV	J7340
Carbocaine with Neo-Cobefrin, *see* Mepivacaine			
Carbocaine, *see* Mepivacaine			
Carboplatin	50 mg	IV	J9045
Carfilzomib	1 mg	IV	J9047
Carmustine	100 mg	IV	J9050
Carnitor, *see* Levocarnitine			
Carticel, *see* Autologous cultured chondrocytes			
Caspofungin acetate	5 mg	IV	J0637
Cayston, *see* Aztreonam			
Cefadyl, *see* Cephapirin Sodium			
Cefazolin sodium	500 mg	IV, IM	J0688, J0690
Cefepime hydrochloride	500 mg	IV	J0692
Cefiderocol	5 mg	IV	J0693
Cefizox, *see* Ceftizoxime sodium			
Cefotaxime sodium	per 1 g	IV, IM	J0698
Cefoxitin sodium	1 g	IV, IM	J0694
Ceftaroline fosamil	1 mg		J0712
Ceftazidime	per 500 mg	IM, IV	J0713
Ceftazidime and Avibactam	0.5 g/0.125 g	IV	J0714
Ceftizoxime sodium	per 500 mg	IV, IM	J0715
Ceftriaxone sodium	per 250 mg	IV, IM	J0696
Ceftolozane 50 mg and tazobactam 25 mg		IV	J0695
Cefuroxime sodium, sterile	per 750 mg	IM, IV	J0697
Celestone Soluspan, *see* Betamethasone acetate and betamethasone sodium phosphate			
CellCept, *see* Mycophenolate mofetil			

DRUG	DOSE	ROUTE	HCPCS
Cel-U-Jec, *see* Betamethasone sodium phosphate			
Cenacort Forte, *see* Triamcinolone diacetate			
Cenacort A-40, *see* Triamcinolone acetonide			
Centruroides Immune F(ab)	up to 120 mg	IV	J0716
Cephalothin sodium	up to 1 g	IM, IV	J1890
Cephapirin sodium	up to 1 g IV,	IM	J0710
Ceredase, *see* Alglucerase			
Cerliponase alfa	1 mg	IV	J0567
Certolizumab pegol	1 mg	SC	J0717
Cerubidine, *see* Daunorubicin HCl			
Cetuximab	10 mg	IV	J9055
Chealamide, *see* Endrate ethylenediamine-tetra-acetic acid			
Chloramphenicol sodium succinate	up to 1 g	IV	J0720
Chlordiazepoxide HCl	up to 100 mg	IM, IV	J1990
Chloromycetin Sodium Succinate, *see* Chloramphenicol sodium succinate			
Chloroprocaine HCl	per 30 ml	VAR	J2400
Chlorpromazine	5 mg	ORAL	Q0161
Chloroquine HCl	up to 250 mg	IM	J0390
Chlorothiazide sodium	per 500 mg	IV	J1205
Chlorpromazine HCl	up to 50 mg	IM, IV	J3230
Chorex-5, *see* Chorionic gonadotropin			
Chorex-10, *see* Chorionic gonadotropin			
Chorignon, *see* Chorionic gonadotropin			
Chorionic gonadotropin	per 1,000 USP		
units	IM	J0725	
Choron 10, *see* Chorionic gonadotropin			
Cidofovir	375 mg	IV	J0740
Cilastatin sodium, Imipenem	per 250 mg	IM, IV	J0743
Cimzia, *see* Certolizumab pegol			
Cinacalcet		ORAL	J0604
Cinryze, *see* C1 Esterase Inhibitor			
Cipro IV, *see* Ciprofloxacin			
Ciprofloxacin	200 mg	IV	J0706
octic suspension 6 mg		OTH	J7342
Cisplatin, powder or solution	per 10 mg	IV	J9060
Cladribine	per mg	IV	J9065
Claforan, *see* Cefotaxime sodium			
Clofarabine	1 mg	IV	J9027
Clonidine Hydrochloride	1 mg	epidural	J0735
Cobex, *see* Vitamin B-12 cyanocobalamin			
Codeine phosphate	per 30 mg	IM, IV, SC	J0745

DRUG	DOSE	ROUTE	HCPCS
Codimal-A, *see* Brompheniramine maleate			
Cogentin, *see* Benztropine mesylate			
Collagenase, Clostridium Histolyticum	0.01 mg	OTH	J0775
Colistimethate sodium	up to 150 mg	IM, IV	J0770
Coly-Mycin M, *see* Colistimethate sodium			
Compa-Z, *see* Prochlorperazine			
Copanlisib	1 mg	IV	J9057
Compazine, *see* Prochlorperazine			
Compounded drug, not otherwise classified			J7999
Cophene-B, *see* Brompheniramine maleate			
Copper contraceptive, intrauterine		OTH	J7300
Cordarone, *see* Amiodarone HCl			
Corgonject-5, *see* Chorionic gonadotropin			
Corticorelin ovine triflutate	1 mcg		J0795
Corticotropin	up to 40 units	IV, IM, SC	J0800
Cortrosyn, *see* Cosyntropin			
Cosmegen, *see* Dactinomycin			
Cosyntropin	per 0.25 mg	IM, IV	J0833, J0834
Cotranzine, *see* Prochlorperazine			
CroFab, *see* Crotalidae Polyvalent Immune Fab			
Cromolyn sodium, unit dose form	per 10 mg	INH	J7631, J7632
Crotalidae immune f(ab')2 (equine)	120 mg	IV	J0841
Crysticillin A.S., *see* Penicillin G procaine			
Cyclophosphamide	100 mg	IV	J9070
Cyclophosphamide, oral	5 mg	ORAL	J9072
	25 mg	ORAL	J8530
Cyclosporine, oral	25 mg	ORAL	J7515
	100 mg	ORAL	J7502
Cyclosporine, parenteral	250 mg	IV	J7516
Cytarabine	100 mg	SC, IV	J9100
Cytarabine liposome	10 mg	IT	J9098
Cytomegalovirus Immune globulin intravenous(human)per vial			
Cytosar-U, *see* Cytarabine			
Cytovene, *see* Ganciclovir sodium			
Cytoxan, *see* Cyclophosphamide; cyclophosphamide, lyophilized; and cyclophosphamide, oral			
D			
D-5-W, infusion	1000 cc	IV	J7070
Dacarbazine	100 mg	IV	J9130
Daclizumab	25 mg	IV	J7513
Dactinomycin	0.5 mg		

DRUG	DOSE	ROUTE	HCPCS
Dalalone, *see* Dexamethasone sodium phosphate			
Dalalone L.A., *see* Dexamethasone acetate			
Dalbavancin	5 mg	IV	J0875
Dalteparin sodium	per 2500 IU	SC	J1645
Daptomycin	1 mg	IV	J0878
	1 mg	IV	J0873
Daratumumab	10 mg	IV	J9144, J9145
Darbepoetin Alfa	1 mcg	IV, SC	J0881, J0882
Daunorubicin citrate, liposomal formulation	10 mg	IV	J9151
Daunorubicin HCl	10 mg	IV	J9150
DaunoXome, *see* Daunorubicin citrate			
DDAVP, *see* Desmopressin acetate			
Decadron Phosphate, *see* Dexamethasone sodium phosphate			
Decadron, *see* Dexamethasone sodium phosphate			
Decadron-LA, *see* Dexamethasone acetate			
Deca-Durabolin, *see* Nandrolone decanoate			
Decaject, *see* Dexamethasone sodium phosphate			
Decaject-L.A., *see* Dexamethasone acetate			
Decitabine	1 mg	IV	J0894
Decolone, *see* Nandrolone decanoate			
De-Comberol, *see* Testosterone cypionate and estradiol cypionate			
Deferoxamine mesylate	500 mg	IM, SC, IV	J0895
Degarelix	1 mg	SC	J9155
Dehist, *see* Brompheniramine maleate			
Deladumone OB, *see* Testosterone enanthate and estradiol valerate			
Delandistrogene moxeparvovec-rokl	per therapeutic dose	IM	J1413
Deladumone, *see* Testosterone enanthate and estradiol valerate			
Delatest, *see* Testosterone enanthate			
Delatestadiol, *see* Testosterone enanthate and estradiol valerate			
Delatestryl, *see* Testosterone enanthate			
Delta-Cortef, *see* Prednisolone, oral			
Delestrogen, *see* Estradiol valerate			
Demadex, *see* Torsemide			
Demerol HCl, *see* Meperidine HCl			
Denosumab	1 mg	SC	J0897
DepAndro, *see* Testosterone cypionate			
DepAndrogyn, *see* Testosterone cypionate and estradiol			

DRUG	DOSE	ROUTE	HCPCS
cypionate			
DepGynogen, *see* Depo-estradiol cypionate			
DepMedalone 40, *see* Methylprednisolone acetate			
DepMedalone 80, *see* Methylprednisolone acetate			
Depo-estradiol cypionate	up to 5 mg	IM	J1000
Depogen, *see* Depo-estradiol cypionate			
Depoject, *see* Methylprednisolone acetate			
Depo-Medrol, *see* Methylprednisolone acetate			
Depopred, *see* Methylprednisolone acetate			
Depo-Provera, *see* Medroxyprogesterone acetate			
Depotest, *see* Testosterone cypionate			
Depo-Testadiol, *see* Testosterone cypionate and estradiol cypionate			
Depotestogen, *see* Testosterone cypionate and estradiol cypionate			
Depo-Testosterone, *see* Testosterone cypionate			
Desferal Mesylate, *see* Deferoxamine mesylate			
Desmopressin acetate	1 mcg	IV, SC	J2597
Dexacen LA-8, *see* Dexamethasone acetate			
Dexacen-4, *see* Dexamethasone sodium phosphate			
Dexamethasone, concentrated form	per mg	INH	J7637
unit form	per mg	INH	J7638
intravitreal Implant	0.1 mg	OTH	J7312
Dexamethasone, lacrimal ophthalmic insert	0.1 mg	OTH	J1095
oral	0.25 mg	ORAL	J8540
Dexamethasone acetate	1 mg	IM	J1094
Dexamethasone sodium phosphate	1 mg	IM, IV, OTH	J1100
Dexasone, *see* Dexamethasone sodium phosphate			
Dexasone L.A., *see* Dexamethasone acetate			
Dexferrum, *see* Iron Dextran			
Dexmedetomidine	1 mcg	ORAL	J1105
Dexone, *see* Dexamethasone sodium phosphate			
Dexone LA, *see* Dexamethasone acetate			
Dexrazoxane hydrochloride	250 mg	IV	J1190
Dextran 40	500 ml	IV	J7100
Dextran 75	500 ml	IV	J7110
Dextrose 5%/normal saline solution,	500 ml = 1 unit	IV	J7042
Dextrose/water (5%)	500 ml = 1 unit	IV	J7060
D.H.E. 45, *see* Dihydroergotamine			
Diamox, *see* Acetazolamide sodium			
Diazepam	up to 5 mg	IM, IV	J3360
Diazoxide	up to 300 mg	IV	J1730
Dibent, *see* Dicyclomine HCl			

DRUG	DOSE	ROUTE	HCPCS
Diclofenac sodium	37.5	IV	J1130
Dicyclomine HCl	up to 20 mg	IM	J0500
Didronel, *see* Etidronate disodium			
Diethylstilbestrol diphosphate	250 mg	IV	J9165
Diflucan, *see* Fluconazole			
Digoxin	up to 0.5 mg	IM, IV	J1160
Digoxin Immune Fab (ovine)	per vial		J1162
Dihydrex, *see* Diphenhydramine HCl			
Dihydroergotamine mesylate	per 1 mg	IM, IV	J1110
Dilantin, *see* Phenytoin sodium			
Dilaudid, *see* Hydromorphone HCl			
Dilocaine, *see* Lidocaine HCl			
Dilomine, *see* Dicyclomine HCl			
Dilor, *see* Dyphylline			
Dimenhydrinate	up to 50 mg	IM, IV	J1240
Dimercaprol	per 100 mg	IM	J0470
Dimethyl sulfoxide, *see* DMSO, Dimethylsulfoxide			
Dinate, *see* Dimenhydrinate			
Dinutuximab	0.1 mg	IM	J1246
Dioval, *see* Estradiol valerate			
Dioval XX, *see* Estradiol valerate			
Diphenacen-50, *see* Diphenhydramine HCl			
Diphenhydramine HCl, Injection	up to 50 mg	IV, IM	J1200
Diphenhydramine HCl, oral	50 mg	ORAL	Q0163
Dipyridamole	per 10 mg	IV	J1245
Disotate, *see* Endrate ethylenediamine-tetra-acetic acid			
Di-Spaz, *see* Dicyclomine HCl			
Ditate-DS, *see* Testosterone enanthate and estradiol valerate			
Diuril Sodium, *see* Chlorothiazide sodium			
D-Med 80, *see* Methylprednisolone acetate			
DMSO, Dimethyl sulfoxide 50%,	50 ml	OTH	J1212
Dobutamine HCl	per 250 mg	IV	J1250
Dobutrex, *see* Dobutamine HCl			
Docetaxel	1 mg	IV	J9172
	20 mg	IV	J9170
Dolasetron mesylate, Injection	10 mg	IV	J1260
Dolasetron mesylate, tablets	100 mg	ORAL	Q0180
Dolophine HCl, *see* Methadone HCl			
Dommanate, *see* Dimenhydrinate			
Donbax, *see* Doripenem			
Dopamine HCl	40 mg		J1265
Doribax, *see* Doripenem			

DRUG	DOSE	ROUTE	HCPCS
Doripenem	10 mg	IV	J1267
Dornase alpha, unit dose form	per mg	INH	J7639
Doxercalciferol	1 mcg	IV	J1270
Doxil, *see* Doxorubicin HCL, lipid			
Doxorubicin HCL	10 mg	IV	J9000
Dramamine, *see* Dimenhydrinate			
Dramanate, *see* Dimenhydrinate			
Dramilin, *see* Dimenhydrinate			
Dramocen, *see* Dimenhydrinate			
Dramoject, *see* Dimenhydrinate			
Dronabinol, oral	2.5 mg	ORAL	Q0167
Droperidol	up to 5 mg	IM, IV	J1790
Drug administered through a metered dose inhaler		INH	J3535
Droperidol and fentanyl citrate	up to 2 ml ampule	IM, IV	J1810
DTIC-Dome, *see* Dacarbazine			
Dua-Gen L.A., *see* Testosterone enanthate and estradiol valerate cypionate			
Duoval P.A., *see* Testosterone enanthate and estradiol valerate			
Durabolin, *see* Nandrolone phenpropionate			
Duraclon, *see* Clonidine Hydrochloride			
Dura-Estrin, *see* Depo-estradiol cypionate			
Duracillin A.S., *see* Penicillin G procaine			
Duragen, *see* Estradiol valerate			
Duralone, *see* Methylprednisolone acetate			
Duralutin, *see* Hydroxyprogesterone Caproate			
Duramorph, *see* Morphine sulfate			
Duratest, *see* Testosterone cypionate			
Duratestrin, *see* Testosterone cypionate and estradiol cypionate			
Durathate-200, *see* Testosterone enanthate			
Durvalumab	10 mg	IV	J9173
Dymenate, *see* Dimenhydrinate			
Dyphylline	up to 500 mg	IM	J1180
Dysport, *see* ABO botulinum toxin type A			
E			
Ecallantide	1 mg	SC	J1290
Eculizumab	10 mg	IV	J1300
Edaravone	1 mg	IV	J1301
Edetate calcium disodium	up to 1000 mg	IV, SC, IM	J0600
Edetate disodium	per 150 mg	IV	J3520
Efgartigimod alfa and hyaluronidase-qvfc	21 mg	IM	J9334

DRUG	DOSE	ROUTE	HCPCS
Elavil, *see* Amitriptyline HCl			
Ellence, *see* Epirubicin HCl			
Elliotts b solution	1 ml	OTH	J9175
Elosulfase alfa	1 mg	IV	J1322
Elotuzumab	1 mg	IV	J9176
Elspar, *see* Asparaginase			
Emapalunab – lzsg	1 mg	IV	J9210
Emend, *see* Fosaprepitant			
Emete-Con, *see* Benzquinamide			
Eminase, *see* Anistreplase			
Emtricitabine and tenofovir alafenamide	200 mg and 25 mg	ORAL	J0751
Emtricitabine and tenofovir disoproxil fumarate	200 mg and 300 mg	ORAL	J0750
Enbrel, *see* Etanercept			
Endrate ethylenediamine-tetra-acetic acid, *see* Edetate disodium			
Enfuvirtide	1 mg	SC	J1324
Enovil, *see* Amitriptyline HCl			
Enoxaparin sodium	10 mg	SC	J1650
Eovist, *see* Gadoxetate disodium			
Epcoritamab-bysp	0.16 mg	IM	J9321
Epinephrine, adrenalin	0.1 mg	SC, IM	J0171
Epirubicin hydrochloride	2 mg		J9178
Epoetin alfa	100 units	IV, SC	Q4081
	100 units	IV, SC	Q5105
	1000 units	IV	Q5106
non-ESRD use	1000 units	IV	J0885
Epoetin alfa–epbx (Retacrit)non-ersd use	1000 units	IV	Q5105
Epoetin alfa–epbx (Retacrit)for-ersd use	100 units	IV	Q5105
Epoetin beta, ESRD use	1 mcg	IV	J0887
non-ESRD use	1 mcg	IV	J0888
Epoprostenol	0.5 mg	IV	J1325
Eptifibatide, Injection	5 mg	IM, IV	J1327
Eravacycline	1 mg	IV	J0122
Ergonovine maleate	up to 0.2 mg	IM, IV	J1330
Eribulin mesylate	0.1 mg	IV	J9179
Ertapenem sodium	500 mg	IM, IV	J1335
Erwinase, *see* Asparaginase			
Erythromycin lactobionate	500 mg	IV	J1364
Estra-D, *see* Depo-estradiol cypionate			
Estra-L, *see* Estradiol valerate			
Estra-Testrin, *see* Testosterone enanthate and estradiol			

DRUG	DOSE	ROUTE	HCPCS
valerate			
Estradiol Cypionate, *see* Depo-estradiol cypionate			
Estradiol L.A., *see* Estradiol valerate			
Estradiol valerate	up to 10 mg	IM	J1380
Estro-Cyp, *see* Depo-estradiol cypionate			
Estrogen, conjugated	per 25 mg	IV, IM	J1410
Estroject LA, *see* Depo-estradiol cypionate			
Estrone	per 1 mg	IM	J1435
Estrone 5, *see* Estrone			
Estrone Aqueous, *see* Estrone			
Estronol, *see* Estrone			
Estronol-L.A., *see* Depo-estradiol cypionate			
Etanercept, Injection	25 mg	IM, IV	J1438
Etelcalcetide	0.1 mg	IV	J0606
Eteplirsen	10 mg	IV	J1428
Ethanolamine	100 mg		J1430
Ethyol, *see* Amifostine			
Etidronate disodium	per 300 mg	IV	J1436
Etonogestrel Implant			J7307
Etopophos, *see* Etoposide			
Etoposide	10 mg	IV	J9181
Etoposide, oral	50 mg	ORAL	J8560
Euflexxa	per dose	OTH	J7323
Everolimus, oral	0.25 mg	ORAL	J7527
Everone, *see* Testosterone Enanthate			
Eylea, *see* Aflibercept			
F			
Factor VIIa (coagulation factor, recombinant)	1 mcg	IV	J7189, J7212
Factor VIII (anti-hemophilic factor, human)	per IU	IV	J7190
Factor VIII (anti-hemophilic factor, porcine)	per IU	IV	J7191
Factor VIII (anti-hemophilic factor, recombinant)	per IU	IV	J7182, J7185, J7192, J7188
Factor VIII (anti-hemophilic factor,	Per IU	IV	J7208
Factor VIII Fc fusion (recombinant)	per IU	IV	J7205, J7207, J7209
Factor VIII (anti-hemophilic factor recombinant)			
(Afstyla)	per IU	IV	J7210
(Kovaltry)	per IU	IV	J7211
Factor IX (anti-hemophilic factor, purified, non-recombinant)	per IU	IV	J7193
Factor IX (anti-hemophilic factor, recombinant)	per IU	IV	J7195, J7200-J7202
Factor IX, complex	per IU	IV	J7194

DRUG	DOSE	ROUTE	HCPCS
Factor X (human)	per IU	IV	J7175
Factor XIII A-subunit (recombinant)	per IU	IV	J7181
Factors, other hemophilia clotting	per IU	IV	J7196
Factrel, *see* Gonadorelin HCl			
Feiba VH Immuno, *see* Factors, other hemophilia clotting			
Fentanyl citrate	0.1 mg	IM, IV	J3010
Feraheme, *see* Ferumoxytol			
Ferric Carboxymaltose	1 mg	IV	J1439
Ferric pyrophosphate citrate powder	0.1 mg of iron	IV	J1444
Ferric pyrophosphate citrate solution	0.1 mg of iron	IV	J1443
Ferrlecit, *see* Sodium ferric gluconate complex in sucrose			
Ferumoxytol	1 mg		Q0138, Q0139
Filgrastim-aafi	1 mcg	IV	Q5110
Filgrastim (G-CSF)	1 mcg	SC, IV	J1442, Q5101
Filgrastim (TBO)	1 mcg	IV	J1447
Firazyr, *see* Icatibant			
Firmagon, *see* Degarelix			
Flebogamma	500 mg	IV	J1572
Flexoject, *see* Orphenadrine citrate			
Flexon, *see* Orphenadrine citrate			
Flolan, *see* Epoprostenol			
Florbetaben f18, diagnostic	per study dose	IV	Q9983
Floxuridine	500 mg	IV	J9200
Fluconazole	200 mg	IV	J1450
Fludara, *see* Fludarabine phosphate			
Fludarabine phosphate	1 mg	ORAL	J8562
	50 mg	IV	J9185
Flunisolide inhalation solution, unit dose form	per mg	INH	J7641
Fluocinolone		OTH	J7311, J7313
Fluocinolone acetonide (Yutiq)	0.01 mg	OTH	J7314
Fluorouracil	500 mg	IV	J9190
Fluphenazine hcl	1.25 mg	IM	J2679
Flutemetamol f18, diagnostic	per study dose	IV	Q9982
Folex, *see* Methotrexate sodium			
Folex PFS, *see* Methotrexate sodium			
Follutein, *see* Chorionic gonadotropin			
Folotyn, *see* Pralatrexate			
Fomepizole	15 mg		J1451
Fomivirsen sodium	1.65 mg	Intraocular	J1452
Fondaparinux sodium	0.5 mg	SC	J1652
Formoterol	12 mcg	INH	J7640

DRUG	DOSE	ROUTE	HCPCS
Formoterol fumarate	20 mcg	INH	J7606
Fortaz, *see* Ceftazidime			
Fosaprepitant	1 mg	IV	J1453
Foscarnet sodium	per 1,000 mg	IV	J1455
Foscavir, *see* Foscarnet sodium			
Fosnetupitant and Palonosetron	235 mg and 0.25 mg	IV	J1454
Fosphenytoin	50 mg	IV	Q2009
Fremanezumab- vfrm	1 mg	IV	J3031
FUDR, *see* Floxuridine			
Fulvestrant	25 mg	IM	J9395
Fungizone Intravenous, *see* Amphotericin B			
Furomide M.D., *see* Furosemide			
Furosemide	up to 20 mg	IM, IV	J1940
G			
Gadoxetate disodium	1 ml	IV	A9581
Gallium nitrate	1 mg	IV	J1457
Galsulfase	1 mg	IV	J1458
GamaSTAN, *see* Gamma globulin and Immune globulin			
Gammagard Liquid	500 mg	IV	J1569
Gamma globulin	1 cc	IM	J1460
	over 10 cc	IM	J1560
Gammaplex	500 mg	IV	J1557
Gammar, *see* Gamma globulin and Immune globulin			
Gammar-IV, *see* Immune globulin intravenous (human)			
Gamulin RH, *see* Rho(D) Immune globulin			
Gamunex	500 mg	IV	J1561
Ganciclovir, Implant	4.5 mg	OTH	J7310
Ganciclovir sodium	500 mg	IV	J1570
Garamycin, gentamicin	up to 80 mg	IM, IV	J1580
Gatifloxacin	10 mg	IV	J1590
Gefitinib	250 mg	ORAL	J8565
Gel-One	per dose	OTH	J7326
Gemcitabine HCl Not otherwise specified	200 mg	IV	J9201
Gemcitabine HCI (Infugem)	200 mg	IV	J9199
Gemcitabine HCl	200 mg	IV	J9201
Gemsar, *see* Gemcitabine HCl			
Gemtuzumab ozogamicin	0.1 mg	IV	J9203
Gentamicin Sulfate, *see* Garamycin, gentamicin			
Gentran, *see* Dextran 40			
Gentran 75, *see* Dextran 75			
Gesterol 50, *see* Progesterone			

DRUG	DOSE	ROUTE	HCPCS
Glassia	10 mg	IV	J0257
Glatiramer Acetate	20 mg	SC	J1595
Glofitamab-gxbm	2.5 mg	IM	J9286
Glucagon HCl	per 1 mg	SC, IM, IV	J1610
Glukor, *see* Chorionic gonadotropin Glycopyrrolate, concentrated form	per 1 mg	INH	J7642
Glycopyrrolate, unit dose form	per 1 mg	INH	J7643
	0.1 mg	INH	J1596
Gold sodium thiomalate	up to 50 mg	IM	J1600
Golimumab	1 mg	IV	J1602
Gonadorelin HCl	per 100 mcg	SC, IV	J1620
Gonic, *see* Chorionic gonadotropin			
Goserelin acetate Implant	per 3.6 mg	SC	J9202
Granisetron, extended release	0.1 mg	IV	J1627
Granisetron HCl, Injection	100 mcg	IV	J1626
Granisetron HCl, oral	1 mg	ORAL	Q0166
Guselkumab	1 mg	IV	J1628
Gynogen L.A. *see* Estradiol valerate			
H			
Halaven, *see* Eribulin mesylate			
Haldol, *see* Haloperidol			
Haloperidol	up to 5 mg	IM, IV	J1630
Haloperidol decanoate			
Hectorol, *see* Doxercalciferol			
Hemin	1 mg		J1640
Hemofil M, *see* Factor VIII			
Hemophilia clotting factors(e.g., anti-inhibitors)	per IU	IV	J7198
Hemophilia clotting factors, NOC	per IU	IV	J7199
HepaGam B	0.5 ml	IM	J1571
	0.5 ml	IV	J1573
Hep-Lock, *see* Heparin sodium (heparin lock flush)			
Hep-Lock U/P, *see* Heparin sodium (heparin lock flush)			
Heparin sodium	1,000 units	IV, SC	J1644
Heparin sodium (heparin lock flush)	10 units	IV	J1642
Herceptin, *see* Trastuzumab			
Hexadrol Phosphate, *see* Dexamethasone sodium phosphate			
Hexaminolevulinate hydrochloride	100 mg	IV	A9589
Histaject, *see* Brompheniramine maleate			
Histerone 50, *see* Testosterone suspension			
Histerone 100, *see* Testosterone suspension			
Histrelin acetate	10 mcg		J1675

DRUG	DOSE	ROUTE	HCPCS
Histrelin Implant	50 mg	OTH	J9225
Hizentra, *see* Immune globulin			
Human fibrinogen concentrate	100 mg	IV	J7178
Human fibrinogen concentrate (fibryga)	1 mg	IV	J7177
Hyalgan, Supartz or VISCO-3		IA	J7321
Hyaluronan or derivative	per dose	IV	J7327
Durolane	1 mg	IA	J7318
Gel-Syn	0.1 mg	IA	J7328
Gelsyn-3	0.1	IV	J7328
Gen Visc 850	1 mg	IA	J7320
Hymovis	1 mg	IA	J7322
Synojoynt	1 mg	VAR	J7331
Triluron	1 mg	IV	J7332
Trivisc	1 mg	IV	J7329
Hyaluronidase	up to 150 units	SC, IV	J3470
Hyaluronidase, ovine	up to 999 units	VAR	J3471
	per 1000 units	VAR	J3472
Hyaluronidase recombinant	1 USP	SC	J3473
Hyate:C, *see* Factor VIII (anti-hemophilic factor (porcine))			
Hybolin Improved, *see* Nandrolone phenpropionate			
Hybolin Decanoate, *see* Nandrolone decanoate			
Hycamtin, *see* Topotecan			
Hydralazine HCl	up to 20 mg	IV, IM	J0360
Hydrate, *see* Dimenhydrinate			
Hydrocortisone acetate	up to 25 mg IV,	IV, IM, SC	J1700
Hydrocortisone sodium phosphate	up to 50 mg	IV, IM, SC	J1710
Hydrocortisone succinate sodium	up to 100 mg	IV, IM, SC	J1720
Hydrocortone Acetate, *see* Hydrocortisone acetate			
Hydrocortone Phosphate, *see* Hydrocortisone sodium phosphate			
Hydromorphone HCl	up to 4 mg	SC, IM, IV	J1170
Hydroxocobalamin	10 mcg	IM	J3425
Hydroxyprogesterone Caproate	1 mg	IM	J1725
Hydroxyprogesterone Caproate, NOS	10 mg	IV	J1729
Hydroxyprogesterone Caproate, (Makena)	10 mg	IV	J1726
Hydroxyzine HCl	up to 25 mg	IM	J3410
Hydroxyzine Pamoate	25 mg	ORAL	Q0177
Hylan G-F	20	OTH	J7322
Hyoscyamine sulfate	up to 0.25 mg	SC, IM, IV	J1980
Hyperstat IV, *see* Diazoxide			
Hyper-Tet, *see* Tetanus Immune globulin, human			
HypRho-D, *see* Rho(D) Immune globulin			

DRUG	DOSE	ROUTE	HCPCS
Hyrexin-50, *see* Diphenhydramine HCl			
Hyzine-50, *see* Hydroxyzine HCl			
I			
Ibalizumab-uiyk	10 mg	IV	J1746
Ibandronate sodium	1 mg	IV	J1740
Ibuprofen	100 mg	IV	J1741
Ibutilide fumarate	1 mg	IV	J1742
Icatibant	1 mg	SC	J1744
Idamycin, *see* Idarubicin HCl			
Idarubicin HCl	5 mg	IV	J9211
Idursulfase	1 mg	IV	J1743
Ifex, *see* Ifosfamide			
Ifosfamide	1 g	IV	J9208
Ilaris, *see* Canakinumab			
Iloprost	20 mcg	INH	Q4074
Ilotycin, *see* Erythromycin gluceptate			
Imferon, *see* Iron dextran			
Imiglucerase	10 units	IV	J1786
Imitrex, *see* Sumatriptan succinate			
Immune globulin			
Bivigam	500 mg	IV	J1556
Flebogamma	500 mg	IV	J1572
Gammagard Liquid	500 mg	IV	J1569
Gammaplex	500 mg	IV	J1557
Gamunex	500 mg	IV	J1561
HepaGam B	0.5 ml	IM	J1571
HepaGam B	0.5 ml	IV	J1573
Hizentra	100 mg	SC	J1559
Hyaluronidase, (hyqvia)	100 mg	IV	J1575
NOS	500 mg	IV	J1566, J1599
Octagam	500 mg	IV	J1568
Privigen	500 mg	IV	J1459
Rhophylac	100 IU	IM	J2791
Subcutaneous	100 mg	SC	J1562
Cuvitru	100 mg	IV	J1555
Immunosuppressive drug, not otherwise classified			J7599
Imuran, *see* Azathioprine			
Inapsine, *see* Droperidol			
Incobotulinumtoxin type A	1 unit	IM	J0588
Inderal, *see* Propranolol HCl			
Inebilizumab-cdon	1 mg	IV	J1823
INFeD, *see* Iron Dextran			

DRUG	DOSE	ROUTE	HCPCS
Infliximab-dyyb	10 mg	IM, IV	Q5103
Infliximab-abda	10 mg	IM, IV	Q5104
Infliximab-qbtx	10 mg	IM, IV	Q5109
Injection factor ix, glycopegylated	1 iu	IV	J7203
Infergen, *see* Interferon alfa-1			
Infliximab, Injection	10 mg	IM, IV	J1745, Q5102
Innohep, *see* Tinzaparin			
Innovar, *see* Droperidol with fentanyl citrate			
Inotuzumab ozogamicin	0.1 mg	IV	J9229
Insulin	5 units	SC	J1815
Insulin lispro	50 units	SC	J1817
Intal, *see* Cromolyn sodium or Cromolyn sodium, compounded			
Integrilin, Injection, *see* Eptifibatide			
Interferon alphacon-1, recombinant	1 mcg	SC	J9212
Interferon alfa-2a, recombinant	3 million units	SC, IM	J9213
Interferon alfa-2b, recombinant	1 million units	SC, IM	J9214
Interferon alfa-n3 (human leukocyte derived)	250,000 IU	IM	J9215
Interferon beta-1a	30 mcg	IM	J1826
	1 mcg	IM	Q3027
	1 mcg	SC	Q3028
Interferon beta-1b	0.25 mg	SC	J1830
Interferon gamma-1b	3 million units	SC	J9216
Intrauterine copper contraceptive, *see* Copper contraceptive, intrauterine			
Invega Sustenna, *see* Paliperidone Palmitate			
Ipilimumab	1 mg	IV	J9228
Ipratropium bromide, unit dose form	per mg	INH	J7644, J7645
Irinotecan	20 mg	IV	J9206, J9205
Iron dextran	50 mg	IV	J1750
Iron sucrose	1 mg	IV	J1756
Irrigation solution for Tx of bladder calculi	per 50 ml	OTH	Q2004
Isavuconazonium	1 mg	IV	J1833
Isocaine HCl, *see* Mepivacaine			
Isoetharine HCl, concentrated form	per mg	INH	J7647, J7648
unit dose form	per mg	INH	J7649, J7650
Isoproterenol HCl, concentrated form	per mg	INH	J7657, J7658
unit dose form	per mg	INH	J7659, J7660
Istodax, *see* Romidepsin			
Isuprel, *see* Isoproterenol HCl			
Itraconazole	50 mg	IV	J1835
Ixabepilone	1 mg	IV	J9207
Ixempra, *see* Ixabepilone			

DRUG	DOSE	ROUTE	HCPCS
J			
Jenamicin, *see* Garamycin, gentamicin			
Jevtana, *see* Cabazitaxel			
K			
Kabikinase, *see* Streptokinase			
Kalbitor, *see* Ecallantide			
Kaleinate, *see* Calcium gluconate			
Kanamycin sulfate	up to 75 mg	IM, IV	J1850
	up to 500 mg	IM, IV	J1840
Kantrex, *see* Kanamycin sulfate			
Keflin, *see* Cephalothin sodium			
Kefurox, *see* Cefuroxime sodium			
Kefzol, *see* Cefazolin sodium			
Kenaject-40, *see* Triamcinolone acetonide			
Keroxx	1 cc	IV	Q4202
Kenalog, *see* Triamcinolone acetonide			
Keppra, *see* Levetiracetam			
Kestrone 5, *see* Estrone			
Ketorolac tromethamine	per 15 mg	IM, IV	J1885
Key-Pred, *see* Prednisolone acetate			
Key-Pred-SP, *see* Prednisolone sodium phosphate			
K-Flex, *see* Orphenadrine citrate			
Khapzory	0.5 mg	IV	J0642
Klebcil, *see* Kanamycin sulfate			
Koate-HP, *see* Factor VIII Kogenate, *see* Factor VIII			
Konakion, *see* Vitamin K, phytonadione, etc.			
Konyne-80, *see* Factor IX, complex			
Krystexxa, *see* Pegloticase			
Kytril, *see* Granisetron HCl			
Kyleena	19.5 mg		
L			
L.A.E. 20, *see* Estradiol valerate			
Laetrile, Amygdalin, vitamin B-17			J3570
Lanadelumab – flyo	1 mg	IV	J0593
Lanoxin, *see* Digoxin			
Lanreotide	1 mg	SC	J1930
Largon, *see* Propiomazine HCl			
Laronidase	0.1 mg	IV	J1931
Lasix, *see* Furosemide			
L-Caine, *see* Lidocaine HCl			
Lepirudin	50 mg		J1945

DRUG	DOSE	ROUTE	HCPCS
Leucovorin calcium	per 50 mg	IM, IV	J0640
Leukine, *see* Sargramostim (GM-CSF)			
Leuprolide acetate (for depot suspension)	per 3.75 mg	IM	J1950
	7.5 mg	IM	J9217
Leuprolide acetate	per 1 mg	IM	J9218
Leuprolide acetate Implant	65 mg	OTH	J9219
Leustatin, *see* Cladribine			
Levalbuterol HCl, concentrated form	0.5 mg	INH	J7607, J7612
Levalbuterol HCl, unit dose form	0.5 mg	INH	J7614, J7615
Levaquin I.U., *see* Levofloxacin			
Levetiracetam	10 mg	IV	J1953
Levocarnitine	per 1 gm	IV	J1955
Levo-Dromoran, *see* Levorphanol tartrate			
Levofloxacin	250 mg	IV	J1956
Levoleucovorin calcium	0.5 mg	IV	J0641
Levonorgestrel Implant		OTH	J7306
Levonorgestrel releasing intrauterine contraceptive	52 mg	OTH	J7297, J7298
KYLEENA	19.5 mg	OTH	J7296
Levorphanol tartrate	up to 2 mg	SC, IV	J1960
Levsin, *see* Hyoscyamine sulfate			
Levulan Kerastick, *see* Aminolevulinic acid HCl			
Lexiscan, *see* Regadenoson			
Librium, *see* Chlordiazepoxide HCl			
Lidocaine HCl	10 mg	IV	J2001
Lidoject, *see* Lidocaine HCl			
Lincocin, *see* Lincomycin HCl			
Lincomycin HCl	up to 300 mg	IV	J2010
Linezolid	200 mg	IV	J2020
Liquaemin Sodium, *see* Heparin sodium			
Lioresal, *see* Baclofen			
Liposomal			
Cytarabine	2.27 mg	IV	J9153
Daunorubicin	1 mg	IV	J9153
LMD (10%), *see* Dextran 40			
Lovenox, *see* Enoxaparin sodium			
Lorazepam	2 mg	IM, IV	J2060
Loxapine	1 mg	OTH	J2062
Lufyllin, *see* Dyphylline			
Luminal Sodium, *see* Phenobarbital sodium			
Lumizyme, *see* Alglucosidase alfa			
Lurbinectedin	0.1 mg	IV	J9223
Lunelle, *see* Medroxyprogesterone acetate/estradiol cypionate			

DRUG	DOSE	ROUTE	HCPCS
Lupron, *see* Leuprolide acetate			
Lyophilized, *see* Cyclophosphamide, lyophilized			
M			
Magnesium sulfate	500 mg		J3475
Makena, *see* Hydroxyprogesterone Caproate			
Mannitol	25% in 50 ml	IV	J2150
	5mg	INH	J7665
Marmine, *see* Dimenhydrinate			
Maxipime, *see* Cefepime hydrochloride			
Mecasermin	1 mg	SC	J2170
Mechlorethamine HCl (nitrogen mustard), HN2	10 mg	IV	J9230
Medralone, *see* Methylprednisolone acetate			
Medrol, *see* Methylprednisolone			
Medroxyprogesterone acetate	1 mg	IM	J1050
Mefoxin, *see* Cefoxitin sodium			
Melphalan HCl	50 mg	IV	J9245
oral	2 mg	ORAL	J8600
Menoject LA, *see* Testosterone cypionate and estradiol cypionate			
Mepergan Injection, *see* Meperidine and promethazine HCl			
Meperidine HCl	per 100 mg	IM, IV, SC	J2175
Meperidine and promethazine HCl	up to 50 mg	IM, IV	J2180
Mepivacaine HCL	per 10 ml	VAR	J0670
Mepolizumab	1 mg	IV	J2182
Meropenem	100 mg	IV	J2185
Mesna	200 mg	IV	J9209
Mesnex, *see* Mesna			
Metaprel, *see* Metaproterenol sulfate			
Metaproterenol sulfate, concentrated form	per 10 mg	INH	J7667, J7668
unit dose form	per 10 mg	INH	J7669, J7670
Metaraminol bitartrate	per 10 mg	IV, IM, SC	J0380
Metastron, *see* Strontium-89 chloride			
Methacholine chloride	1 mg	INH	J7674
Methadone HCl	up to 10 mg	IM, SC	J1230
Methergine, *see* Methylergonovine maleate			
Methocarbamol	up to 10 ml	IV, IM	J2800
Methotrexate, oral	2.5 mg	ORAL	J8610
Methotrexate sodium	5 mg	IV, IM, IT, IA	J9250
	50 mg	IV, IM, IT, IA	J9260
not therapeutically equivalent to J9250 and J9260	50 mg	IV, IM, IT, IA	J9255
Methotrexate LPF, *see* Methotrexate sodium			

DRUG	DOSE	ROUTE	HCPCS
Methyldopate HCl	up to 250 mg	IV	J0210
Methylnaltrexone	0.1 mg	SC	J2212
Methylprednisolone, oral	per 4 mg	ORAL	J7509
Methylprednisolone acetate	20 mg	IM	J1020
	40 mg	IM	J1030
	80 mg	IM	J1040
Methylprednisolone sodium succinate	up to 40 mg	IM, IV	J2920
	up to 125 mg	IM, IV	J2930
Metoclopramide HCl	up to 10 mg	IV	J2765
Metvixia, *see* Aminolevulinate			
Miacalcin, *see* Calcitonin-salmon			
Micafungin sodium	1 mg		J2248
Midazolam HCl	per 1 mg	IM, IV	J2250
Milrinone lactate	5 mg	IV	J2260
Minocin, *see* Minocycline Hydrochloride			
Minocycline Hydrochloride	1 mg	IV	J2265
Mirena, *see* Levonorgestrel releasing intrauterine contraceptive			
Mithracin, *see* Plicamycin			
Mitomycin	0.2 mg	Ophthalmic	J7315
	5 mg	IV	J9280, J9281
Mitosol, *see* Mitomycin			
Mitoxantrone HCl	per 5 mg	IV	J9293
Mogamulizumab – kpkc	1 mg	IV	J9204
Monocid, *see* Cefonicid sodium			
Monoclate-P, *see* Factor VIII			
Monoclonal antibodies, parenteral	5 mg	IV	J7505
Mononine, *see* Factor IX, purified, non-recombinant			
Morphine sulfate	up to 10 mg	IM, IV, SC	J2270
Morphine sulfate, preservative-free	10 mg	SC, IM, IV	J2274
Moxetumomab Pasudotox - tdfk	0.01 mg	IV	J9313
Moxifloxacin	100 mg	IV	J2280
Mozobil, *see* Plerixafor			
M-Prednisol, *see* Methylprednisolone acetate			
Mucomyst, *see* Acetylcysteine or Acetylcysteine, compounded			
Mucosol, *see* Acetylcysteine			
Muromonab-CD3	5 mg	IV	J7505
Muse, *see* Alprostadil			
Mustargen, *see* Mechlorethamine HCl			
Mutamycin, *see* Mitomycin			
Mycophenolic acid	180 mg	ORAL	J7518
Mycophenolate Mofetil	250 mg	ORAL	J7517

DRUG	DOSE	ROUTE	HCPCS
Myleran, *see* Busulfan			
Mylotarg, *see* Gemtuzumab ozogamicin			
Myobloc, *see* RimabotulinumtoxinB			
Myochrysine, *see* Gold sodium thiomalate			
Myolin, *see* Orphenadrine citrate			
N			
Nabilone	1 mg	ORAL	J8650
Nalbuphine HCl	per 10 mg	IM, IV, SC	J2300
Naloxone HCl	per 1 mg	IM, IV, SC	J2310
Naltrexone, depot form	1 mg	IM	J2315
Nandrobolic L.A., *see* Nandrolone decanoate			
Nandrolone decanoate	up to 50 mg	IM	J2320
Narcan, *see* Naloxone HCl			
Naropin, *see* Ropivacaine HCl			
Nasahist B, *see* Brompheniramine maleate			
Nasal vaccine inhalation		INH	J3530
Natalizumab	1 mg	IV	J2323
Navane, *see* Thiothixene			
Navelbine, *see* Vinorelbine tartrate			
ND Stat, *see* Brompheniramine maleate			
Nebcin, *see* Tobramycin sulfate			
NebuPent, *see* Pentamidine isethionate			
Necitumumab	1 mg	IV	J9295
Nelarabine	50 mg	IV	J9261
Nembutal Sodium Solution, *see* Pentobarbital sodium			
Neocyten, *see* Orphenadrine citrate			
Neo-Durabolic, *see* Nandrolone decanoate			
Neoquess, *see* Dicyclomine HCl			
Neosar, *see* Cyclophosphamide			
Neostigmine methylsulfate	up to 0.5 mg	IM, IV, SC	J2710
Neo-Synephrine, *see* Phenylephrine HCl			
Nervocaine, *see* Lidocaine HCl			
Nesacaine, *see* Chloroprocaine HCL			
Nesacaine-MPF, *see* Chloroprocaine HCl			
Nesiritide	0.1 mg	IV	J2325
Neumega, *see* Oprelvekin			
Neupogen, *see* Filgrastim (G-CSF)			
Neutrexin, *see* Trimetrexate glucuronate			
Nicardipine	0.1 mg	IM	J2404
Nipent, *see* Pentostatin			
Nivolumab	1 mg	IV	J9299
Nordryl, *see* Diphenhydramine HCl			

DRUG	DOSE	ROUTE	HCPCS
Norflex, *see* Orphenadrine citrate			
Norzine, *see* Thiethylperazine maleate			
Not otherwise classified drugs			J3490
Not otherwise classified drugs other than administered thru DME		INH	J7799
Not otherwise classified drugs administered thru DME		INH	J7699
Not otherwise classified drugs, anti-neoplastic			J9999
Not otherwise classified drugs, chemotherapeutic		ORAL	J8999
Not otherwise classified drugs, Immunosuppressive			J7599
Not otherwise classified drugs, non-chemotherapeutic		ORAL	J8499
Novantrone, *see* Mitoxantrone HCl			
Novo Seven, *see* Factor VIIa NPH, *see* Insulin			
Nplate, *see* Romiplostim			
Nubain, *see* Nalbuphine HCl			
Nulicaine, *see* Lidocaine HCl			
Nulojix, *see* Belatacept			
Numorphan, *see* Oxymorphone HCl			
Nusinersen	0.1 mg	IV	J2326
O			
Ocriplasmin	0.125 mg	IV	J7316
Octagam	500 mg	IV	J1568
Ocrelizumab	1 mg	IV	J2350
Octreotide Acetate, Injection	1 mg	IM	J2353
	25 mcg	IV, SQ	J2354
Oculinum, *see* Botulinum toxin type A			
Ofatumumab	10 mg	IV	J9302
Ofirmev, *see* Acetaminophen			
O-Flex, *see* Orphenadrine citrate			
Oforta, *see* Fludarabine phosphate			
Olanzapine	1 mg	IM	J2358
Olaratumab	10 mg	IV	J9285
Omadacycline	1 mg	IV	J0121
Omacetaxine Mepesuccinate	0.01 mg	IV	J9262
Omalizumab	5 mg	SC	J2357
Omnipen-N, *see* Ampicillin			
Omontys, *see* Peginesatide			
OnabotulinumtoxinA	1 unit	IM	J0585
Oncaspar, *see* Pegaspargase			
Oncovin, *see* Vincristine sulfate			
Ondansetron HCI	1 mg	IV	J2405
Ondansetron HCl, oral	1 mg	ORAL	Q0162
Oprelvekin	5 mg	SC	J2355

DRUG	DOSE	ROUTE	HCPCS
Oraminic II, *see* Brompheniramine maleate			
Oritavancin	10 mg	IV	J2407
Ormazine, *see* Chlorpromazine HCl			
Orphenadrine citrate	up to 60 mg	IV, IM	J2360
Orphenate, *see* Orphenadrine citrate			
Orthovisc		OTH	J7324
Or-Tyl, *see* Dicyclomine			
Oxacillin sodium	up to 250 mg	IM, IV	J2700
Oxaliplatin	0.5 mg	IV	J9263
Oxymorphone HCl	up to 1 mg	IV, SC, IM	J2410
Oxytetracycline HCl	up to 50 mg	IM	J2460
Oxytocin	up to 10 units	IV, IM	J2590
Ozurdex, *see* Dexamethasone, intravitreal Implant			
P			
Paclitaxel	1 mg	IV	J9267
Paclitaxel protein-bound particles	1 mg	IV	J9264
not therapeutically equivalent to J9264	1 mg	IV	J9258
Palifermin	50 mcg	IV	J2425
Paliperidone Palmitate	1 mg	IM	J2426
Palonosetron HCl	25 mcg	IV	J2469
Netupitant 300 mg and palonosetron	0.5 mg	ORAL	J8655
Pamidronate disodium	per 30 mg	IV	J2430
Panitumumab	10 mg	IV	J9303
Papaverine HCl	up to 60 mg	IV, IM	J2440
ParaGard T 380 A, *see* Copper contraceptive, intrauterine			
Paraplatin, *see* Carboplatin			
Paricalcitol, Injection	1 mcg	IV, IM	J2501
Pasireotide, long acting	1 mg	IV	J2502
Patisiran	0.1 mg	IV	J0222
Pegademase bovine	25 iu		J2504
Pegaptanib	0.3 mg	OTH	J2503
Pegaspargase	per single dose vial	IM, IV	J9266
Pegfilgrastim	6 mg	SC	J2505
Pegfilgrastim-jmdb	0.5 mg	SC	J2506, Q5122
Peginesatide	0.1 mg	IV, SC	J0890
Pegloticase	1 mg	IV	J2507
Pegunigalsidase alfa-iwxj	1 mg	IM	J2508
Pemetrexed	10 mg	IV	J9305
Pembrolizumab	1 mg	IV	J9271
Pemetrexed (pemrydi rtu)	10 mg	IM	J9324

DRUG	DOSE	ROUTE	HCPCS
Penicillin G benzathine	100,000 units	IM	J0561
Penicillin G benzathine and penicillin G procaine	100,000 units	IM	J0558
Penicillin G potassium	up to 600,000 units	IM, IV	J2540
Penicillin G procaine, aqueous	up to 600,000 units	IM, IV	J2510
Pentamidine isethionate	per 300 mg	INH	J2545,J7676
Pentastarch, 10%	100 ml		J2513
Pentazocine HCl	30 mg	IM, SC, IV	J3070
Pentobarbital sodium	per 50 mg	IM, IV, OTH	J2515
Pentostatin	per 10 mg	IV	J9268
Perforomist, *see* Formoterol fumarate			
Peramivir	1 mg	IV	J2547
Permapen, *see* Penicillin G benzathine			
Perphenazine, Injection	up to 5 mg	IM, IV	J3310
Perphenazine, tablets	4 mg	ORAL	Q0175
Persantine IV, *see* Dipyridamole			
Pertuzumab	1 mg	IV	J9306
Pet Imaging			
Gallium Ga-68, dotatate, diagnostic	0.1 millicurie	IV	A9587
Fluciclovine F-18, diagnostic	1 millicurie	IV	A9588
Pfizerpen, *see* Penicillin G potassium			
Pfizerpen A.S., *see* Penicillin G procaine			
Phenazine, *see* Promethazine HCl			
Phenergan, *see* Promethazine HCl			
Phenobarbital sodium	up to 120 mg	IM, IV	J2560
Phentolamine mesylate	up to 5 mg	IM, IV	J2760
Phenylephrine HCl	up to 1 ml	SC, IM, IV	J2370
Phenylephrine 10.16 mg/Ketorolac 2.88	1 ml	VAR	J1097
Phenytoin sodium	per 50 mg	IM, IV	J1165
Photofrin, *see* Porfimer sodium			
Phytonadione (Vitamin K)	per 1 mg	IM, SC, IV	J3430
Piperacillin/Tazobactam Sodium, Injection	1.125 g	IV	J2543
Pitocin, *see* Oxytocin			
Platinol AQ, *see* Cisplatin			
Plas+SD, *see* Plasma, pooled multiple donor			
Plasma, cryoprecipitate reduced	each unit	IV	P9044
Plasma, pooled multiple donor, frozen, each unit		IV	P9023, P9070
Plasma (single donor), pathogen reduced, frozen each unit		IV	P9071
Platelets, pheresis, pathogen reduced each unit		IV	P9073
Pathogen(s) test for platelets		OTH	P9100
Platinol, *see* Cisplatin			

DRUG	DOSE	ROUTE	HCPCS
Plazomicin	5 mg	IV	J0291
Plerixafor	1 mg	SC	J2562
Plicamycin	2,500 mcg	IV	J9270
Polatuzumab vedotin	1 mg	IV	J9309
Polocaine, *see* Mepivacaine			
Polycillin-N, *see* Ampicillin			
Porfimer Sodium	75 mg	IV	J9600
Positron emission tomography radiopharmaceutical, diagnostic			
for tumor identification, NOC		IV	A9597
for non-tumor identification, NOC		IV	A9598
Potassium chloride	per 2 mEq	IV	J3480
Pralatrexate	1 mg	IV	J9307
Pralidoxime chloride	up to 1 g	IV, IM, SC	J2730
Predalone-50, *see* Prednisolone acetate			
Predcor, *see* Prednisolone acetate			
Predicort-50, *see* Prednisolone acetate			
Prednisone, Immediate release or delayed release	1 mg	ORAL	J7512
Prednisolone, oral	5 mg	ORAL	J7510
Prednisolone acetate	up to 1 ml	IM	J2650
Predoject-50, *see* Prednisolone acetate			
Pregnyl, *see* Chorionic gonadotropin			
Premarin Intravenous, *see* Estrogen, conjugated			
Prescription, chemotherapeutic, not otherwise specified		ORAL	J8999
Prescription, non-chemotherapeutic, not otherwise specified		ORAL	J8499
Primacor, *see* Milrinone lactate			
Primaxin, *see* Cilastatin sodium, Imipenem			
Priscoline HCl, *see* Tolazoline HCl			
Privigen	500 mg	IV	J1459
Pro-Depo, *see* Hydroxyprogesterone Caproate			
Procainamide HCl	up to 1 g	IM, IV	J2690
Prochlorperazine	up to 10 mg	IM, IV	J0780
Prochlorperazine maleate, oral	5 mg	ORAL	Q0164
Profasi HP, *see* Chorionic gonadotropin			
Profilnine Heat-Treated, *see* Factor IX			
Progestaject, *see* Progesterone			
Progesterone	per 50 mg	IM	J2675
Prograf, *see* Tacrolimus, oral or parenteral			
Prokine, *see* Sargramostim (GM-CSF)			
Prolastin, *see* Alpha 1-proteinase inhibitor, human			
Proleukin, *see* Aldesleukin			
Prolixin Decanoate, *see* Fluphenazine decanoate			

DRUG	DOSE	ROUTE	HCPCS
Promazine HCl	up to 25 mg	IM	J2950
Promethazine HCl, Injection	up to 50 mg	IM, IV	J2550
Promethazine HCl, oral	12.5 mg	ORAL	Q0169
Pronestyl, *see* Procainamide HCl			
Proplex T, *see* Factor IX			
Proplex SX-T, *see* Factor IX			
Propofol	10 mg	IV	J2704
Propranolol HCl	up to 1 mg	IV	J1800
Prorex, *see* Promethazine HCl			
Prostaphlin, *see* Procainamide HCl			
Prostigmin, *see* Neostigmine methylsulfate			
Protamine sulfate	per 10 mg	IV	J2720
Protein C Concentrate	10 IU	IV	J2724
Protirelin	per 250 mcg	IV	J2725
Prothazine, *see* Promethazine HCl			
Prothrombin complex concentrate (human)	per i.u.	IM	C9159
Protopam Chloride, *see* Pralidoxime chloride			
Proventil, *see* Albuterol sulfate, compounded			
Prozine-50, *see* Promazine HCl			
Pulmicort Respules, *see* Budesonide			
Pyridoxine HCl	100 mg		J3415
Q			
Quelicin, *see* Succinylcholine chloride			
Quinupristin/dalfopristin	500 mg (150/350)	IV	J2770
Qutenza, *see* Capsaicin patch			
R			
Ramucirumab	5 mg	IV	J9308
Ranibizumab	0.1 mg	OTH	J2778
Ranitidine HCL, Injection	25 mg	IV, IM	J2780
Rapamune, *see* Sirolimus			
Rasburicase	0.5 mg	IV	J2783
Recombinate, *see* Factor VIII			
Redisol, *see* Vitamin B-12 cyanocobalamin			
Regadenoson	0.1 mg	IV	J2785
Regitine, *see* Phentolamine mesylate			
Reglan, *see* Metoclopramide HCl			
Regular, *see* Insulin			
Relefact TRH, *see* Protirelin			
Relistor, *see* methylnaltrexone			
Remicade, *see* Infliximab, Injection			
Reo Pro, *see* Abciximab			

DRUG	DOSE	ROUTE	HCPCS
Rep-Pred, *see* Methylprednisolone acetate			
Reslizumab	1 mg	IV	J2786
RespiGam, *see* Respiratory Syncytial Virus			
Retavase, *see* Reteplase			
Reteplase	18.8 mg	IV	J2993
Retrovir, *see* Zidovudine			
Revefenacin inhalation solution		INH	J7677
Ravulizumab – cwvz	10 mg	IV	J1303
Rheomacrodex, *see* Dextran 40			
Rhesonativ, *see* Rho(D) Immune globulin, human			
Rheumatrex Dose Pack, *see* Methotrexate, oral			
Rho(D) Immune globulin		IM, IV	J2791
Rho(D) Immune globulin, human 1 dose package,	300 mcg	IM	J2790
	50 mg	IM	J2788
Rho(D)immune globulin, human, solvent detergent	100 IU	IV	J2792
RhoGAM, *see* Rho(D) Immune globulin, human			
Rhophylac	100 IU	IM, IV	J2791
RiaSTAP, *see* Human Fibrinogen concentrate			
Rilonacept	1 mg	SC	J2793
RimabotulinumtoxinB	100 units	IM	J0587
Ringers lactate infusion	up to 1,000 cc	IV	J7120, J7121
Risperidone	0.5 mg	IM	J2794
Risperidone (perseris)	0.5 mg	IV	J2798
Risperidone (uzedy)	1 mg	IM	J2799
Rituxan, *see* Rituximab			
Rituximab	100 mg	IV	J9310
Rituximab – abbs	10 mg	IV	Q5115
Robaxin, *see* Methocarbamol			
Rocephin, *see* Ceftriaxone sodium			
Roferon-A, *see* Interferon alfa-2A, recombinant			
Rolapitant	0.5 mg	IV	J2797
Rolapitant, oral, 1 mg	1 mg	ORAL	J8670
Romidepsin	1 mg	IV	J9315
Romiplostim	10 mcg	SC	J2796
Romosozumab – aqqg	1 mg	IV	J3111
Ropivacaine Hydrochloride	1 mg	OTH	J2795
Rozanolixizumab-noli	1 mg	IM	J9333
Rubex, *see* Doxorubicin HCl			
Rubramin PC, *see* Vitamin B-12 cyanocobalamin			
S			
Saline solution	5% dextrose, 500 ml	IV	J7042

DRUG	DOSE	ROUTE	HCPCS
	infusion, 250 cc	IV	J7050
	infusion, 1,000 cc	IV	J7030
Saline solution, sterile	500 ml = 1 unit	IV, OTH	J7040
Sandimmune, *see* Cyclosporine			
Sandoglobulin, *see* Immune globulin intravenous (human)			
Sandostatin Lar Depot, *see* Octreotide			
Sargramostim (GM-CSF)	50 mcg	IV	J2820
Sculptra	0.5 mg	IV	Q2028
Sebelelipase alfa	1 mg	IV	J2840
Selestoject, *see* Betamethasone sodium phosphate			
Sermorelin acetate	1 mcg	SC	Q0515
Siltuximab	10 mg	IV	J2860
Sincalide	5 mcg	IV	J2805
Sinusol-B, *see* Brompheniramine maleate			
Sirolimus	1 mg	ORAL	J7520
Skyla	13.5 mg	OTH	J7301
Sodium ferric gluconate in sucrose	12.5 mg		J2916
Sodium Hyaluronate			
Euflexxa			J7323
Hyalgan, Supartz, Visco-3			J7321
Orthovisc			J7324
Solganal, *see* Aurothioglucose			
Solu-Cortef, *see* Hydrocortisone sodium phosphate (J1710)			
Solu-Medrol, *see* Methylprednisolone sodium succinate			
Solurex, *see* Dexamethasone sodium phosphate			
Solurex LA, *see* Dexamethasone acetate			
Somatrem	1 mg	SC	J2940
Somatropin	1 mg	SC	J2941
Somatuline Depot, *see* Lanreotide			
Sparine, *see* Promazine HCl			
Spasmoject, *see* Dicyclomine HCl			
Spectinomycin HCl	up to 2 g	IM	J3320
Sporanox, *see* Itraconazole			
Staphcillin, *see* Methicillin sodium			
Stelara, *see* Ustekinumab			
Stilphostrol, *see* Diethylstilbestrol diphosphate			
Streptase, *see* Streptokinase			
Streptokinase	per 250,000 IU	IV	J2995
Streptomycin Sulfate, *see* Streptomycin			
Streptomycin	up to 1 g	IM	J3000

DRUG	DOSE	ROUTE	HCPCS
Streptozocin	1 gm		
Strontium-89 chloride	per millicurie		
Sublimaze, *see* Fentanyl citrate			
Succinylcholine chloride	up to 20 mg	IV, IM	J0330
Injection, sulfur hexafluoride lipid microspheres	per ml	IV	Q9950
Sumatriptan succinate	6 mg	SC	J3030
Supartz		OTH	J7321
Sucostrin, *see* Succinylcholine chloride			
Sus-Phrine, *see* Adrenalin, epinephrine			
Synercid, *see* Quinupristin/dalfopristin			
Synkavite, *see* Vitamin K, phytonadione, etc.			
Syntocionon, *see* Oxytocin			
Synvisc and Synvisc-One	1 mg	OTH	J7325
Sytobex, *see* Vitamin B-12 cyanocobalamin			
T			
Tacrolimus, oral, extended release	0.1 mg	ORAL	J7508
(Envarsus XR)	0.25 mg	ORAL	J7503
Tacrolimus, oral, Immediate release	per 1 mg	ORAL	J7507
Tacrolimus, parenteral	5 mg	IV	J7525
Tagraxofusp – erzs	10 mcg	IV	J9269
Taliglucerase Alfa	10 units	IV	J3060
Talimogene laherparepvec	per 1 million plaque forming units	IV	J9325
Talquetamab-tgvs	0.25 mg	IM	C9163
Talwin, *see* Pentazocine HCl			
Taractan, *see* Chlorprothixene			
Taxol, *see* Paclitaxel			
Taxotere, *see* Docetaxel			
Tazidime, *see* Ceftazidime			
Technetium TC Sestamibi	per dose		A9500
Tedizolid phosphate	1 mg	IV	J3090
TEEV, *see* Testosterone enanthate and estradiol valerate			
Teflaro, *see* Ceftaroline fosamil			
Telavancin	10 mg	IV	J3095
Temozolomide	1 mg	IV	J9328
	5 mg	ORAL	J8700
Temsirolimus	1 mg	IV	J9330
Tenecteplase	1 mg	IV	J3101
Teniposide	50 mg		Q2017
Tequin, *see* Gatifloxacin			
Terbutaline sulfate	up to 1 mg	SC, IV	J3105

DRUG	DOSE	ROUTE	HCPCS
Terbutaline sulfate, concentrated form	per 1 mg	INH	J7680
unit dose form	per 1 mg	INH	J7681
Teriparatide	10 mcg	SC	J3110
Terramycin IM, *see* Oxytetracycline HCl			
Testa-C, *see* Testosterone cypionate			
Testadiate, *see* Testosterone enanthate and estradiol valerate			
Testadiate-Depo, *see* Testosterone cypionate			
Testoject-LA, *see* Testosterone cypionate			
Testaqua, *see* Testosterone suspension			
Test-Estro Cypionates, *see* Testosterone cypionate and estradiol cypionate			
Test-Estro-C, *see* Testosterone cypionate and estradiol cypionate			
Testex, *see* Testosterone propionate			
Testoject-50, *see* Testosterone suspension			
Testoject-LA, *see* Testosterone cypionate			
Testone LA, *see* Testosterone enanthate			
Testosterone Aqueous, *see* Testosterone suspension			
Testosterone enanthate	1 mg	IM	J3121
Testosterone cypionate	1 mg	IM	J1071
Testosterone undecanoate	1 mg	IM	J3145
Testradiol 90/4, *see* Testosterone enanthate and estradiol valerate			
Testrin PA, *see* Testosterone enanthate			
Tetanus Immune globulin, human	up to 250 units	IM	J1670
Tetracycline	up to 250 mg	IM, IV	J0120
Thallous Chloride TL 201	per MCI		A9505
Theelin Aqueous, *see* Estrone			
Theophylline per MCI	per 40 mg	IV	J2810
TheraCys, *see* BCG live			
Thiamine HCl	100 mg		J3411
Thiethylperazine maleate, Injection	up to 10 mg	IM	J3280
Thiethylperazine maleate, oral	10 mg	ORAL	Q0174
Thiotepa	15 mg	IV	J9340
Thorazine, *see* Chlorpromazine HCl			
Thymoglobulin, also *see* Immune globulin			
anti-thymocyte globulin, equine	250 mg	IV	J7504
anti-thymocyte globulin, rabbit	25 mg	IV	J7511
Thypinone, *see* Protirelin			
Thyrogen, *see* Thyrotropin Alfa			
Thyrotropin Alfa, Injection	0.9 mg	IM, SC	J3240
Tice BCG, *see* BCG live			

DRUG	DOSE	ROUTE	HCPCS
Ticon, *see* Trimethobenzamide HCl			
Tigan, *see* Trimethobenzamide HCl			
Tigecycline	1 mg	IV	J3243
Tiject-20, *see* Trimethobenzamide HCl			
Tinzaparin	1000 IU	SC	J1655
Tirofiban Hydrochloride, Injection	0.25 mg	IM, IV	J3246
TNKase, *see* Tenecteplase			
TOBI, *see* Tobramycin, inhalation solution			
Tobramycin, inhalation solution	300 mg	INH	J7682, J7685
Tobramycin sulfate	up to 80 mg	IM, IV	J3260
Tocilizumab	1 mg	IV	J3262
Tofersen	1 mg	IM	J1304
Tofranil, *see* Imipramine HCl			
Tolazoline HCl	up to 25 mg	IV	J2670
Topotecan	0.25 mg	ORAL	J8705
	0.1 mg	IV	J9351
Toradol, *see* Ketorolac tromethamine			
Torecan, *see* Thiethylperazine maleate			
Torisel, *see* Temsirolimus			
Tornalate, *see* Bitolterol mesylate			
Torsemide	10 mg/ml	IV	J3265
Totacillin-N, *see* Ampicillin			
Trabectedin	0.1 mg	IV	J9352
Trastuzumab	10 mg	IV	J9355
Trastuzumab – anns (kanjinti)	10 mg	IV	Q5117
Trastuzumab - dkst	10 mg	IV	Q5114
Trastuzumab - dttb	10 mg	IV	Q5112
Trastuzumab- pkrb	10 mg	IV	Q5113
Trastuzumab- qyyp (trazimera)	10 mg	IV	Q5116
Trastuzumab and Hyaluronidase	10 mg	IV	J9356
Treanda, *see* Bendamustine HCl			
Treprostinil	1 mg		J3285
Tri-Kort, *see* Triamcinolone acetonide			
Triam-A, *see* Triamcinolone acetonide			
Triamcinolone, concentrated form	per 1 mg	INH	J7683
Triamcinolone, unit dose	per 1 mg	INH	J7684
Triamcinolone acetonide	1 mg		J3300
	1 mg per 10 mg	IM	J3300 J3301
Triamcinolone diacetate	per 5 mg	IM	J3302
Triamcinolone hexacetonide	per 5 mg	VAR	J3303
Triesence, *see* Triamcinolone acetonide			
Triflupromazine HCl	up to 20 mg	IM, IV	J3400

DRUG	DOSE	ROUTE	HCPCS
Trilafon, *see* perphenazine			
Trilog, *see* Triamcinolone acetonide			
Trilone, *see* Triamcinolone diacetate			
Trimethobenzamide HCl, Injection	up to 200 mg	IM	J3250
Trimethobenzamide HCl, oral	250 mg	ORAL	Q0173
Trimetrexate glucuronate	per 25 mg	IV	J3305
Triptorelin Pamoate Trisenox, *see* Arsenic trioxide			
Triptorelin XR	3.75 mg	SC	J3316
Trobicin, *see* Spectinomycin HCl			
Trovan, *see* Alatrofloxacin mesylate			
Tysabri, *see* Natalizumab	3.75 mg	SC	J3315
U			
Ultrazine-10, *see* Prochlorperazine			
Unasyn, *see* Ampicillin sodium/sulbactam sodium			
Unclassified drugs (see also Not elsewhere classified)			J3490
Unclassified drug or biological used for ESRD on dialysis		IV	J3591
Unspecified oral antiemetic			Q0181
Urea	up to 40 g	IV	J3350
Ureaphil, *see* Urea			
Urecholine, *see* Bethanechol chloride			
Urofollitropin	75 iu	IV	J3355
Urokinase	5,000 IU vial	IV	J3364
	250,000 IU vial	IV	J3365
Ustekinumab	1 mg	SC	J3357
V			
V-Gan, *see* Promethazine HCl			
Valergen, *see* Estradiol valerate			
Valertest, *see* Testosterone enanthate and estradiol valerate			
Valium, *see* Diazepam			
Valoctocogene roxaparvovec-rvox	per ml	IM	J1412
Valrubicin, intravesical	200 mg	OTH	J9357
Valstar, *see* Valrubicin			
Vancocin, *see* Vancomycin HCl			
Vancoled, *see* Vancomycin HCl			
Vancomycin HCl	500 mg	IV, IM	J3370
Vasoxyl, *see* Methoxamine HCl			
Vedolizumab	1 mg	IV	J3380
Velaglucerase alfa	100 units	IV	J3385
Velban, *see* Vinblastine sulfate			
Velmanase alfa-tycv	1 mg	IM	J0217

DRUG	DOSE	ROUTE	HCPCS
Velsar, *see* Vinblastine sulfate			
Venofer, *see* Iron sucrose			
Ventolin, *see* Albuterol sulfate			
VePesid, *see* Etoposide and Etoposide, oral			
Versed, *see* Midazolam HCl			
Verteporfin	0.1 mg	IV	J3396
Vesprin, *see* Triflupromazine HCl			
Vestronidase alfa-vjbk	1 mg	IV	J3397
Viadur, *see* Leuprolide acetate Implant			
Vibativ, *see* Telavancin			
Vinblastine sulfate	1 mg	IV	J9360
Vincasar PFS, *see* Vincristine sulfate			
Vincristine sulfate	1 mg	IV	J9370
Vincristine sulfate Liposome	1 mg	IV	J9371
Vinorelbine tartrate	per 10 mg	IV	J9390
Vistaject-25, *see* Hydroxyzine HCl			
Vistaril, *see* Hydroxyzine HCl			
Vistide, *see* cidofovir			
Visudyne, *see* Verteporfin			
Vitamin K, phytonadione, menadione, menadiol sodium diphosphate	per 1 mg	IM, SC, IV	J3430
Vitamin B-12 cyanocobalamin	up to 1,000 mcg	IM, SC	J3420
Von Willebrand Factor Complex, human	per IU VWF:RCo	IV	J7187
	per IU VWF:RCo	IV	J7183
Vonvendi	per IU VWF:RCp	IV	J7179
Voretigene neparvovec-rzyl	1 billion vector genomes	IV	J3398
Voriconazole	10 mg	IV	J3465
Vpriv, *see* Velaglucerase alfa			
W			
Wehamine, *see* Dimenhydrinate			
Wehydryl, *see* Diphenhydramine HCl			
Wellcovorin, *see* Leucovorin calcium			
Wilate, *see* Von Willebrand Factor complex (human)			
Win Rho SD, *see* Rho(D) immunoglobulin, human, solvent detergent			
Wyamine Sulfate, *see* Mephentermine sulfate			
Wycillin, *see* Penicillin G procaine			
Wydase, *see* Hyaluronidase			

DRUG	DOSE	ROUTE	HCPCS
X			
Xeloda, *see* Capecitabine			
Xeomin, *see* Incobotulinumtoxin type A			
Xgeva, *see* Denosumab			
Xiaflex, *see* Collagenase			
Xopenex, *see* Albuterol			
Xylocaine HCl, *see* Lidocaine HCl			
Xyntha, *see* Factor VIII (anti-hemophilic factor, recombinant)			
Y			
Yervoy, *see* Ipilimumab			
Z			
Zanosar, *see* Streptozocin			
Zantac, *see* Ranitidine HCL			
Zemplar, *see* Paricalcitol			
Zenapax, *see* Daclizumab			
Zetran, *see* Diazepam Ziconotide	1 mcg	OTH	J2278
Zidovudine	10 mg	IV	J3485
Zinacef, *see* Cefuroxime sodium			
Ziprasidone Mesylate	10 mg	IM	J3486
Zithromax, *see* Azithromycin dihydrate			
Zithromax I.V., *see* Azithromycin, Injection			
Ziv-Aflibercept	1 mg	IV	J9400
Zofran, *see* Ondansetron HCl			
Zoladex, *see* Goserelin acetate Implant			
Zoledronic Acid	1 mg	IV	J3489
Zolicef, *see* Cefazolin sodium			
Zortress, *see* Everolimus			
Zosyn, *see* Piperacillin			
Zyprexa Relprevv, *see* Olanzapine			
Zyvox, *see* Linezolid			